POISONING - FROM SPECIFIC TOXIC AGENTS TO NOVEL RAPID AND SIMPLIFIED TECHNIQUES FOR ANALYSIS

Edited by **Ntambwe Malangu**

Poisoning - From Specific Toxic Agents to Novel Rapid and Simplified Techniques for Analysis
http://dx.doi.org/10.5772/65817
Edited by Ntambwe Malangu

Contributors

Edit Gara Dr, Virginie Lattard, Sébastien Lefebvre, Isabelle Fourel, Etienne Benoit, Stéphane Queffélec, Bruno Megarbane, Dominique Vodovar, Virginie Siguret, Hiroshi Kinoshita, Naoko Tanaka, Elif Bozcal, Melih Dagdeviren, Tatiana Mogilnaya, Graciela Castro-Escarpulli, Cecilia Hernández-Cortez, Ingrid Palma-Martinez, Luis Uriel González-Avila, Andrea Guerrero-Mandujano, Ntambwe Malangu, Murat Darçın, Murat Alkan, E. Selcen Darçın, Gürdoğan Doğrul, Nicolai Nistor, Otilia Frasinariu, Violeta Streanga, Ameera Seyedzadeh, Asel Mwafy, Francisco Sánchez-Bayo, Francisco Sanchez-Bayo, Luis De Almeida, Robert Williams, Graeme Wright, Ivan Kennedy, Angus Crossan

Published by InTech

Janeza Trdine 9, 51000 Rijeka, Croatia

Publishing Process Manager Dajana Pemac
Technical Editor SPi Global
Cover InTech Design team

First published December, 2017
Printed in Croatia
Legal deposit, Croatia: National and University Library in Zagreb

Additional hard copies can be obtained from orders@intechopen.com

Poisoning - From Specific Toxic Agents to Novel Rapid and Simplified Techniques for Analysis, Edited by Ntambwe Malangu
p. cm.
Print ISBN 978-953-51-3681-1
Online ISBN 978-953-51-3682-8

For EU product safety concerns:
IN TECH d.o.o., Prolaz Marije Krucifikse Kozulić 3, 51000 Rijeka, Croatia,
info@intechopen.com or visit our website at intechopen.com.

Meet the editor

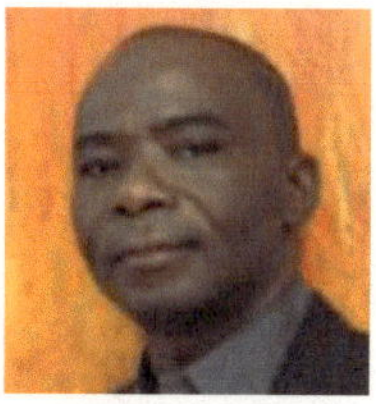

Prof. Ntambwe Malangu, born in Kabinda, Congo (DRC), is a pharmacoepidemiologist with public health expertise in drug safety issues. He is currently the head of the Department of Epidemiology and Biostatistics at the School of Public Health at Sefako Makgatho Health Sciences University, Pretoria, South Africa, and the production editor for *PULA: Botswana Journal for African Studies* as well as a reviewer for a handful of international peer-reviewed journals. From 2006, he has been working as an international health consultant and technical advisor with major development partners. Malangu holds a bachelor's degree in Pharmacy from the University of Kinshasa (1991), a Master of Medical Science degree from the Medical University of Southern Africa (2003), and a PhD degree (2007) and a Doctor of Medical Science degree from the University of Limpopo (2012). Malangu has over 60 publications including scientific abstracts and letters, books, book chapters, and full papers.

Contents

Preface

Poisoning, whether acute or chronic and whether accidental or deliberate, is one of the major causes of morbidity and mortality worldwide. This book is a collection of papers about some common causes of poisoning in humans and animals. Given the fact that applied toxicology, in its various forms (clinical, occupational, forensic, etc.), is not commonly and effectively taught as a subject in its own right, the aim of this book is to provide both theoretical and practical information on the specified toxic agents and analytical techniques discussed.

The materials presented here can be categorized into two groups. The first group of papers deals with clinical toxicology topics including poisoning by anticoagulant rodenticides, food toxins, carbon monoxide, and the toxicity of beta-lactam antibiotics. The second group of papers deals with forensic or analytical toxicology topics such as simplified methods for the analysis of gaseous toxic agents, rapid methods for the analysis and monitoring of pathogens in drinking water and water-based solutions, as well as the linkages between clinical and forensic toxicology. Each chapter presents new information on the topic discussed based on authors' experience while summarizing existing knowledge.

The introductory chapter provides an overview on issues, challenges, and resources for the establishment and running of clinical and forensic toxicological assessment services and concludes with a statement on how the two disciplines relate. The second chapter is a comprehensive monograph on the use and utility of anticoagulants, their chemical properties, pharmacokinetics, mechanisms of action, human and animal exposures, and management of poisoning incidents. The third chapter discusses food poisoning caused by bacteria-emitting toxins and elaborates on its epidemiological characteristics including food-borne diseases, pathogens involved, and other risk factors. The fourth chapter is also a monograph on carbon monoxide poisoning with emphasis with a case study illustrating a novel management approach implemented in Hungary. The fifth chapter is a detailed description on toxicological aspects of beta-lactam antibiotics including their structure-activity relationships, pathophysiology, molecular biology, and strategies to address their toxicity. The sixth chapter elaborates on acute poisoning by neonicotinoids, while the seventh chapter discusses occupational risk factors for acute pesticide poisoning. The eight chapter reports on how activating carbon fibers and date pits can be useful in the management of liver toxicity. The ninth chapter describes novel simplified techniques for forensic analysis of gaseous substances suchas carbon monoxide, hydrogen cyanide, hydrogen sulfide, and helium. The techniques used include color testing, gas chromatography, detector tube, oximeter, and spectrophotometric method. The tenth chapter elaborates on novel apparatus and methods for real-time detection and monitoring of viruses and pathogenic organisms in drinking water and aqueous solutions based on nonlinear effects. The final chapter describes a practical tool for ensuring safety in agricultural produces, the Aflatoxin QuicktestTM.

Taken together, this book will be a good teaching aid and can be a prescribed or recommended reading for postgraduate students and professionals in the fields of public health, medicine, pharmacy, nursing, biology, toxicology, and forensic sciences. The materials presented by a team of international experts and authors make an enriching reading geared at improving the prevention, detection, and management of both acute and chronic poisoning due to the toxic agents described.

Many individuals have contributed to the preparation and production of this book; their dedication and selfless contribution are humbly acknowledged here. In particular, professors and scientists Moguilnaya Tatiana and Sheryshev Aleksey from Moscow Aviation Institute, Russia; Hiroshi Kinoshita, Naoko Tanaka, Ayaka Takakura, Mostofa Jamal, Asuka Ito, Mitsuru Kumihashi, Shoji Kimura, Kiyoshi Ameno, Kunihiko Tsutsui, and Shuji Matsubara from Kagawa University, Japan; Elif Bozcal from Istanbul University, Turkey; Melih Dagdeviren from Ege University, Turkey; Edit Gara from Semmelweis University, Hungary; Cecilia Hernández-Cortez, Ingrid Palma-Martínez, Luis Uriel Gonzalez-Avila, Andrea Guerrero-Mandujano, Raúl Colmenero Solís, and Graciela Castro-Escarpulli from the National Institute of Biological Sciences (Escuela Nacional de Ciencias Biológicas), Mexico; Sébastien Lefebvre, Isabelle Fourel, Etienne Benoit, and Virginie Lattard from the Universite de Lyon, France; Stéphane Queffélec from the Centre National d'Informations Toxicologiques Vétérinaires (CNITV), France; Virginie Siguret from the Université Paris Descartes, France; Dominique Vodovar and Bruno Mégarbane from the Université Paris-Diderot, France; Francisco Sánchez-Bayo and his team from the School of Life and Environmental Sciences from the University of Sydney, Australia; Ameereh Seyedzadeh, Asel Mwafy, Waleed Khalil Ahmed, Kamala Pandurangan, and Ali Hilal-Alnaqbi from the Department of Mechanical Engineering, United Arab Emirates University; Nicolai Nistor, Otilia Elena Frăsinariu and Violeta Ştreangă from Grigore T. Popa University of Medicine and Pharmacy, Iasi, Romania; and Selcen Darçın E, Murat Darçın, Murat Alkan, and Gürdoğan Doğrul from Gazi University, Ankara, Turkey. Moreover, my personal assistant Ornela Lofulo Niangi Malangu and Martina Blečić, Dajana Pemac, and the production and editorial teams from InTechOpen have all played a major role in ensuring that this book is published.

Prof. Ntambwe Malangu
Sefako Makgatho Health Sciences University,
Pretoria, South Africa

Section 1

Introduction

Chapter 1

Introductory Chapter: Linkages Between Clinical and Forensic Toxicology

Ntambwe Malangu

Additional information is available at the end of the chapter

http://dx.doi.org/10.5772/intechopen.70303

1. Overview on interconnections between sciences and professionals in case of poisoning

Poisoning, whether acute or chronic, and whether accidental or deliberate, is one of the major causes of morbidity and mortality worldwide. International data gathered by the World Health Organization (WHO) suggest that at least an estimated over 100.000 people died worldwide from poisoning every year [1]. Of the factors contributing to this high loss of lives, is the misdiagnosing of poisoning due to lack of qualified personnel and lack of appropriate medical equipment for conducting relevant investigations.

Strictly speaking studying poisoning incidents, how they occur, their symptoms and signs, the toxic agents involved, the diagnosis and management thereof as well as the outcomes of treatment, is a multi-disciplinary endeavour that requires skills and competences in injury epidemiology, clinical and forensic, or analytical toxicology.

Although epidemiologists painstakingly work to study, describe, and quantify the determinants of both acute and chronic poisoning incidents, medical clinicians and clinical toxicologists, clinical pharmacists and nurses are the professionals who are confronted on a daily basis with cases of acute poisoning requiring their immediate attention to save or preserve the lives of victims of such incidents.

Clinicians, particularly, emergency and critical care doctors, ought to decide on the basis of symptoms and signs, often not unique to the incident, whether it is a case of acute poisoning or not. The history related by patients themselves, their relatives and or sometimes by paramedics or police personnel who brought the victim constitutes more often the main evidence clinicians may get about the circumstances of the acute poisoning incident. Understandably, where such history is lacking or incomplete, forensic toxicological assessment of the victim's specimen is another tool capable of providing clues to what may have happened [2].

In settings where published and widely publicized treatment guidelines exist, clinicians may have algorithms to guide their assessments and presumptions. In settings where such guidelines do not exist, the clinicians' instincts and experiences are the valuable tools for making a correct presumptive diagnosis and crafting a management care plan.

2. Importance of guidelines and algorithms in diagnosis and management of a poisoning incident

Several studies have reported the usefulness of treatment guidelines in general and for specific diseases notably epidemics such as HIV and noncommunicable diseases [3–6]. In summary, treatment guidelines and algorithms for management of specific diseases and conditions:

a. facilitate the choice of appropriate medicines and prescribing of correct doses;

b. provide guidance in establishing differential diagnosis;

c. speed the consultation process as clinicians are guided on what tests to perform and what to look for.

Unfortunately, with regard to poisoning incidents, national treatment guidelines of several countries have shortcomings as guidance and algorithms on specific poisoning agents are not presented there in [7]. It should be noted that the International Programme on Chemical Safety (IPCS) has published guidelines concerning the prevention and clinical management of poisoning including a manual on "Basic Analytical Toxicology" which provides practical guidance on clinical aspects and detailed monographs on tests to be conducted for specified chemicals [8].

3. Role of forensic toxicology and medical laboratory in the diagnosis and monitoring of treatment in case of a poisoning incident

Medical laboratory and forensic toxicological assessments are important in establishing the diagnosis and identifying the toxic agents involved in a poisoning incident, and possibly the doses ingested. In case of deliberate poisoning, suicide or para-suicide as well as in case of intoxication or criminal poisoning, the identification of the toxic agents help not only in the management of the victim but also in providing clues that may lead to the possible culprit [9, 10].

Although, medical laboratory testing plays a crucial role in the detection, diagnosis and treatment of disease in patients; and that laboratory tests help determine the presence of a disease and monitor the effectiveness of treatment; in case of poisoning, detecting biochemical parameters modified as a result of the effects of the toxic agent is an important contribution for the purposes of making a diagnosis. Classical cases include the determination of acetylcholinesterase in case of acute poisoning due to pesticides as well as the identification of toxins produced by bacteria involved in food poisoning incidents [11–13].

With regard to forensic or analytical toxicology, its role in the detection, identification, and quantification of drugs, chemicals, and other foreign compounds (xenobiotics) in biological and related specimens such as blood, saliva, hair, urine, etc., is of utmost importance in the diagnosis, treatment, prognosis, and prevention of poisoning. Sometimes, a forensic toxicological assessment is the only means by which objective evidence of the nature and magnitude of exposure to a particular toxic agent or a group of toxicants can be obtained [14].

4. Limitations of medical and forensic laboratory services

There are several obstacles and limitations with regard to the existence and operation of forensic laboratory services. In several countries, firstly, the lack of properly trained clinical and forensic toxicologists is the main obstacle to the establishment and use of forensic laboratory services. The competences required for a trained analytical toxicologist include a fundamental knowledge of principles of emergency medicine and intensive care, a good grasp of pharmacology and clinical toxicology as well as a practical mastery of clinical chemistry and basic laboratory operations, including aspects of medical laboratory health and safety. Secondly, the lack of appropriate funding for the training and establishment of such services further compound the problem. Thirdly, it is noteworthy that even where relevant clinical personnel such as clinical pharmacists exist, equipment needed to run the services are lacking. It should be noted that several types of equipment are required for providing analytical toxicological assessments, this include:

a. A carbon monoxide (CO)-Oximeter: normally very necessary for determining carboxyhaemoglobin and methaemoglobin measurements in case of a suspected incident by carbon monoxide [15].

b. Standard clinical chemistry analysers and assay kits: for use in determining basic biochemical parameters such as glucose, total bilirubin, ALT, AST, cholesterol, triglycerides, creatinine, urea, uric acid, fibrinogen, calcium and phosphorus, aminotransferases, etc [16].

c. Machines for UV-visible spectrophotometry, thin-layer chromatography (TLC), high performance liquid chromatography (HPLC), and gas chromatography-mass spectrometry (GC-MS), and possibly high performance liquid chromatography-tandem mass spectrometry (HPLC-MS-MS): for use in the identification and quantification of a wide variety of medicines, drugs, chemicals, and pollutants [17].

d. Machines for atomic absorption spectrophotometry or inductively coupled mass spectrometry (ICP-MS): for use for metals analysis [18].

5. Necessity for rapid methods in forensic toxicology

The need to treat the victim of acute poisoning as well as the need to apprehend the perpetrators of deliberate or criminal intoxication dictates the need for rapid methods for identifying poisons involved in a poisoning incident. This is a subject of ongoing research and it requires massive investments particularly in developing countries where funding for research is scarce.

Moreover, some of the methods mentioned above such as GC, HPLC and TLC require the presence of reference chemicals to be used for the identification and quantitation of toxicants [19]. However, the availability and access to these references and other reagents pose several challenges particularly to developing countries that may not have sufficient funds to purchase these products [14].

For the above reasons, newer and simpler methods, techniques, equipments, and devices that are more affordable and easy to operate are urgently required to develop and establish forensic toxicology services in several developing countries.

6. Concluding remarks

Clinical toxicology and forensic toxicology share a mutually beneficial partnership; these two sciences support both the management of the patients who have been victims of poisoning; and the identification of the causative agent that may have inflicted toxicity, injury or death as a result of an acute accidental or deliberate poisoning incident. Several initiatives are required to develop and establish analytical toxicology services. These include educational interventions to train people with required competencies; and funding to establish and equip laboratories capable of assisting clinicians with meaningful findings to guide the management of victims of poisoning incidents.

Author details

Ntambwe Malangu

Address all correspondence to: gustavmalangu@gmail.com

Sefako Makgatho Health Sciences University, Pretoria, South Africa

References

[1] WHO. Summary Tables of Mortality Estimates by Cause, Age and Sex, by Country, 2000-2015. Available at: http://www.who.int/healthinfo/global_burden_disease/estimates/en/index1.html [Accessed 05-July-2015]

[2] Cooper G, Negrusz A. Clarke's Analytical Forensic Toxicology. Pharmaceutical Press; 2013

[3] Davis DA, Taylor-Vaisey A. Translating guidelines into practice: A systematic review of theoretic concepts, practical experience and research evidence in the adoption of clinical practice guidelines. Canadian Medical Association Journal.1997;**157**(4):408-416

[4] Dybul M, Fauci AS, Bartlett JG, Kaplan JE, Pau AK. Guidelines for using antiretroviral agents among HIV-infected adults and adolescents. Recommendations of the panel on clinical practices for treatment of HIV. MMWR. Recommendations and reports: Morbidity and mortality weekly report. Recommendations and Reports. 2002;**51**(RR-7):1-55

[5] Weber MA, Schiffrin EL, White WB, Mann S, Lindholm LH, Kenerson JG,... Cohen DL. Clinical practice guidelines for the management of hypertension in the community. The Journal of Clinical Hypertension. 2014;**16**(1):14-26

[6] Amoakoh-Coleman M, Klipstein-Grobusch K, Agyepong IA, Kayode GA, Grobbee DE, Ansah EK. Provider adherence to first antenatal care guidelines and risk of pregnancy complications in public sector facilities: A Ghanaian cohort study. BMC Pregnancy and Childbirth. 2016;**16**(1):369

[7] Malangu N. Contribution of plants and traditional medicines to the disparities and similarities in acute poisoning incidents in Botswana, South Africa and Uganda. African Journal of Traditional, Complementary and Alternative Medicines. 2014;**11**(2):425-438

[8] IPCS. Basic Analytical Toxicology. Available at: http://www.who.int/ipcs/publications/training_poisons/basic_analytical_tox/en/index1.html [Accessed 05-July-2017]

[9] Baker FJ, Silverton RE. Introduction to Medical Laboratory Technology. Butterworth-Heinemann; 2014

[10] Masters SB, Trevor AJ. Basic & Clinical Pharmacology. In: Katzung BG, editor. McGraw-Hill Medical; 2016

[11] Roberts DM, Brett J. Clinical management of acute OP pesticide poisoning. In: Basic and Clinical Toxicology of Organophosphorus Compounds. London: Springer; 2014. pp. 141-175

[12] Marxen S, Stark TD, Frenzel E, Rütschle A, Lücking G, Pürstinger G, Pohl EE, Scherer S, Ehling-Schulz M, Hofmann T. Chemodiversity of cereulide, the emetic toxin of Bacillus cereus. Analytical and Bioanalytical Chemistry. DOI: 10.1007/s00216-015-8511-y

[13] Ballantyne B, Marrs TC. Clinical and Experimental Toxicology of Organophosphates and Carbamates. Elsevier; 2017

[14] Flanagan RJ. Role of the laboratory in the diagnosis and management of poisoning. In: Dart RC, editor. Medical Toxicology. 3rd ed. Baltimore: Lippincott, Williams & Wilkins; 2003: pp. 337-58

[15] Jang DH, Kelly M, Hardy K, Lambert DS, Shofer FS, Eckmann DM. A preliminary study in the alterations of mitochondrial respiration in patients with carbon monoxide poisoning measured in blood cells. Clinical Toxicology. 2017;**55**(6):579-584

[16] Zunic L, Skrbo A, Causevic A, Prnjavorac B, Sabanovic Z, Pandza H, Masic I. Role of laboratory diagnostic medical biochemistry services-analysis of requirements for the laboratory test in the laboratory of primary health care center. Medicinski Arhiv. 2011;**65**(4):202-206

[17] Peters FT. Recent advances of liquid chromatography–(tandem) mass spectrometry in clinical and forensic toxicology. Clinical Biochemistry. 2011;**44**(1):54-65

[18] Goyer RA. Metal Toxicology: Approaches and Methods. Elsevier; 2016

[19] Maurer HH. Current role of liquid chromatography–mass spectrometry in clinical and forensic toxicology. Analytical and Bioanalytical Chemistry. 2007;**388**(7):1315-1325

Section 2

Clinical Toxicology Topics

Chapter 2

Poisoning by Anticoagulant Rodenticides in Humans and Animals: Causes and Consequences

Sébastien Lefebvre, Isabelle Fourel,
Stéphane Queffélec, Dominique Vodovar,
Bruno Mégarbane, Etienne Benoit,
Virginie Siguret and Virginie Lattard

Additional information is available at the end of the chapter

http://dx.doi.org/10.5772/intechopen.69955

Abstract

Anticoagulant rodenticides (ARs) are a keystone of the management of rodent populations in the world. The widespread use of these molecules raises questions on exposure and intoxication risks, which define the safety of these products. Exposures and intoxications can affect humans, domestic animals and wildlife. Consequences are different for each group, from the simple issue of intoxication in humans to public health concern if farm animals are exposed. After a rapid presentation of the mechanism of action and the use of anticoagulant rodenticides, this chapter assesses the prominence of poisoning by anticoagulant rodenticides in humans, domestic animals and wildlife.

Keywords: anticoagulant, rodent, poisoning

1. Introduction

The management of rodents around the world is a great concern, in many aspects. Rodents are ubiquitous and opportunistic animals, some such as the brown rats (*Rattus norvegicus*) and the black rats (*Rattus rattus*) are present at all continents except Antarctic [1]. These rodent populations are an ecological and an economic issue in the islands where they are not indigenous [2]. Agriculture is also affected by rodents; in France, for instance, water voles (*Arvicola terrestris*) devastate some lands [3]. Finally, rodents are a major nuisance in cities where their proximity to and interactions with human populations and infrastructure can cause impairments and become a hazard for the public health as they are reservoirs of many diseases. In

China, rodents destroyed the rice stock that would be sufficient to feed 200 millions of people [4] and the estimation of the cost induced by rodents' damage is about 19 billions of dollars [5]. Many similar cases have been recorded around the world [1, 6].

To deal with these concerns, rodent populations have to be controlled. One of the most used management methods is the chemical method based on the use of anticoagulant rodenticides (ARs). Anticoagulant rodenticides (ARs) have been used since the 1940s to control rodent populations. Warfarin was the first molecule used. But after its use for more than one decade, resistant strains of rodents to ARs have emerged [7]. To deal with resistance, this first generation of ARs has been supplemented by a second generation. ARs of the second generation are frequently named 'superwarfarins' or long-acting anticoagulant rodenticides. Indeed, these molecules are more potent than the first generation due to their longer half-life, which implies longer tissue-persistence and better efficacy.

Indeed, the consequence of the widespread use of ARs and more specifically the second generation of ARs, that are more efficient and more persistent, has been an increase of the exposure risks and the intoxication risks for non-target species such as pets, wildlife as well as humans. Nevertheless, anticoagulant rodenticides are renowned as a safe method to manage rodent populations. This safety is due to their mechanism of action as well as on the implementation of good practices in their use and by the respect of related regulations. Beyond this renown, it is important to monitor the impact of using ARs regarding the risk of untargeted species poisoning and to discuss on the remaining grey area in our knowledge on anticoagulant rodenticides.

Hence, after a rapid presentation of the mechanism of action and the use of anticoagulant rodenticides, this chapter assesses the importance of the exposure and the intoxication by anticoagulant rodenticides.

2. Anticoagulant rodenticides

The current anticoagulant rodenticide molecules belong to the family of vitamin K antagonist (VKA) molecules. The effects of VKAs have been observed in the 'sweet clover' poisoning of bovines, which results in a haemorrhagic disease and often the death of the animal [8–10]. Clover (*Melilotus officinalis*), used as fodder, contains coumarin a precursor of dicoumarol which is a VKA (**Figure 1E**). If clover fodders are not stored under proper conditions, fermentations may occur. These fermentations change clover coumarin in dicoumarol. Thus, clover fodder become toxic [10]. Dicoumarol was synthesised by Paul and Stahmann in 1941, opening the opportunity of use VKA as medicine and rodenticide [11]. Then other VKA molecules have been synthesised, including the famous warfarin (**Figure 1D**) and all other products that are more potent than dicoumarol [12].

The main molecules used in the rodent population management are presented in **Figure 1**. VKA molecules are derived from a coumarin (**Figure 1A**), thiocoumarin (**Figure 1B**) or 1,3-indandione (**Figure 1C**) core. The distinction of the second generation of AR from the first generation is the radical. In second generation, radical includes three benzene structures,

http://dx.doi.org/10.5772/intechopen.69955

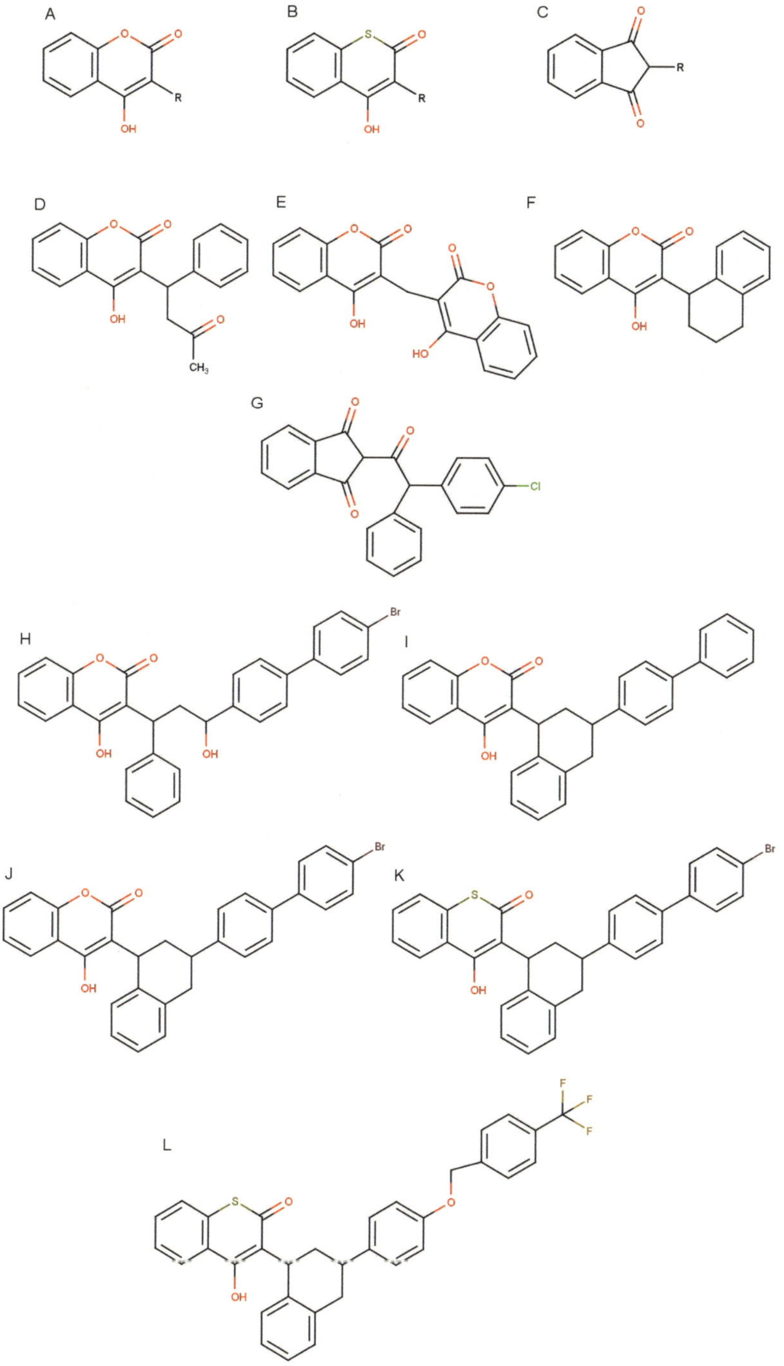

Figure 1. Chemical structure of: (A) coumarin core; (B) thiocoumarin core; (C) 1,3-indandione core; (D) warfarin; (E) dicoumarol; (F) coumatetralyl; (G) chlorophacinone; (H) bromadiolone; (I) difenacoum; (J) brodifacoum; (K) difethialone; and (L) flocoumafen.

which increase the fat solubility of the molecules and influence their pharmacokinetic properties. In order to understand the interest of VKAs and the key issue of their safety, it is important to present their mechanism of action and their pharmacokinetics.

2.1. Mechanism of action

Vitamin K antagonists (VKA) are non-competitive inhibitors of the vitamin K epoxide reductase enzyme (VKORC1) [13, 14]. This membrane enzyme of endoplasmic reticulum is responsible for the recycling of vitamin K. Vitamin K is a cofactor essential to many biotransformations of proteins and more specifically to obtain an active form of some clotting factors, the factors II, VII, IX and X. These factors, called vitamin K-dependent clotting factors, have to go through a post-translational gamma-carboxylation of their glutamate residues into gamma-carboxyglutamic acid to be able to chelate calcium and have their physiological activity [15, 16]. This reaction is done by gamma-glutamyl carboxylase (GGCX), which is another membrane enzyme of endoplasmic reticulum, and needs the oxidation of vitamin K hydroquinone to vitamin K epoxide to provide the required reducing power [17, 18]. Then VKORC1 recycles vitamin K epoxides to vitamin K hydroquinones (**Figure 2**) [19].

The amount of vitamin K provided by the majorities of food is not sufficient to offset the complete arrest of vitamin K cycle. Consequently, when VKORC1 is inhibited by VKA, a sufficient amount of vitamin K hydroquinone cannot be recycled from vitamin K epoxides to ensure the gamma-carboxylation of vitamin K-dependent proteins, and more especially the vitamin K-dependent clotting factors. Consequently, the blood concentrations of active vitamin K-dependent clotting factors decrease and lead to an increase of clotting times then, with time, to the death by haemorrhages.

2.2. Pharmacokinetics properties

Vitamin K antagonists are reputed to be highly and rapidly absorbed after *per os* administration. Then they are mainly stocked in liver. Their liver storage and their elimination are

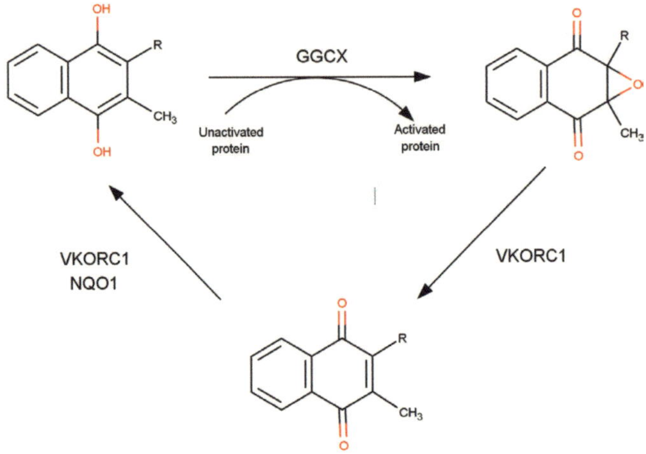

Figure 2. Vitamin K cycle.

http://dx.doi.org/10.5772/intechopen.69955

key factors, which determine a part of their efficiency and their persistence. The elimination pathway depends on the molecule and on its enantiomeric form [20]. For example, enantiomers of warfarin are eliminated differently. The (S)-enantiomer is metabolised exclusively by the hepatic cytochrome P450 isoform 2C9 (CYP2C9) while (R)-enantiomer is metabolised by isoforms CYP1A2, CYP2C19, CYP3A and hepatic ketoreductase [21, 22]. Although the (R)-enantiomer has a longer half-life, it is less efficient and the modulation of its elimination does not have a significant impact on the coagulation [23–25]. There is a great discrepancy between tissue persistence of first generation and second generation of ARs. First-generation molecules have tissue persistence of few days while the second generation has tissue persistence of few weeks [26]. This point is a major concern for AR ecotoxicity.

Moreover, second-generation ARs (i.e. bromadiolone, difenacoum, brodifacoum, flocoumafen and difethialone) contain two asymmetric carbons systematically. Therefore, commercial second-generation ARs are a mixture of two diastereoisomeric forms (1R,3R)(1S,3S)-isomers and (1R,3S)(1S,3R)-isomers with different pharmacokinetic properties. For each second-generation AR, there is systematically one diastereoisomeric form with a shorter half-life than the other one (**Table 1**) [20, 27]. Proportion between stereoisomers in commercial baits is defined by regulatory documents. For example, bromadiolone must be a mixture of more than 70 of trans-isomers and fewer than 30% of cis-isomers. These differences in half-life between stereoisomers could be a fundamental point in the development of future more eco-friendly AR with modification of regulatory defined ratios.

2.3. Interest of anticoagulants in rodent population management

The first methods used to control rodent populations aim to kill them immediately. They were based on physical traps or on rapid killer molecules like strychnine. However, the neophobic behaviour of some rodents such as rats and their social organisation make these molecules ineffective. Indeed, the precocity of symptoms or death after a bait eating by congeners induces

Molecules	$T_{1/2}$ (h)
Brodifacoum cis	120.8
Brodifacoum trans	68.7
Bromadiolone cis	26.9
Bromadiolone trans	75.6
Difenacoum cis	78.3
Difenacoum trans	24.2
Difethialone cis	71.6
Difethialone trans	52.9
Flocoumafene cis	76.7
Flocoumafene trans	177.4

Table 1. Half-lives of some anticoagulant rodenticide enantiomers.

bait aversion in the rodent population [28, 29]. Conversely, the time to onset of anticoagulant action is sufficient to avoid that rodents link their symptoms and death to bait eating [29].

Moreover, the delay and the mechanism of action of ARs are the keystone of their safety of use comparatively to other rodenticides. Indeed, the delay allows the possibility to implement a treatment after an exposure to ARs and the mechanism of action can be easily bypassed which offers an efficient and safe antidotes, the vitamin K.

Nevertheless, some issues exist with anticoagulant rodenticides, first the resistance of some population to some AR molecules. This issue has led to the creation of the second generation of ARs, which are more efficient against resistant strains [30]. However, this generation is more persistent which involves other issues. This persistence extends the duration of antidote treatment after exposure. Moreover, it entails a greater concentration of AR molecules in rodents after its death; thus, it might increase the risk of secondary poisoning of predators or scavenger animals. Consequently, to prevent poisoning of humans and animals, many actions have been implemented in the use of ARs.

2.4. Prevention of poisoning

In Europe, an anticoagulant rodenticide product can be registered either as a plant protection product or as a biocide. According to the kind of registration, restriction and modality of use are defined in order to prevent human and animal intoxication. Nevertheless, there are important differences on the modality and restriction among the European Member States. Here, we present some member state (MS) actions to prevent poisoning.

The majority of MS distinguishes the individual use of ARs and the professional use. Professional users are mainly the pest control operator, they have to be trained. In some countries like France or Italy, the sale of ARs is restricted for the individual user, thus, in France, individuals cannot buy more than 1.5 kg of AR bait. In other countries, like Germany, only trained professionals are allowed to use the second generation of ARs. Moreover, some molecules can be allowed as biocides and be forbidden as plant protection products.

The presentation of ARs is also regulated. Baits are presented as poisoned seed, paste or foam. Previously concentred products like tracking powder and oil concentrate were used but they have been forbidden in many states. Thus, concentrations of the current AR baits are of the order of few dozen to few hundred milligrams of active product per kilogram of bait. The concentration depends on the efficiency of the active molecule. The main consequence of the use of products with low concentration is that it is difficult to reach the lethal dose at once for mammal heavier than rodents such as cats, dogs or humans. Nevertheless, the high half-life of some anticoagulants allows to reach this dose after a multi-exposure. The use of a bitter agent in bait is mandatory notably to avoid and limit exposure.

Finally, to avoid the exposure of untargeted species, in many states, baits have to be placed in secured bait stations. These stations have to be labelled to inform people on their content and on the action to perform in the case of exposure. Moreover, stations avoid the dispersion of baits which allows to control the consumption and they are waterproof, which prevent water pollution. Nevertheless, some rodents are reluctant to enter in bait stations which might involve failing in pest control. In spite of all described elements to prevent exposures and intoxications of human and untargeted animals to ARs, many cases have been reported.

Therefore, some recent research makes effort to implement a third generation of ARs which is based on the stereochemistry concept, which would be efficient against resistant strains of rodents and be less persistent and thus less involved in secondary poisoning [20, 27].

3. Human exposures and intoxications

Intoxication with anticoagulant rodenticides is a major public health concern. The involvement of poison control centres is crucial in the record of poisoning cases in both rural and urban areas. Besides, emergency departments report rare cases of intoxication by suicide or homicide. Most of these poisonings occur following accidental exposure, especially ingestion in children. Bleeding severity is highly variable, depending on the rodenticide exposure and on the delay between the exposure and patient management. The diagnosis relies on simple coagulation tests. Emergency department physicians should be aware of anticoagulant poisonings since management differs according to the anticoagulant rodenticide including warfarin or long-acting superwarfarin types.

3.1. Epidemiology

The incidence of poisoning with anticoagulant rodenticides is difficult to assess, mostly based on national registries. In the literature, cases associated with bleeding are published as case reports or small series, probably corresponding to the most severe ones.

In the annual report based on the US National Poison Data System and published by the American Association of Poison Control Centers, data related to long-acting superwarfarin- or warfarin-type rodenticides intoxication are given separately. Over the last 5-year period (2011–2015), the cumulated number of exposures is 44,095 for long-acting superwarfarin-type and 1029 for warfarin-type drugs, with a single exposure in 97.3 and 95.6% of the cases, respectively [31–35]. Interestingly, the number of reported cases has slightly decreased since 2008 (**Figure 3**) [36–38]. The mean prevalence of exposure over the last 5 years is 3.4% for long-acting superwarfarin-type and 4.9% for warfarin-type drugs. The age distribution shows that children, especially those of less than 5 years old, are the most involved (**Figure 4**); only 9% of the reported cases are adults. Finally, clinical outcomes are reported (**Figure 5**). Remarkably, outcome is favourable in 93.6% of the cases, probably due to the limited ingested doses in relation to the bad taste of numerous rodenticides. The bitterness brought by the excipients in the currently marketed rodenticides considerably limits the ingested amounts, especially in young children. In cases associated with significant complications, severe bleedings are observed in less than 10% of cases, with fatal bleedings occurring in only eight patients among the 44,095 exposed patients during the last 5-year period in the USA. Overall, poisoning with rodenticides remains a rare cause of morbidities and fatalities [31–35].

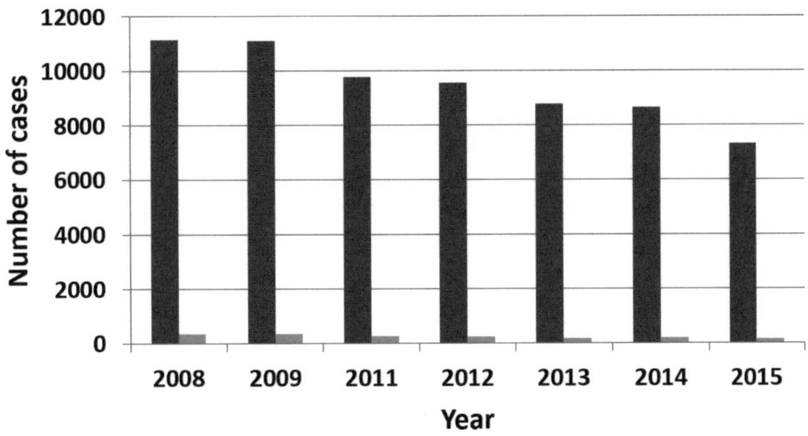

Figure 3. Number of poisonings with anticoagulant rodenticides reported by the American Association of Poison Control Centers from 2008 to 2015. Black bars: intoxications with long-acting anticoagulant-type rodenticides; grey bars: intoxications with warfarin-type rodenticides.

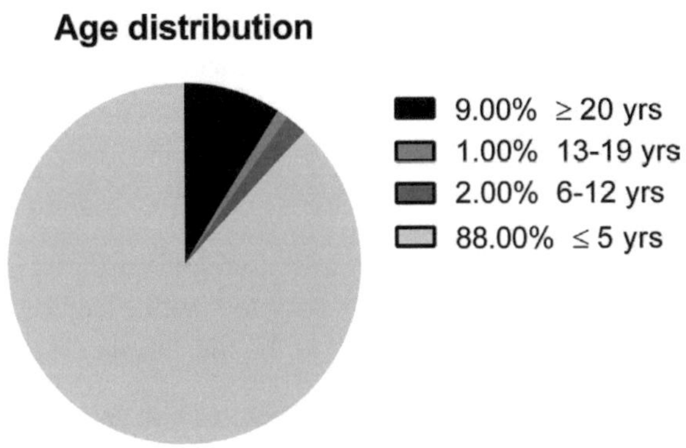

Figure 4. Distribution of the cases of poisoning with anticoagulant rodenticides reported by the American Association of Poison Control Centers in 2011–2015 according to the patient age.

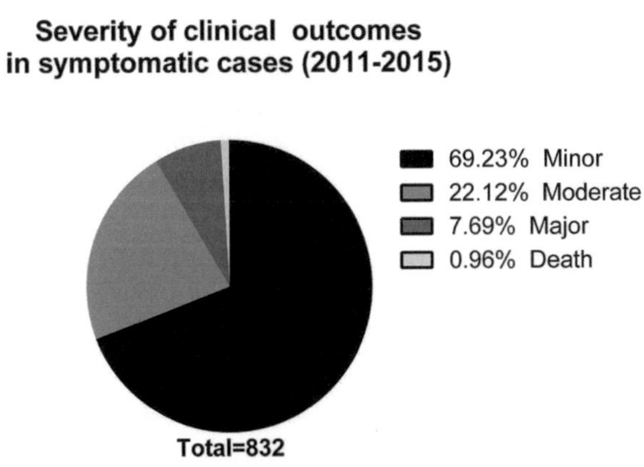

Figure 5. Distribution of the cases of poisoning with anticoagulant rodenticides reported by the American Association of Poison Control Centers in 2011–2015 according to the outcome.

http://dx.doi.org/10.5772/intechopen.69955

3.2. Clinical outcomes and laboratory diagnosis

The threat in poisoning with rodenticides is the onset of severe bleeding. In humans like in rodents, anticoagulant rodenticides inhibit the enzyme vitamin K epoxide reductase complex (VKORC1) leading to the absence of vitamin K recycling, which is essential for the gamma-carboxylation of vitamin K-dependent proteins in the hepatocytes, especially clotting prothrombin, factors VII, IX and X. This leads to impaired functioning of gamma-carboxylated vitamin-K-dependent factors due to their inability to bind activated platelets. Given the half-lives of coagulation in humans, i.e. from 6 hours for FVII to ~60 hours for prothrombin, the onset of hypocoagulability and the risk of bleeding are delayed after the exposure to rodenticides. The risk of bleeding depends on the severity of the hypocoagulability state induced by rodenticides and on the duration of hypocoagulability. The spectrum of bleeding is wide: extended unexplained spontaneous ecchymosis, epistaxis, hematoma, bleeding from the gastro-intestinal or the genitourinary tract as well as intra-cerebral bleeding are reported [39–46].

The diagnosis of rodenticide intoxication has to be considered for any patient with prolonged prothrombin time (increased INR), prolonged activated partial prothrombin time; the vitamin K-dependent factor II, VII, X, IX coagulant activities are decreased while factor V coagulant activity and the fibrinogen level are normal [41, 43, 47, 48]. Liver dysfunction, cholestasis and severe starvation can be ruled out by normal liver enzymes and serum albumin concentration. Moderate to severe anaemia can be present, depending on the severity of bleeding. Special attention and high clinical suspicion are required in patients with apparent negative history of warfarin treatment. The diagnosis of rodenticide intoxication should be suspected when the international normalised ratio (INR) strongly fluctuates on vitamin K therapy, especially while high doses of vitamin K are required. The accessibility to anticoagulant rodenticides should be checked; monitoring of persons who deal with rodenticides in their home or workplace, especially those suffering from dementia or psychiatric disorders, is necessary [49]. The intoxication can be confirmed by the identification and measurement of the rodenticides in plasma by specific assays [42, 45, 50].

3.3. Principles of poisoning management

Acute life-threatening complications can be prevented with timely intervention. Immediate administration of high doses of phytomenadione (vitamin K1) and/or factor prothrombin complex concentrate (30 UI/kg FIX) can successfully reverse the anticoagulant effects of anticoagulant rodenticides. With tissue half-lives estimated at between 16 and 220 days, reversal of superwarfarin toxicity is a long-term issue. Therefore, long-term daily treatment for several weeks of phytomenadione is necessary. Treatment courses averaged 168 days. To avoid re-bleeding, close monitoring of INR is necessary. Adjunctive haemostatic therapy with recombinant factor VIIa and prothrombin complex concentrate has been used [50–54].

4. Overview on animal exposures and intoxications

To assess the importance of animal intoxications, it is important to discriminate two situations: the domestic animals and the wildlife. Concerning wildlife, the evaluations of exposures and intoxications are often realised during focused scientific campaign and are often based on contamination studies or after an important mortality in wildlife. In domestic animal, besides the scientific campaign, there are, in some countries, animal specialised poison control centres, which can provide data on exposure, intoxications and linked symptoms.

In this part, it is important to take account of the differences between exposure and intoxication. Concerning exposure, it is the fact to take a dose of anticoagulants, it can be suspected by an owner who sees its animal eating baits, sometimes without knowing what the active substance is, or find in wildlife by pinpointing the presence of VKA in the sample. Intoxication is when the active substance induced clinical signs. This distinction is fundamental in the study of VKA toxicology. Indeed, to observe intoxication, the exposure dose and the delay of action has to be sufficient. This issue is discussed further concerning the wildlife exposure/intoxication studies.

4.1. Domestic animals

In France, two control poison centres are specialised in animals. The most important in terms of call number is the 'Centre National d' Informations Toxicologiques Vétérinaires (CNITV)' which responds to questions from owners or veterinarians on a 24-hour/7 day basis. We used this important database to assess the importance of VKA exposures and intoxications in domestic animals.

The data of the last 9 years have been analysed. During this period, the CNITV has received about 150,000 calls. Each month, 10.73% (CI 10.41-11.06) of solicitations are about VKA exposure or intoxication. Moreover, about whole VKA appeal is on domestic animals (99.2%). Appeals accrue from veterinary (69%) and owner (29%) mainly.

During the analysis of data, an important seasonality of the calls concerning VKAs has been pinpointed (**Figure 6**). Significant ($p < 0.05$) increases of the number of calls for VKA exposure are observed during the months of August, September and October followed by a significant decrease of appeal numbers from December to April, which is surprising. Indeed, based on our experience, the periods when people apply rodenticides in cities are at the beginning of winter (late November) and at the beginning of spring (March), when rodents are active and when the scarcity of food encourages rodents to eat baits. Conversely, during summer and the beginning of autumn, rodents can find many sources of food; consequently, they are less likely to eat baits, which increase the risk that baits are eaten by untargeted animals, notably dogs. However, summer is also the time when there is less human in cities and this element with a lenient weather encourages the presence of rodents outside where they are more visible. In response, cities and individuals might increase the number of baits, which is unfavourable for the rodent population management and rocket up the risk of pet exposures to VKA.

More generally, data pinpoint a trend reversal; before September 2013, the number of cases has significantly increased with a slope of 3.9% per annum ($p < 0.0001$) whereas after this date it has significantly decreased of 10.5% per annum ($p < 0.0001$). The increase trend has to be relativised as the total number of calls significantly increases during this period. However, after 2013, the total number of calls was stable ($p = 0.13$). Consequently, a significant decrease in the number of calls for VKAs after 2013 is confirmed. We hypothesise that the source of this diminution is the evolution of the regulation. Indeed, regulation has enforced the use of secured bait station since 2013, which seems to reduce the exposure of domestic species.

http://dx.doi.org/10.5772/intechopen.69955

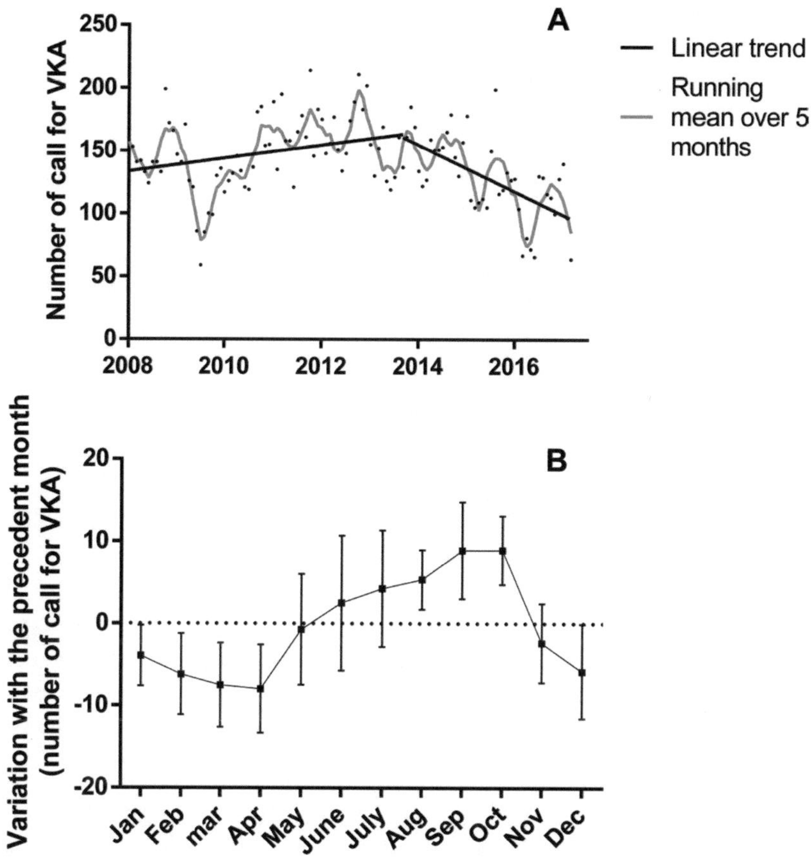

Figure 6. (A): Evolution of monthly calls for VKA exposure over time. Grey curve is the running means over 5 months. Dark lines are linear regression from January 2008 to September 2013 and from September 2013 to February 2017. (B) Variation of the number of calls for VKA exposure with the precedent month, values are represented as the mean of observed variations for the concerned month over the period 2008–2016 and its 95% confidence interval.

Pets and more specifically dogs are over represented (**Figure 7**). This might be explained by the lack of use of secured bait station by private individuals and by the behaviour of dogs. Poisoning is mainly accidental even if some malicious poisoning are reported (2.03%). The proportion of suspected malicious case concerning cats is significantly higher than for the general case. Indeed, cats and dogs represent, respectively, 19.14 and 63.64% of malicious reports. These uses of anticoagulant rodenticides with harmful intent against animals but also against humans have led to restrict the sale of rodenticides in some countries such as Italy [55].

Concerning molecules, in 22% of calls, the exact molecule is not identified. Nevertheless, exposures or intoxications with one of the six molecules authorised are reported, they are difenacoum, difethialone, brodifacoum, bromadiolone, chlorophacinone and coumatetralyl, which represent, respectively, 23, 18, 10, 9, 3 and 2% of the calls for AR. It is significant that the four main anticoagulants are second-generation ARs. This was predictable because first-generation ARs are less efficient on resistant strains of rodents consequently main ARs sold belong to the second generation.

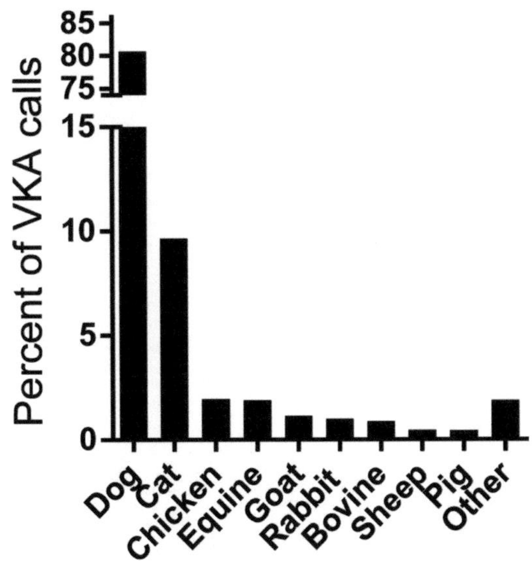

Figure 7. Percentage of species concerned by calls on VKA.

The consequences of an exposure without intoxication are completely different for pets and farm animals. Indeed, for pets when an exposure occurs, the aim is to prevent intoxication. In farm animals, more than intoxication prevention, the presence of anticoagulant molecules in products such as meat, eggs or milk has to be considered. Further, we discuss issues of ARs in pets then in farm animals.

In pets, depending on caller, the circumstances of appeal are different. Indeed, 90% of calls from individuals report exposure without intoxication, whereas the proportion of this circumstance drops significantly to 75% when it is a call from a veterinary ($p < 0.0001$). This can be easily understood, if an animal shows a symptom, the owner priority is to bring it to the veterinarian to be healed. Differences according to species are also pinpointed. In dogs, 81% of calls for AR exposure do not report symptoms versus 62% in cats ($p < 0.0001$). The source of this distinction may be the detection of the exposure, which is earlier in dogs. Moreover, cats may be more prone to be secondary exposed to ARs from intoxicated rodents and this kind of exposure is not visible by the owner. It should be noted that according to the low doses of bait and to the difference between the toxic doses for a rodent versus a cat, a large number of intoxicated rodents should be eaten to induce intoxication.

In dogs and cats, when an exposure is suspected and when it is possible, the best way to prevent intoxication is to induce vomiting in the first hour after the exposure. If medicines are not available, it is possible to use 10 volume hydrogen peroxide. Hydrogen peroxide solution can be given orally to animals at 1 mL for every 5 kg of weight. Be careful, salt must not be used to induce vomiting. Indeed, excess of salt can cause fatal hypernatremia [56].

Sometimes, even the exposure is uncertain or the absorption of VKA after vomiting is unknown, to confirm exposure, two means are currently tested by our team: the dosing of VKAs in plasma and their dosing in faeces. The difficulty of dosing in plasma is that for some VKAs, the presence in the plasma is temporary then VKAs are stored in liver. Therefore, dosing in plasma is often associated with false-negatives. The dosing of VKA in faeces seems to be more reliable with an excretion that can be detected for several weeks.

As there is not any well-described toxicity dose, it is important to follow the possible effect of AR in order to prevent serious intoxication. Moreover, there is no correlation between the dose of VKA and the symptom severity [57]. Today, the gold standard to diagnose VKA intoxication is the prothrombin time [58]. It is advised realising a prothrombin time about 48 hours after the suspected exposure [59]. If the prothrombin time is elevated then a treatment has to be initiated. Other methods such as vitamin K clotting factor concentration measurement are explored to detect AR effects sooner. Factor VII seems to be a good candidate as its half-life after a VKA administration is the shorter [60].

If no treatment is given, symptoms may appear after 2–6 days [57, 58]. Symptoms are the classic signs of coagulopathy, which may be pinpointed by owner as bleeding, pale mucous membrane, haematomas, haematuria or haematemesis as well as their consequences on animal general condition as lameness, depression or lethargy [57, 58, 61]. Owing to intrathoracic bleeding, respiratory distress occurs frequently in anticoagulant intoxications [62–64].

Animals exposed with an elevation of prothrombin time after exposure or with AR-linked symptoms have to receive vitamin K_1 supplementation as long as the recycling mechanism is inhibited. Vitamin K_1 is given *per os* daily with a dose of 5 mg/kg of body weight. The duration of the VKA inhibition depends on the pharmacokinetics of AR molecule with huge differences between molecules. Thus, the duration of treatment after an exposure to the first-generation AR is estimated to 3 weeks versus 5–7 for the second generation. Nevertheless, there is a lack of studies to support these durations of treatment. Thus, a treatment can be initiated during at least 1 month then stopped during 48 hours. After 2 days of treatment discontinuation, the vitamin K regeneration mechanism can be assessed by measuring prothrombin time. If prothrombin time is elevated, treatment has to be replicated until a new assessment of regeneration mechanism else, the treatment can be arrested. Vitamin K_3 is inefficient to treat VKA intoxication. The treatment of symptomatic animals may require fresh plasma to reconstitute the pool of clotting factors urgently, moreover, in this case, it is recommended initiating the vitamin K treatment by an intravenous administration. If there is a proper compliance of the vitamin K treatment, the prognostic is excellent [57].

In farm animals, when an AR exposure occurs, the safety of the product has to be considered. Little information is available on the contamination of food following AR exposure. Nevertheless, many methods have been implemented to assess the residues in foodstuffs [65, 66]. Concerning meat, it has been shown that VKA molecules are present in muscle after exposure and that the cooking does not influence their activities [67]. Likewise, VKA molecules are also present in eggs after hen exposure, and are still detected in eggs 14 days after exposure [68]. Concerning the milk, it has been observed an excretion of VKA in human milk when a VKA is used as medication for the mother [69]. Consequently, it might be supposed that the same occurs in animals. Thus, when an animal is exposed, its litter should be separated of its mother and fed with relevant artificial milk. If separation is not possible or if diagnostic is late, litter should be supplemented with vitamin K_1. Concerning foodstuffs provided by an exposed animal, their management would be done in accordance with relevant authority.

4.2. Wildlife exposures and intoxication

Wildlife expositions or intoxications to ARs have been reported around the world for many mammals such as minks [70], bobcats [71], stoats and weasels [72], foxes [73, 74] and boars [67] and as well for many birds [75–77]. Exposition of fish was reported near an island where an eradication of rodent with brodifacoum was performed and the risk for human through the consumption appeared very low [78].

These intoxications may be primary when non-target species eat directly the bait. It is the case when baits are directly available without protection or when they are washed away and diluted in sea or river. In Spain, a study on water and soil samples revealed no imminent environmental risk in treated areas with chlorophacinone and brodifacoum [79]. However, the use of secured bait stations prevents this kind of exposition.

The secondary exposition occurs when a scavenger or a predator eats an exposed rodent. It is the most described exposition of wildlife to ARs and the most difficult to prevent. Many factors may influence the level of secondary exposition. First, due to the bait appetence, rodents can eat more AR than necessary to lead to their death, which might increase their concentration in AR. Moreover, if rodent is resistant to ARs, this phenomenon might be amplified. Indeed, a resistant rodent eats twice to fivefold more AR than susceptible rodent [1]. After the onset of symptoms in rodents, their behaviour evolves. They increase their activity during the day and stay longer in uncovered area, which enhances the risk to be hunted by predators [1]. The delayed action of ARs, inherent to its mechanism, allows rodents to eat several times the LD50 dose between the first bait intake and the death [1] and may as well increase the risk of secondary exposition. Pesticide usage has been correlated with non-target wildlife exposition [74, 75], and the intensity of treatment was related to incidence on local fox populations in France [80]. Finally, the diet is certainly going to influence secondary exposition and species like raptors, foxes and mustelids largely feeding on rodents when abundant are consequently the most at risk, as demonstrated for the red kite (Milvus milvus) [81]. The removal of visible rodent bodies helps to reduce the risk of secondary exposition [82] but is not always possible because of landscape limited access and in the case of aerial application [1]. Mitigation measures have been considered to protect predatory species but new approaches are still required [82].

Persistence and toxicity of the molecule are key factors. They depend on the used active ingredient [26, 83]. Historically, second-generation ARs had been designed to be more persistent and toxic on resistant strain. Thus, secondary poisonings of wildlife associated with the use of second generation are more often reported. But the development of new ARs recently proposed is based on the stereochemistry of second-generation ARs with reduced persistence but equivalent toxicity might greatly decrease the level of secondary exposition [20].

They are two types of consequences of the exposition of wildlife to ARs. First, if the species is eaten by human [67, 78], the consequences are comparable to those discussed for farm animals. Second, if the exposition is sufficiently important, it might lead to intoxication of the animals and to its death, which can be problematic mainly for endangered species. The rate of exposure of non-target species has often been evaluated, and summed liver concentrations above a limit of 0.2 mg/kg associated with clinical signs (i.e. macroscopic haemorrhages with no trauma) have been statistically characterised as representative of a high-risk toxic threshold

http://dx.doi.org/10.5772/intechopen.69955

[84]. According to these criteria, hepatic concentrations above 0.2 mg/kg have been associated with mortalities in raptors and small mustelids from Denmark [85], in raptors and hedgehogs from Mediterranean region of Spain [86], in six raptor species from Canary Islands, Spain [77].

It is difficult to discriminate a simple exposition and intoxication in wildlife. Indeed, as well as in domestic animal, toxic doses are not well described for all species. Moreover, the majorities of exposition studies are performed on dead animal, and as the lesion induced by ARs is not specific, so it might be difficult to conclude to its implications. Less than 10% of exposed and dead birds have been confirmed to be intoxicated by ARs [1, 87]. Currently, there are no reports of a significant incidence of ARs on non-targeted species populations [82]. Nevertheless, impact of ARs on wildlife has to be more monitored in order to limit the impact of rodent population management. The probable future design of eco-friendly baits with new isomer ratio will change the need the way AR hepatic residues are monitored. The recently described multi-residue LC-MS/MS method [88] is an appropriate tool to start investigating second-generation AR diastereoisomer proportions in non-target wildlife and to evaluate their respective persistence in predators.

5. Conclusion

Anticoagulant rodenticides are a keystone of the rodent population management. Like other poisons, there is a risk of human or non-targeted species poisoning. The wide use of anticoagulant rodenticides near human living space and agriculture space involves an important exposure of humans and domestic animals. Nevertheless, since few years, many risk mitigation measures have been taken and the number of exposure in humans and domestic animals has decreased. Moreover, in contrast to the majority of chemical biocide, anticoagulant rodenticides have an effective antidote, the vitamin K. Consequently, anticoagulant poisoning is rarely fatal. However, the impact of anticoagulant rodenticides on wildlife is least well known and deserves more investigation.

Author details

Sébastien Lefebvre[1], Isabelle Fourel[1], Stéphane Queffélec[2], Dominique Vodovar[4], Bruno Mégarbane[4], Etienne Benoit[1], Virginie Siguret[3] and Virginie Lattard[1]*

*Address all correspondence to: virginie.lattard@vetagro-sup.fr

1 USC 1233 RS2GP, VetAgro Sup, INRA, Univ Lyon, Marcy l'étoile, France

2 Centre National d'Informations Toxicologiques Vétérinaires (CNITV), Marcy l'étoile, France

3 Université Paris Descartes, INSERM UMR-S1140 and Service d'hématologie biologique, Hôpital Lariboisière (AP-HP), Paris, France

4 Université Paris-Diderot, INSERM UMRS-1144 and Réanimation Médicale et Toxicologique, Hôpital Lariboisière (AP-HP), Paris, France

References

[1] Buckle AP, Smith RH, editors. Rodent Pests and their Control. 2nd ed. Boston, MA: CAB; 2015. 422p.

[2] Russell JC, Holmes ND. Tropical island conservation: Rat eradication for species recovery. Biological Conservation. May 2015;**185**:1-7

[3] Truchetet D, Couval G, Michelin Y, Giraudoux P. Genèse de la problématique du campagnol terrestre en prairies. Fourrages [Internet]. 9 Dec 2016; (220, 220). Available from: http://prodinra.inra.fr/?locale=fr#!ConsultNotice:287077 [Accessed: 9 March 2017]

[4] Singleton GR. Impacts of Rodents on Rice Production in Asia. Discuss Pap [Internet]. 2003. Available from: http://www.academia.edu/29606094/Impacts_of_rodents_on_rice_production_in_Asia [Accessed: 28 March 2017]

[5] Pimentel D, Lach L, Zuniga R, Morrison D. Environmental and economic costs of nonindigenous species in the United States. BioScience. 1 Jan 2000;**50**(1):53-65

[6] Stenseth NC, Leirs H, Skonhoft A, Davis SA, Pech RP, Andreassen HP, et al. Mice, rats, and people: The bio-economics of agricultural rodent pests. Frontiers in Ecology and the Environment. 1 Sep 2003;**1**(7):367-375

[7] Boyle CM. Case of apparent resistance of *Rattus norvegicus* berkenhout to anticoagulant poisons. Nature. 1960;**188**(4749):517-517

[8] Alstad AD, Casper HH, Johnson LJ. Vitamin K treatment of sweet clover poisoning in calves. Journal of the American Veterinary Medical Association. Oct 1985;**187**(7):729-731

[9] Goplen BP. Sweetclover production and agronomy. The Canadian Veterinary Journal. May 1980;**21**(5):149-151

[10] Huebner CF, Link KP. Studies on the hemorrhagic sweet clover disease VI. The synthesis of the δ-diketone derived from the hemorrhagic agent through alkaline degradation. Journal of Biological Chemistry. 1941;**138**(2):529-534

[11] Link KP, Mark S. Di-esters of 3,3′-methylenebis (4-hydroxycoumarin) and process of making them. US2345635 A, 1942

[12] Miyoshi I, Paul LK, Stahmann MA. 3-Substituted 4-hydroxycoumarin and process of making it. US2427578 A, 1947

[13] Lasseur R, Longin-Sauvageon C, Videmann B, Billeret M, Berny P, Benoit E. Warfarin resistance in a French strain of rats. Journal of Biochemical and Molecular Toxicology. 1 Jan 2006;**19**(6):379-385

[14] Thijssen HHW, Baars LGM. Microsomal warfarin binding and vitamin K 2,3-epoxide reductase. Biochemical Pharmacology. 1 Apr 1989;**38**(7):1115-1120

[15] Esmon CT, Sadowski JA, Suttie JW. A new carboxylation reaction. The vitamin K-dependent incorporation of H-14-CO3- into prothrombin. Journal of Biological Chemistry. 25 Jun 1975;**250**(12):4744-4748

[16] Suttie JW. Vitamin K-dependent carboxylase. Annual Review of Biochemistry. 1985; **54**:459-477

[17] Friedman PA, Shia MA, Gallop PM, Griep AE. Vitamin K-dependent gamma-carbon-hydrogen bond cleavage and nonmandatory concurrent carboxylation of peptide-bound glutamic acid residues. Proceedings of the National Academy of Sciences of the United States of America. Jul 1979;**76**(7):3126-3129

[18] Larson AE, Suttie JW. Vitamin K-dependent carboxylase: Evidence for a hydroperoxide intermediate in the reaction. Proceedings of the National Academy of Sciences of the United States of America. Nov 1978;**75**(11):5413-5416

[19] Jin D-Y, Tie J-K, Stafford DW. The conversion of vitamin K epoxide to vitamin K quinone and vitamin K quinone to vitamin K hydroquinone uses the same active site cysteines. Biochemistry (Moscow). 19 Jun 2007;**46**(24):7279-7283

[20] Damin-Pernik M, Espana B, Lefebvre S, Fourel I, Caruel H, Benoit E, et al. Management of Rodent Populations by Anticoagulant Rodenticides: Toward Third-Generation Anticoagulant Rodenticides. Drug Metab Dispos. 2017 Feb 1;**45**(2):160-5

[21] Kaminsky LS, Zhang Z-Y. Human P450 metabolism of warfarin. Pharmacology & Therapeutics. 1997;**73**(1):67-74

[22] Rettie AE, Korzekwa KR, Kunze KL, Lawrence RF, Eddy AC, Aoyama T, et al. Hydroxylation of warfarin by human cDNA-expressed cytochrome P-450: A role for P-4502C9 in the etiology of (S)-warfarin-drug interactions. Chemical Research in Toxicology. 1 Jan 1992;**5**(1):54-59

[23] Breckenridge A, Orme M, Wesseling H, Lewis RJ, Gibbons R. Pharmacokinetics and pharmacodynamics of the enantiomers of warfarin in man. Clinical Pharmacology & Therapeutics. Apr 1974;**15**(4):424-430

[24] O'Reilly RA. Studies on the optical enantiomorphs of warfarin in man. Clinical Pharmacology & Therapeutics. Aug 1974;**16**(2):348-354

[25] Takahashi DH, Echizen H. Pharmacogenetics of warfarin elimination and its clinical implications. Clinical Pharmacokinetics. 14 Sep 2012;**40**(8):587-603

[26] Vandenbroucke V, Bousquet-Melou A, De Backer P, Croubels S. Pharmacokinetics of eight anticoagulant rodenticides in mice after single oral administration. Journal of Veterinary Pharmacology and Therapeutics. Oct 2008;**31**(5):437-445

[27] Damin-Pernik M, Espana B, Besse S, Fourel I, Caruel H, Popowycz F, et al. Development of an ecofriendly anticoagulant rodenticide based on the stereochemistry of difenacoum. Drug Metabolism and Disposition: The Biological Fate of Chemicals. Dec 2016;**44**(12):1872-1880

[28] Nachman M, Hartley PL. Role of illness in producing learned taste aversions in rats: A comparison of several rodenticides. Journal of Comparative and Physiological Psychology. 1975;**89**(9):1010-1018

[29] Parshad VR, Kochar JK. Potential of three rodenticides to induce conditioned aversion to their baits in the Indian mole rat, Bandicota bengalensis. Applied Animal Behaviour Science. 1 Nov 1995;**45**(3):267-276

[30] Lefebvre S, Benoit E, Lattard V. Comparative biology of the resistance to vitamin K antagonists: An overview of the resistance mechanisms. In: Basaran O, Biteker M, editors. Anticoagulation Therapy [Internet]. InTech; 2016. Available from: http://www.intechopen.com/books/anticoagulation-therapy/comparative-biology-of-the-resistance-to-vitamin-k-antagonists-an-overview-of-the-resistance-mechani [Accessed: 11 January 2017]

[31] Bronstein AC, Spyker DA, Cantilena Jr LR, Rumack BH, Dart RC. 2011 Annual Report of the American Association of Poison Control Centers' National Poison Data System (NPDS): 29th Annual Report. Clinical Toxicology. 1 Dec 2012;**50**(10):911-1164

[32] Mowry JB, Spyker DA, Brooks DE, Zimmerman A, Schauben JL. 2015 Annual Report of the American Association of Poison Control Centers' National Poison Data System (NPDS): 33rd Annual Report. Clinical Toxicology. 25 Nov 2016;**54**(10):924-1109

[33] Mowry JB, Spyker DA, Brooks DE, McMillan N, Schauben JL. 2014 Annual Report of the American Association of Poison Control Centers' National Poison Data System (NPDS): 32nd Annual Report. Clinical Toxicology. 26 Nov 2015;**53**(10):962-1147

[34] Mowry JB, Spyker DA, Cantilena Jr LR, McMillan N, Ford M. 2013 Annual Report of the American Association of Poison Control Centers' National Poison Data System (NPDS): 31st Annual Report. Clinical Toxicology. 1 Dec 2014;**52**(10):1032-1283

[35] Mowry JB, Spyker DA, Cantilena Jr LR, Bailey JE, Ford M. 2012 Annual Report of the American Association of Poison Control Centers' National Poison Data System (NPDS): 30th Annual Report. Clinical Toxicology. 1 Dec 2013;**51**(10):949-1229

[36] Bronstein AC, Spyker DA, Cantilena LR, Green JL, Rumack BH, Dart RC. 2010 Annual Report of the American Association of Poison Control Centers' National Poison Data System (NPDS): 28th Annual Report. Clinical Toxicology. 1 Dec 2011;**49**(10):910-941

[37] Bronstein AC, Spyker DA, Cantilena LR, Green JL, Rumack BH, Giffin SL. 2008 Annual Report of the American Association of Poison Control Centers' National Poison Data System (NPDS): 26th Annual Report. Clinical Toxicology (Philadelphia, Pa). Dec 2009;**47**(10):911-1084

[38] Bronstein AC, Spyker DA, Cantilena LR, Green JL, Rumack BH, Giffin SL. 2009 Annual Report of the American Association of Poison Control Centers' National Poison Data System (NPDS): 27th Annual Report. Clinical Toxicology (Philadelphia, Pa). Dec 2010;**48**(10):979-1178

[39] Spahr JE, Maul JS, Rodgers GM. Superwarfarin poisoning: A report of two cases and review of the literature. American Journal of Hematology. 1 Jul 2007;**82**(7):656-660

[40] Kamijo Y, Sato C, Yoshimura K, Soma K. Notable pink excreta and severe myocardial suppression in superwarfarin (difethialone) intoxication. Internal Medicine. 2011;**50**(22):2819-2822

[41] Zheng F, Jin Y, Wang M, Niu Z, Xu P, Xie H. Congenital combined deficiency of factor VII and X in a patient due to accidental diphacinone intoxication. Thrombosis and Haemostasis. 2011;**106**(1):180-181

[42] Hong J, Yhim H-Y, Bang S-M, Bae SH, Yuh YJ, Yoon S-S, et al. Korean patients with superwarfarin intoxication and their outcome. Journal of Korean Medical Science. Dec 2010;**25**(12):1754-1758

[43] Boettcher S, Wacker A, Moerike K, Kopp H-G, Jaschonek K, Grobosch T, et al. Acquired coagulopathy caused by intoxication with the superwarfarin-type anticoagulant rodenticide flocoumafen. European Journal of Haematology. 1 Feb 2011;**86**(2):173-175

[44] Kim SY, Cho SY, Lee HJ, Suh J-T, Oh SH, Lee W-I, et al. Superwarfarin Intoxication of unknown etiology accompanying hemoperitoneum in a patient on fluconazole therapy. Annals of Clinical & Laboratory Science. 20 Jun 2010;**40**(3):300-303

[45] Zolcinski M, Padjas A, Musial J. Intoxication with three different superwarfarin compounds in an adult woman. Thrombosis and Haemostasis. Jul 2008;**100**(1):156-157

[46] Papin F, Clarot F, Vicomte C, Gaulier JM, Daubin C, Chapon F, et al. Lethal paradoxical cerebral vein thrombosis due to suspicious anticoagulant rodenticide intoxication with chlorophacinone. Forensic Science International. 2 Mar 2007;**166**(2-3):85-90

[47] Grobosch T, Angelow B, Schönberg L, Lampe D. Acute bromadiolone intoxication. Journal of Analytical Toxicology. May 2006;**30**(4):281-286

[48] King N, Tran M-H. Long-acting anticoagulant rodenticide (superwarfarin) poisoning: A review of its historical development, epidemiology, and clinical management. Transfusion Medicine Reviews. Oct 2015;**29**(4):250-258

[49] Lee H-J, You M-R, Moon W-R, Sul H, Chung C-H, Park C-Y, et al. Evaluation of risk factors in patients with vitamin K-dependent coagulopathy presumed to be caused by exposure to brodifacoum. Korean Journal of Internal Medicine. Jul 2014;**29**(4):498-508

[50] Lo VMH, Ching CK, Chan AYW, Mak TWL. Bromadiolone toxicokinetics: Diagnosis and treatment implications. Clinical toxicology (Philadelphia, PA). Sep 2008;**46**(8):703-710

[51] Card DJ, Francis S, Deuchande K, Harrington DJ. Superwarfarin poisoning and its management. BMJ Case Reports. 13 Oct 2014;**2014**

[52] Haesloop O, Tillick A, Nichol G, Strote J. Superwarfarin ingestion treated successfully with prothrombin complex concentrate. The American Journal of Emergency Medicine. Jan 2016;**34**(1):116.e1-116.e12

[53] Wang Y, Kotik V, Fahim G, Alagusundaramoorthy S, Eltawansy SA, Mathis S, et al. Treatment of brodifacoum overdose with prothrombin complex concentrate. The American Journal of Health-System Pharmacy AJHP: American Journal of Health-System Pharmacy. 1 Jan 2016;**73**(1):e14-e17

[54] Park J. Can we more efficiently save patients with vitamin K-dependent coagulopathy caused by superwarfarin intoxication? Korean Journal of Internal Medicine. Jul 2014;**29**(4):430-433

[55] Muscarella M, Armentano A, Iammarino M, Palermo C, Amorena M. Anticoagulant rodenticide poisoning in animals of Apulia and Basilicata, Italy. Veterinaria Italiana. 30 Jun 2016;**52**(2):153-159

[56] Khanna C, Boermans H, Wilcock B. Fatal hypernatremia in a dog from salt ingestion. Journal of the American Animal Hospital Association. 1 Mar 1997;**33**(2):113-117

[57] Waddell LS, Poppenga RH, Drobatz KJ. Anticoagulant rodenticide screening in dogs: 123 cases (1996-2003). Journal of the American Veterinary Medical Association. 15 Feb 2013;**242**(4):516-521

[58] Murphy MJ. Rodenticides. Veterinary Clinics of North America: Small Animal Practice. Mar 2002;**32**(2):469-484, viii

[59] Woody BJ, Murphy MJ, Ray AiC, Green RA. Coagulopathic effects and therapy of brodifacoum toxicosis in dogs. Journal of Veterinary Internal Medicine. 1 Jan 1992;**6**(1):23-28

[60] Lefebvre S, Hascoët C, Damin-Pernik M, Rannou B, Benoit E, Lattard V. Monitoring of antivitamin K-dependent anticoagulation in rodents – towards an evolution of the methodology to detect resistance in rodents. Pesticide Biochemistry and Physiology [Internet]. 2017. Available from: http://www.sciencedirect.com/science/article/pii/S004835751730072X [Accessed: 28 February 2017]

[61] Sheafor SE, Couto CG. Anticoagulant rodenticide toxicity in 21 dogs. Journal of the American Animal Hospital Association. Feb 1999;**35**(1):38-46

[62] Blocker TL, Roberts BK. Acute tracheal obstruction associated with anticoagulant rodenticide intoxication in a dog. Journal of Small Animal Practice. 1 Dec 1999;**40**(12):577-580

[63] Berry CR, Gallaway A, Thrall DE, Carlisle C. Thoracic radiographic features of anticoagulant rodenticide toxicity in fourteen dogs. Veterinary Radiology & Ultrasound. 1 Nov 1993;**34**(6):391-396

[64] Bergh MS, Silverstein DC. What Is your diagnosis? Journal of the American Veterinary Medical Association. 15 Apr 2006;**228**(8):1193-1194

[65] Shimshoni JA, Soback S, Cuneah O, Shlosberg A, Britzi M. New validated multiresidue analysis of six 4-hydroxy-coumarin anticoagulant rodenticides in hen eggs. Journal of Veterinary Diagnostic Investigation. Nov 2013;**25**(6):736-743

[66] Pouliquen H, Fauconnet V, Morvan ML, Pinault L. Determination of warfarin in the yolk and the white of hens' eggs by reversed-phase high-performance liquid chromatography. Journal of Chromatography B Biomedical Sciences and Applications. 21 Nov 1997;**702**(1-2):143-148

[67] Pitt WC, Higashi M, Primus TM. The effect of cooking on diphacinone residues related to human consumption of feral pig tissues. Food and Chemical Toxicology. Sep 2011; **49**(9):2030-2034

[68] Kammerer M, Pouliquen H, Pinault L, Loyau M. Residues depletion in egg after warfarin ingestion by laying hens. Veterinary and Human Toxicology. Oct 1998;**40**(5):273-275

[69] De Swiet M, Lewis PJ. Excretion of anticoagulants in human milk. The New England Journal of Medicine. 29 Dec 1977;**297**(26):1471

[70] Fournier-Chambrillon C, Berny PJ, Coiffier O, Barbedienne P, Dassé B, Delas G, et al. Evidence of secondary poisoning of free-ranging riparian mustelids by anticoagulant rodenticides in France: Implications for conservation of European mink (Mustela lutreola). Journal of Wildlife Diseases. Oct 2004;**40**(4):688-695

[71] Serieys LEK, Armenta TC, Moriarty JG, Boydston EE, Lyren LM, Poppenga RH, et al. Anticoagulant rodenticides in urban bobcats: Exposure, risk factors and potential effects based on a 16-year study. Ecotoxicology (London, England). May 2015;**24**(4):844-862

[72] Elmeros M, Christensen TK, Lassen P. Concentrations of anticoagulant rodenticides in stoats Mustela erminea and weasels Mustela nivalis from Denmark. Science of the Total Environment. 15 May 2011;**409**(12):2373-2378

[73] Geduhn A, Jacob J, Schenke D, Keller B, Kleinschmidt S, Esther A. Relation between intensity of biocide practice and residues of anticoagulant rodenticides in Red Foxes (Vulpes vulpes). Spanoghe P, editor. PLoS One. 29 Sep 2015;**10**(9):e0139191

[74] Sage M, Fourel I, Cœurdassier M, Barrat J, Berny P, Giraudoux P. Determination of bromadiolone residues in fox faeces by LC/ESI-MS in relationship with toxicological data and clinical signs after repeated exposure. Environmental Research. Oct 2010;**110**(7):664-674

[75] Hughes J, Sharp E, Taylor MJ, Melton L, Hartley G. Monitoring agricultural rodenticide use and secondary exposure of raptors in Scotland. Ecotoxicology. Aug 2013;**22**(6):974-984

[76] Langford KH, Reid M, Thomas KV. The occurrence of second generation anticoagulant rodenticides in non-target raptor species in Norway. Science of the Total Environment. 15 Apr 2013;**450-451**:205-208

[77] Ruiz-Suárez N, Henríquez-Hernández LA, Valerón PF, Boada LD, Zumbado M, Camacho M, et al. Assessment of anticoagulant rodenticide exposure in six raptor species from the Canary Islands (Spain). Science of the Total Environment. 1 Jul 2014;**485-486**:371-376

[78] Masuda BM, Fisher P, Beaven B. Residue profiles of brodifacoum in coastal marine species following an island rodent eradication. Ecotoxicology and Environmental Safety. Mar 2015;**113**:1-8

[79] Hernández AM, Bernal J, Bernal JL, Martín MT, Caminero C, Nozal MJ. Simultaneous determination of nine anticoagulant rodenticides in soil and water by LC-ESI-MS. Journal of Separation Science. Aug 2013;**36**(16):2593-2601

[80] Jacquot M, Coeurdassier M, Couval G, Renaude R, Pleydell D, Truchetet D, et al. Using long-term monitoring of red fox populations to assess changes in rodent control practices. Journal of Applied Ecology. 1 Dec 2013;**50**(6):1406-1414

[81] Coeurdassier M, Poirson C, Paul J-P, Rieffel D, Michelat D, Reymond D, et al. The diet of migrant Red Kites Milvus milvus during a Water Vole Arvicola terrestris outbreak in eastern France and the associated risk of secondary poisoning by the rodenticide bromadiolone. Ibis. 1 Jan 2012;**154**(1):136-146

[82] Rattner BA, Lazarus RS, Elliott JE, Shore RF, van den Brink N. Adverse outcome pathway and risks of anticoagulant rodenticides to predatory wildlife. Environmental Science & Technology. Aug 2014;**48**(15):8433-8445

[83] Erickson WA, Urban DJ. Potential Risks of Nine Rodenticides to Birds and Nontarget Mammals: A Comparative Approach [Internet]. US Environmental Protection Agency, Office of Prevention, Pesticides and Toxic Substances Washington, DC; 2004. Available from: http://pesticideresearch.com/site/docs/bulletins/EPAComparisonRodenticideRisks.pdf [Accessed: 10 April 2017]

[84] Thomas PJ, Mineau P, Shore RF, Champoux L, Martin PA, Wilson LK, et al. Second generation anticoagulant rodenticides in predatory birds: Probabilistic characterisation of toxic liver concentrations and implications for predatory bird populations in Canada. Environment International. Jul 2011;**37**(5):914-920

[85] Christensen TK, Lassen P, Elmeros M. High exposure rates of anticoagulant rodenticides in predatory bird species in intensively managed landscapes in Denmark. Archives of Environmental Contamination and Toxicology. Oct 2012;**63**(3):437-444

[86] López-Perea JJ, Camarero PR, Molina-López RA, Parpal L, Obón E, Solá J, et al. Interspecific and geographical differences in anticoagulant rodenticide residues of predatory wildlife from the Mediterranean region of Spain. Science of the Total Environment. Apr 2015;**511**:259-267

[87] Murray M. Anticoagulant rodenticide exposure and toxicosis in four species of birds of prey presented to a wildlife clinic in Massachusetts, 2006-2010. Journal of Zoo and Wildlife Medicine, Official Publication of American Association of Zoo Veterinarians. Mar 2011;**42**(1):88-97

[88] Fourel I, Damin-Pernik M, Benoit E, Lattard V. Core-shell LC–MS/MS method for quantification of second generation anticoagulant rodenticides diastereoisomers in rat liver in relationship with exposure of wild rats. Journal of Chromatography. Jan 2017;**1041-1042**: 120-132

Chapter 3

Food Poisoning Caused by Bacteria (Food Toxins)

Cecilia Hernández-Cortez, Ingrid Palma-Martínez,
Luis Uriel Gonzalez-Avila,
Andrea Guerrero-Mandujano,
Raúl Colmenero Solís and Graciela Castro-Escarpulli

Additional information is available at the end of the chapter

http://dx.doi.org/10.5772/intechopen.69953

Abstract

In the environment, there are polluting substances that can cause adverse reactions in human beings when entering the body through different ways (ingestion, inhalation, injection, or absorption). The main pollutants can be poisons, chemical compounds, toxic gases, and bacterial toxins. These can be found in different places and their effects depend on the dose and exposure time. Furthermore, foodborne diseases (FBDs) can cause disability; these diseases can be caused by toxins produced by bacteria or other toxic substances in the food, which can cause severe diarrhea, toxic shock syndrome, debilitating infections such as meningitis and even death. FBDs are transmitted through food contaminated with pathogenic microorganisms that have multiple factors of virulence, which gives them the ability to cause an infection; some bacterial genres can produce toxins directly in the food, but other genres can produce them once they have colonized the intestine. Among the pathogens involved in FBDs that are also considered to be toxigenic are Salmonella spp., *Vibrio parahaemolyticus, Vibrio cholerae, Staphylococcus aureus, Clostridium botulinum, Clostridium perfringens, Bacillus cereus, Listeria monocytogenes*. Foodborne diseases can be prevented and acute diarrhea syndromes, fever and even death from dehydration can be avoided, especially in children under the age of 5 and in immunocompromised people.

Keywords: toxins, bacteria, food poisoning, food-borne disease

1. Introduction

The main pollutants can be poisons, chemical compounds, toxic gases, and bacterial toxins. There are several diseases that human beings can acquire by ingesting some type of pollutants, for example, chemical contamination can lead to acute poisoning or long-term diseases such as cancer. Furthermore, foodborne diseases (FBDs) can cause disability; these diseases can be caused by the toxins produced by the bacteria or other toxic substances in food [1].

It is important to know that poisoning is the cause of morbidity and mortality worldwide. There are different types of intoxication: (a) intoxication caused by chemical substances (such as drugs, pesticides, heavy metals, gases, and solvents) where the patient has direct contact with the toxic substance, and (b) food poisoning, of which the transmission vehicle is contaminated food with pathogens or chemical products. Nowadays, chemical poisoning is a health problem; about six million chemicals are known, of which 80,000 to 100,000 are commonly used in different daily products. In 2006, the World Health Organization (WHO) estimated that more than 25% of poisonings and 5% of cases of cancer, neuropsychiatric disorders, and vascular diseases worldwide were caused by chemical exposure [1, 2].

It is difficult to diagnose chemical poisoning, since a chronological record of the patient's life is required, considering the exposure routes, dose, and time of exposure to the chemical. However, there are protocols that facilitate the diagnosis of chemical poisoning and how to treat incidents from chemical poisoning [1].

Furthermore, food poisoning or foodborne disease (FBD) is one of the main problems in public health worldwide. According to the WHO, each year 600 million people around the world, or 1 out of 10, become ill after consuming contaminated food. Among all these people, 420,000 die, including 125,000 children under 5 years of age, due to the vulnerability of this population to develop a diarrheal syndrome, about 43% of FBDs occur in these patients. About 70% of FBDs result from food contaminated with a microorganism [2–4].

Among the microorganisms causing FBDs are bacteria that have different virulence factors that give them the ability to cause a disease; among these factors, we can find toxins that can be produced in food or once the pathogen has colonized the digestive tract.

It is to be noted that the aim of this chapter is to convey information about some characteristics of the main pathogens producing toxins in food, the diseases they can cause, their complications and treatment options as well as the main sources of contamination in restaurants or street markets.

1.1. Types of bacterial toxins

A bacterial toxin is a macromolecule mainly of protein origin, which can cause toxic damage in a specific organ of the host [5]. Toxins can be divided in endotoxins and exotoxins:

- Endotoxins or lipopolysaccharides (LPS): These are the components of the outer membrane of the Gram-negative bacteria; they are considered the most important antigen of the bacteria; they are released into the medium after different processes such as lysis and cell division. This endotoxin is capable of causing endotoxic shock and tissue damage [5–7].

LPS are formed by three regions [7]:

- Lipid A is a glycolipid formed by a disaccharide (glucosamine) bound to fatty acids, that are usually capric, lauric, myristic, palmitic, and stearic acids, which are inserted in the outer membrane of the bacterium.
- The nucleus a heteropolysaccharide derived from hexoses and heptoses.
- Lipid A and the nucleus are bound by the sugar acid 2-keto-3-deoxyoctanate (KDO).
- The O chain is a repeating unit polymer of 1–8 glycosidic residues; this polymer is highly variable among bacterial species and genus.

In addition to the pyrogenicity of the endotoxin, an important role has been attributed to the adherence mechanism of the bacteria to the host cell; since in previous studies, it has been observed that when LPS is modified or not expressed, the adherence observed is modified or inhibited.

- Exotoxins: These are the macromolecules of protein origin, which are produced and later released to the medium by the microorganism. Depending on their mechanism of action, exotoxins are divided as follows:
  - Toxins Type I. These toxins modify the host's cells without internalizing in the cells; for example, the superantigens produced by *Staphylococcus aureus* and *Streptococcus pyogenes*.
  - Toxins Type II. Within this group there are hemolysins and phospholipases; this group of toxins is characterized by pore formation and/or destroying the membranes of the host cells. With this virulence factor, the pathogen can invade the host cell; for example, aerolysin and GCAT protein produced by *Aeromonas* spp.
  - Toxins Type III. These toxins are known as A/B due to their binary structure. Fraction B has the function of binding to the receptor of the cell and fraction A is the unit that possesses enzymatic activity, which, depending on the toxin and its mechanism of action, will be the damage to the cell; for example, the Shiga toxin produced by *Escherichia coli* O157:H7, the Cholera toxin (Ctx) produced by *Vibrio cholerae*, and the Anthrax toxin produced by *Bacillus anthracis* [5, 6].

Exotoxins of Gram-negative enteropathogenic bacteria play an important role in the pathogenesis of diarrheal disease, causing hypersecretion of liquids without the destruction and death of intestinal mucosal cells. These toxins are generically referred to as enterotoxins that are different from cytotoxins [8].

There are also two other groups of toxins, those that alter the cytoskeleton and those with neurotoxic activity; however, some toxins may present activity corresponding to more than one of the groups described in **Table 1**.

Toxin type	Definition
Enterotoxin	It produces a net secretion in ligated intestinal segments without histological evidence of intestinal lesion or damage to nonerythrocytic cells in *in vitro* tests. It stimulates the increase in the short circuit current (Isc) and the potential difference (PD) in the using chamber without evidence of intestinal damage; this result involves the secretion of (active) electrogenic anions. Additionally, a toxin can impair electrically neutral NaCl absorption, which also results in a net secretion of ions.
Cytoskeleton-altering toxin	It alters the cellular form and has been frequently shown to be caused by the F-actin rearrangement. The toxin can cause limited cell damage but is not lethal, and it may or may not be associated with the evidence of net secretion in *in vivo* or *in vitro* disease models in intestinal epithelial cells.
Cytotoxin	It causes cell or tissue damage, usually ending with cell death. The toxin may or may not be associated with net secretion in *in vivo* or *in vitro* disease models in intestinal epithelial cells.
Neurotoxins	It involves the release of one or more neurotransmitters from the enteric nervous system. It alters the activity of smooth muscle in the intestine.

Source: Adapted from Sears et al. [8].

Table 1. Classification of enteric toxins.

Toxins produced by pathogens involved in foodborne diseases are as follows:

Cholera toxin (Ctx) (*Vibrio cholerae*), Thermolabile toxin (LT) Thermostable toxin (ST) (Enterotoxigenic *E. coli*), Shiga Toxin (*Shigella dysenteriae* and *E. coli* O157:H7) Botulinum toxin (BTX) (*Clostridium botulinum*), CPE Enterotoxin (*Clostridium perfringens*), Alpha-Toxin, Beta-Toxin, Epsilon-Toxin and Iota-Toxin (*C. perfringens*), Toxin A/Toxin B (*Clostridium difficile*), Enterotoxins (A, B, C1, C2, D and E, G, H, I, J), Toxic Shock Syndrome Toxin (TSST-1), Cereulide, and hemolysin BL (HBL), nonhemolytic enterotoxin (NHE) (*S. aureus*), Citotoxin K or CytK (*Bacillus cereus*) [9–15].

1.2. Epidemiology

The high population growth and the food marketing, have generated pathogens causing FBDs to be quickly transported, this has produced outbreaks in different regions, affecting the morbidity, mortality, and economy of the population involved. The trend seen in the United States, the United Kingdom, and Europe indicates that the incidence of FBDs is increasing; this will be a health problem in the following years [4, 16].

There are different types of genus commonly associated with FBDs such as *Campylobacter* spp., enterotoxigenic *E. coli* (ETEC), enteropathogenic *E. coli* (EPEC), *Salmonella* spp., *Shigella* spp., Shiga toxin-producing *E. coli* (STEC) and *V. cholerae* [4, 17].

A total of 66% of foodborne diseases is caused by bacteria. Major diseases include botulism caused by *C. botulinum*, gastroenteritis caused by *E. coli* strains, Salmonellosis and Staphylococcal poisoning. Moreover, *B. cereus* and *V. cholerae* are bacteria frequently reported as causative agents of toxicoinfection by food [18, 19].

http://dx.doi.org/10.5772/intechopen.69953

In some countries, food poisoning caused by *S. aureus* is the most prevalent; reports indicate that *S. aureus* can be responsible for up to 41% of food poisoning outbreaks. Although it can affect people of any age, the range with the highest incidence goes from 20 to 49 years of age, where up to 48% of the cases can be concentrated. The main food products related to food poisoning caused by *S. aureus* are chicken and eggs, cakes, pastas, sauces, milk, and its derived products [20].

Globally, the highest number of cases is caused by ETEC, 233 million cases, and *Shigella* spp., 188 million cases; however, the highest numbers of deaths are caused by EPEC, 121,455 deaths; ETEC, 73,041 deaths, and *Shigella* spp., 64,993 deaths. In total, 40% of the cases and 43% of the deaths caused by FBDs occurred in children under the age of 5 years old [17].

Food poisoning caused by *B. cereus* can occur any time of the year; it does not present a defined geographical distribution, and because it is naturally found in the environment, its distribution in various types of food occurs easily, especially in those of plant origin such as cereals and rice. Reports about food poisoning outbreaks caused by *B. cereus* are underestimated due to the lack of diagnostic tools; however, globally, there are figures where food poisoning caused by this pathogen occupies from 1 to 17.5% of the total cases of food poisoning caused by bacteria [21, 22].

Food poisoning caused by *C. botulinum* is less frequent and the epidemiological information about it is scarce; outbreaks of food poisoning caused by this pathogen usually include members of one family, that is, they do not involve a large number of individuals and the main cause of such outbreaks is the consumption of canned food at home [23, 24].

Food poisoning caused by *C. perfringens* occurs at any time of the year, but it is more frequent in the last months of the year. It does not present a geographical distribution; in some countries like the United States, the outbreaks caused by this pathogen occupy the second place in foodborne diseases. Generally, this type of outbreaks affect a large number of individuals, therefore, they have a high range of morbidity. In total, 90% of the cases are caused by the intake of meat and poultry products; the contamination of meat and other food products occurs by the contact of pipelines with feces or contaminated surfaces [24, 25].

Nevertheless, the distribution of pathogens varies depending on the region, due to cultural and economic factors that allow both incidence and mortality to be different for each pathogen associated with FBDs. For example, in Europe, *Campylobacter* and *Salmonella* are reported pathogens; their reservoirs are livestock and domestic animals, and food contamination is produced due to bad practices in the food production chain and by cross-contaminations; however, although they play an important role in enteric diseases, they are less frequent than in countries defined by the World Health Organization (WHO) as high-mortality countries (Western Pacific Region and Africa Region), where the sanitary conditions and food and water contamination are factors that increase the incidence and mortality of these genera [17].

In 2010, WHO wrote a report about the main pathogens involved in FBDs, dividing all countries in regions; these regions were grouped based on adult and infant mortality (**Figure 1**).

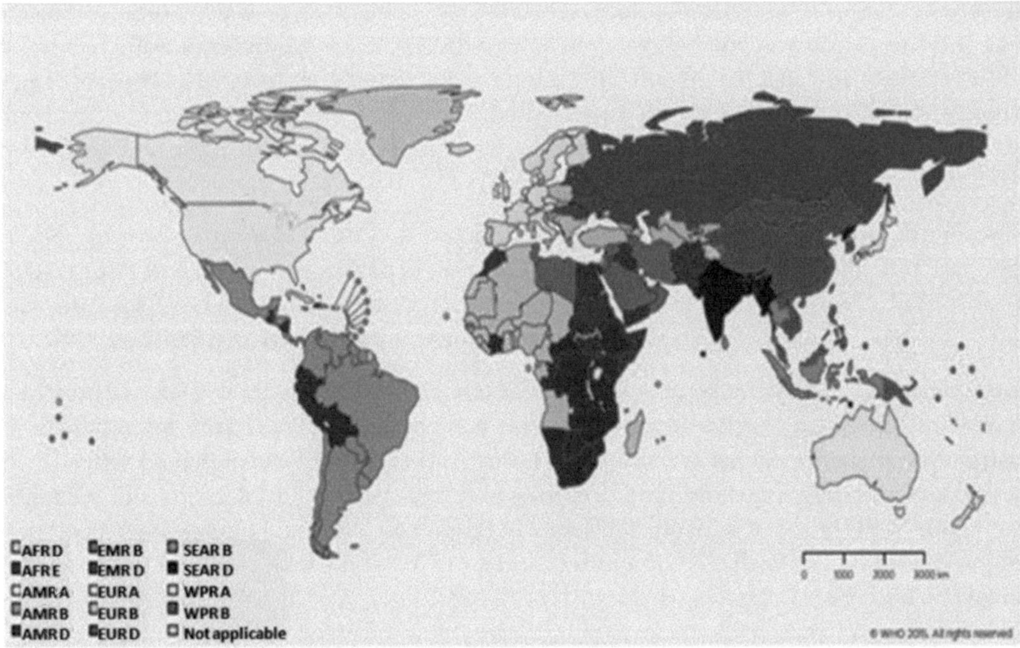

Figure 1. Geographical distribution of countries by region. Subregions are defined on the basis of infant and adult mortality. Stratum/Layer A = very low infant and adult mortality; stratum B = low infant mortality and very low adult mortality; stratum C = low infant mortality and high adult mortality; stratum D = high infant and adult mortality; and stratum E = high infant mortality and very high adult mortality. AFR: African subregion, AMR: American subregion, EMR: Eastern Mediterranean, EUR: European subregion, SEAR: South-East Asian subregions, WPR: Western Pacific subregion. Adapted from World Health Organization [26].

The risk group causing FBDs depends on the region, in developing countries such as African regions, South America, and South Asia, pathogens causing diarrheal diseases and the invasive pathogens causing infectious diseases and bacteria are the group that causes FBDs, followed by some cestodes and helminths; nevertheless, African regions, cestodes, and helminths are the group that causes FBDs because health and economic conditions limit proper food handling and preservation [17, 26].

With the above, as each risk group is different for each region, in the same way, the distribution of the main pathogens involved in FBDs depends on each region, as well as their incidence; however, developing countries continue to show a great number of cases of FBDs. In addition, the prevalence of pathogens in these countries is higher than in developed countries (**Figure 2**) [4, 26].

Additionally, each region has different socioeconomic characteristics, this creates an impact on the incidence and the mortality of FBDs associated with different bacterial pathogens; the *Shigella* genus occupies the first place in deaths in all regions; however, each region shows a different distribution among the genus that produce the highest number of deaths; this is due to the fact that medical care is different in each region, which means that in some regions a genus causes high mortality and in other regions it is only of medical relevance (**Figure 3**) [4, 17, 26].

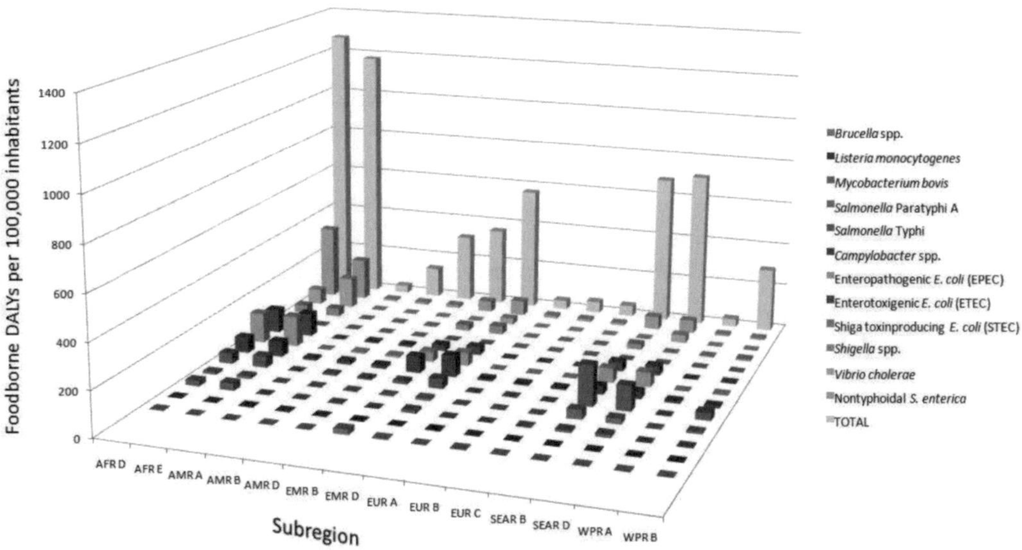

Figure 2. Global burden of FBDs by subregion (DALYS per 100,000 inhabitants) caused by major pathogens. DAYLs: Disability-adjusted life years metric, AFR: African subregion, AMR: American subregion, EMR: Eastern Mediterranean, EUR: European subregion, SEAR: South-East Asian subregions, WPR: Western Pacific subregion. Adapted from World Health Organization [26].

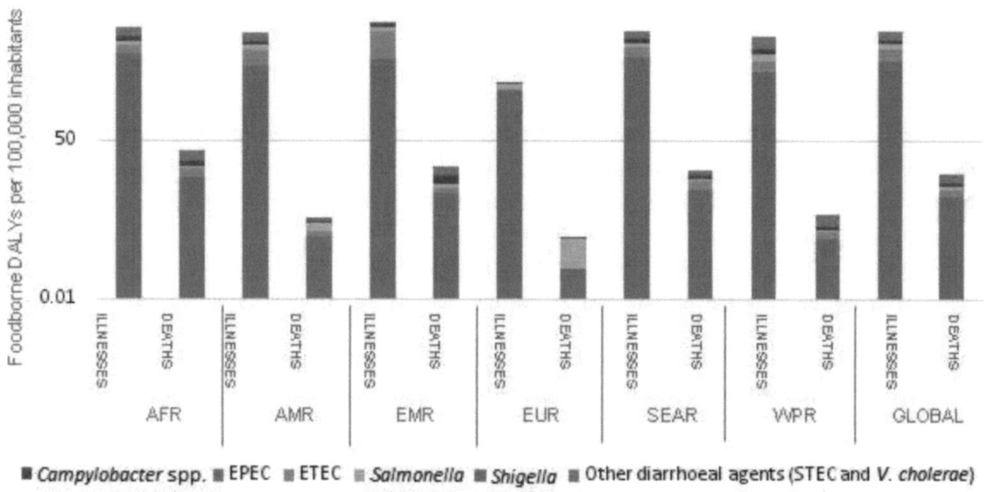

Figure 3. Median rate per 100,000 of diarrheal illnesses and deaths by region. The scale is on logarithmic basis 10. Adapted from Pires et al. [17].

In accordance with the above, it is emphasized the importance of medical authorities to know the incidence of the pathogens causing FBDs that circulate in their regions; not only to know the morbidity and mortality rate, but also to provide the population with the appropriate medical care directed to the pathogen causing FBDs.

2. Risk factors and prevention measures associated with food poisoning

The main risk factor involved in bacterial food poisoning is food contamination by pathogenic bacteria that produce toxins; such contamination can occur at any time, that is, from the crop, in the case of vegetables or, just before eating them, due to the consumer's manipulation; in this way, all the people living on the earth are susceptible to food poisoning. Therefore, food poisoning is a worldwide public health problem, generally the most affected are children, the elderly, pregnant women, and immunocompromised people. As expected, individual factors such as age, gender, place of residence, socioeconomic factors, among others, are crucial in food poisoning acquisition and development [27–29].

Food contamination can occur from primary production to the final consumer, consequently, there are different contamination risks according to the practices carried out in the different stages such as agricultural, livestock, and fish production; industrialization (in the case of processed food); marketing (points of sale), and transportation to the final consumer (homes, community dining rooms, and restaurants) [30].

During the primary production, producers should consider the particular characteristics of the environment where they grow or breed and reproduce livestock, by applying measures to prevent any pollution caused by the air, water, or natural fertilizers. In general, the main risk of contamination in primary production is the unsafe agricultural practices such as the use of manure as natural fertilizer and irrigation with sewage, which violates the fundamental principle of preventing, at all costs and contamination of raw materials from fecal matter [31, 32].

Additionally, another important factor to ensure food safety and good quality is the adequate control of time and temperature when cooking, processing, cooling, and storing food. To achieve a good control of such parameters, it is necessary to consider the physical, chemical, and microbiological characteristics of each type of food, for example, water activity, pH and type, and the initial number of microorganisms presented there. Similarly, other aspects need to be taken into account such as shelf life and usage, that is, whether it is a raw, processed, packaged, or ready-to-eat food [33, 34].

Microbiological contamination can occur through direct contact or through air, utensils, contact surfaces, or the handler's hands; therefore, ready-to-eat foods must be separated in space and time from raw or unprocessed foods. In addition, the latter must always be washed or disinfected. In all stages of the food chain, it is indispensable to use water; hence, this could be the main source of food contamination. It is then necessary to control and monitor the type and the source of the water used at each stage; however, when it is used for food handling, water has to be drinkable water that meets the physical, chemical, and microbiological criteria that its name requires [29, 31, 35].

In terms of facilities, it is important to establish and monitor systems that ensure their maintenance, cleaning, and sanitation. These systems also include an adequate waste management and an effective pest control. The latter constitute a potential risk of any type of contamination; that is why it is necessary to implement measures that prevent the entrance of any type of pests, as well as measures to avoid their nesting and proliferation. Finally, pest eradication must be carried out by any physical, chemical, or biological method that does not represent a threat to health and food safety [27, 31].

Within the food chain, food transportation plays an important role in preventing contamination and proliferation of microorganisms in food; thus, it is necessary to consider measures to prevent any type of contamination and to provide an environment to control the proliferation of pathogenic microorganisms and the production of bacterial toxins. Some important factors to consider during food transportation are temperature, direct exposure to sunlight, humidity, and airflows. At this stage, the type of containers and the type of packaging also play an important role; the aforementioned and transport conditions should be chosen based on the characteristics of the food that is being transported [36].

Another important measure is the information that producers and suppliers offer to consumers regarding the characteristics and proper handling of prepackaged foods; this is why, generally, food must be packaged and labeled in such a way that the consumer has enough information to handle, store, and prepare the products appropriately without threatening his or her health. Labels should also include a batch number allowing rapid identification and market recalls of products potentially being dangerous for human consumption [37, 38].

In general, microorganisms, more specifically bacteria, can proliferate under very different conditions; that is why they can be found in any type of environment. Even though bacteria are good at adapting to the environments they are in, there are certain conditions that promote bacterial growth more than others. These conditions include food, humidity, acidity, temperature, time, and oxygen; all of these are grouped in what is known as FATTOM (Food, Acidity, Time, Temperature, Oxygen, and Moisture). Knowing and avoiding these optimal conditions can help to prevent bacterial growth, bacterial infections, and food poisoning [39–41].

Most foods contain nutrients required for microbial growth, which makes them easy targets for the microorganisms to develop; therefore, perishable. To reduce the breakdown of food and to prevent foodborne diseases, the proliferation of microorganisms under certain conditions must be controlled, as well as the conditions that must be used to reduce food spoilage to lengthen the time during which physicochemical and organoleptic characteristics must be kept under minimum acceptance parameters. Factors affecting the proliferation rate of microorganisms can be considered as intrinsic and extrinsic [42, 43].

2.1. Intrinsic parameters

Intrinsic factors affecting the proliferation rate are more related to the internal characteristics of food products, and the way in which these characteristics maintain or affect the growth of microorganisms; these factors include water activity, pH, oxidation-reduction potential, content and type of nutrients, inhibiting substances, and biological structures [44, 45].

2.1.1. Water activity

It is defined as the amount of water available for the growth of microorganisms; microbial proliferation decreases when water availability also decreases. The water available for metabolic activity determines the degree of microbial growth instead of the total moisture content. The unit of measurement for the water that microorganisms require is usually expressed as water activity (A_w), which is defined as the water vapor pressure of food substrate, divided by the water vapor pressure of pure water, at the same temperature. This concept is related to relative humidity (RH), thus: RH = 100 × A_w. The approximate optimal A_w for the growth of most microorganisms is 0.99; most bacteria require an A_w greater than 0.91 to grow. Gram-negative bacteria require higher values than Gram-positive bacteria. Most of the natural food products have an A_w of 0.99 or more. Generally, bacteria have the highest requirements of water activity, fungi have the lowest, and yeasts have intermediate requirements. Most bacteria that decompose food do not grow with an A_w less than 0.91, but fungi and yeasts can grow with values of 0.80 or less, including surfaces partially dehydrated. The lowest value reported for bacteria in food is 0.75 for halophytes, while xerophilic fungi and osmophilic yeasts have shown growth at A_w values of 0.65 and 0.61, respectively [46, 47].

2.1.2. pH

The pH is defined as the negative logarithm of hydronium ions concentration; it is considered as a unit of measure to establish acidity or alkalinity levels of a substance, in this case food, and it is determined by the number of free hydrogen ions (H^+). The effects of adverse pH affect at least two aspects of the microbial cell-functioning of its enzymes and nutrients transportation to the cell.

The cytoplasmic membrane of microorganisms is relatively impermeable to H^+ and OH^- ions; its concentration in the cytoplasm remains reasonably constant, despite the wide variations that may occur in the pH of the surrounding medium. When microorganisms are in an environment below or above the neutral level, their ability to proliferate depends on their ability to change the environmental pH to a more appropriate range, since key components like DNA or ATP require a neutral medium [42, 43, 47].

The pH for the optimal growth of most microorganisms is close to neutrality (pH = 6.6–7.5). Yeasts can grow in an acid environment and thrive in an intermediate range (4.0–4.5), although they survive in values between 1.5 and 8.5. Fungi tolerate a wide range (0.5–11.0), but their growth is generally higher in an acid pH (too acid for bacteria and yeast). Bacterial growth is usually favored by pH values closer to the neutral level. Nevertheless, acidophilic bacteria grow on substrates with a pH of up to 5.2 and below that point the growth reduces dramatically [42, 48].

In general, fruits, vinegars, and wines have pH values lower than those required for bacterial growth, so they can usually be decomposed by fungi and yeasts. Most vegetables have pH values lower than those from fruits, and consequently, vegetables are more exposed to bacterial or fungi decomposition. In contrast, most meats and sea products have pH values equal or greater than 5.6, making them susceptible to decomposition by bacteria, fungi, and yeasts [44, 48, 49].

2.1.3. Oxidation-reduction potential

The oxidation-reduction potential (O/R) is an indicator of the oxidizing and reducing power of a substrate; that is, the O/R potential of a substrate can be generally defined as the ease with which a substrate loses or gains electrons (when a food product loses electrons, it oxidizes, whereas, when it gains electrons it is reduced; thus, a food product that easily gives electrons is a good reducing agent and the one that receives electrons is a good oxidizing agent). To achieve optimum growth, some microorganisms require reducing conditions and others require oxidizing conditions. The O/R potential of a system is expressed with the Eh symbol (when electrons are transferred from one compound to another, a potential difference is created between the two compounds; this difference can be measured and expressed as millivolts [mV]). The more oxidized a substance is, the more positive the electrical potential will be; and the more reduced a substance is, the more negative the electrical potential will be. When the concentration of oxidant and reducer is equal, there is an electrical potential of zero [39].

Saprophytes that are capable of transferring hydrogen as H^+ and e^- (electrons) to molecular oxygen are aerobic; that is, aerobic microorganisms require positive Eh values (oxidized) for their growth, whereas anaerobic microorganisms require negative values of Eh (reduced). Facultative microorganisms can grow under any of the conditions. It has to be considered that maximum and minimum Eh values (in mV) necessary for aerobic and anaerobic growth could be lethal to the other group. Among food substances that help to maintain reducing conditions are the –SH groups in meats and the ascorbic acid, as well as, reducing sugars in fruits and vegetables. Some aerobic bacteria grow better under slightly reducing conditions being known as microaerophiles such as *Lactobacillus* and *Campylobacter*. Most of fungi and yeasts found in food are aerobic, although a few tend to be facultative anaerobes. Regarding the Eh value of food, vegetables, especially juices, tend to have Eh values of +300 to +400 mV; so, it is not surprising to find that aerobic bacteria and fungi are the common cause of decomposition in this type of products. Meats have Eh values around −200 mV; in ground meats, Eh is usually around +200 mV. Various types of cheese show Eh values between −20 and −200 mV [46].

2.1.4. *Content of nutrients*

Microorganisms have nutritional requirements, most of them need external sources of nitrogen, energy, minerals, as well as vitamins, and related growth factors; these requirements are found in our food, so if they have the right conditions to develop, they will. In general, fungi have the lowest nutrient requirement, followed by Gram-negative bacteria, then yeasts and finally, Gram-positive bacteria, which have the highest requirements [46, 50].

The primary sources of nitrogen used by heterotrophic microorganisms are amino acids. A great number of other nitrogen compounds may serve for this function for several types of organisms. For example, some of them can use free nucleotides and amino acids, while others can be capable of using peptides and proteins. In general, simple compounds like amino acids will be used by almost all of the organisms before attacking more complex compounds such as high molecular weight proteins. The same applies to polysaccharides and lipids [39, 51].

Microorganisms in food tend to use as energy sources, sugars, alcohols, and amino acids. Fungi are the most efficient in the use of proteins, complex carbohydrates, and lipids because they contain enzymes capable of hydrolyzing these molecules into simpler components; many bacteria have a similar capacity, but most yeasts require simpler molecules. All microorganisms need minerals, although vitamin requirements vary. Fungi and some bacteria can synthesize enough B vitamins to meet their needs, while others need to have a source of vitamins, food products being an excellent source of them [39, 50].

Gram-positive bacteria are the ones that have lower synthesized capacity, so they need one or more of these components to grow. In contrast, Gram-negative bacteria and fungi are capable of synthesizing the most, if not all, of their requirements and consequently, these two groups of organisms can grow in food products with low content of B vitamins [46, 52, 53].

2.2. Extrinsic parameters

Food factors are very important for the development of microorganisms; there are external or extrinsic factors. This term refers to environmental factors that affect the growth rate of microorganisms; these factors include temperature, oxygen availability, and relative humidity, as well as, the presence and activities of other microorganisms [46].

2.2.1. Storage temperature

Microorganisms have an optimal range, as well as a minimum and maximum temperature to grow. Therefore, ambient temperature determines not only the proliferation rate, but also the genera of microorganisms that are going to be developed, along with the microbial activity degree that is registered. The change in only a few degrees in temperature will favor the growth of completely different organisms, and it will result in a different type of food decomposition and/or foodborne disease. Due to these characteristics, thermal treatment is employed as a method to control microbial activity [46, 54].

The optimal temperature for the proliferation of most microorganisms ranges from 14 to 40°C, although some genera develop below 0°C, and other genera grow at temperatures above 100°C. Nevertheless, food quality must be taken into account when selecting storage temperature. Although it can be desirable to storage all food products at temperatures equal or less to those of refrigeration, this is not the best thing to do to maintain a desirable quality in some food products such as banana, whose quality is best maintained in storage at 13–17°C than at 5–7°C. Similarly, many vegetables are favored at temperatures near 10°C such as potatoes, celery, cabbage, and many others. In each case, the success of storage temperature depends, to a large extent, on the relative humidity and the presence or absence of gases such as carbon dioxide and ozone [46, 55].

2.2.2. Oxygen availability and presence of other gases in the environment

Like temperature, the oxygen availability determines the microorganisms that will be active. Some have an absolute requirement for oxygen, while others grow in total absence of it, and others may grow with or without oxygen. Microorganisms that require free oxygen are called aerobic microorganisms, while those that thrive in the absence of oxygen are called anaerobic; and those that grow both in presence or absence of free oxygen are known as facultative microorganisms [43, 46, 56].

Carbon dioxide is the most important atmospheric gas that is used to control food microorganisms. Along with oxygen, it is used in packaged food with modified atmosphere. Ozone is another atmospheric gas with antimicrobial properties, and for decades, it has been used as an agent to lengthen shelf life of certain types of food. Although being effective against a variety of microorganisms, it is a highly oxidizing agent;thus, it cannot be used in food products with high lipid content, as it could accelerate rancidity. Normally, ozone levels of 0.15–5.00 ppm in the air inhibit the growth of some bacteria that decompose food as well as yeast growth [46, 57].

2.2.3. *Relative humidity in the environment*

Relative humidity (RH) of the environment is important from the point of view of water activity within food and the growth of microorganisms on surfaces. This extrinsic factor affects microbial growth and can be influenced by temperature. All microorganisms have a high-water requirement, this being needed for their growth and activity [46, 54].

When the A_w of a food product is set at 0.60, it is important that this food is stored under RH conditions that do not allow food to draw humidity from the air and, therefore, it increases its own A_w from the surface and subsurface to an extent where microbial growth can occur. A high relative humidity can cause humidity condensation in food, equipment, walls, and ceilings. Condensation causes wet surfaces, which lead to microbial growth and decomposition. Microbial growth is inhibited by a low relative humidity. When food products with low A_w values are placed in high RH environments, food takes in moisture until they reach balance. Similarly, food products with high A_w lose moisture when placed in an environment with low RH. There is a relationship between RH and temperature that must be taken into account when selecting the appropriate storage environments for food products. Overall, the higher the temperature, the less the RH, and vice versa [46, 54, 58].

Bacteria require higher humidity than yeasts and fungi. The optimal relative humidity for bacteria is 92% or higher, while yeasts prefer 90% or higher, and fungi thrive if the relative humidity is between 85 and 90%. Food products suffering superficial decomposition by fungi, yeasts, and specific bacteria, should be stored under low RH conditions. Poorly packed meats such as whole chickens and beef cuts, tend to suffer a lot of superficial decomposition inside the refrigerator before internal decomposition occurs, usually, due to high RH in refrigerators, and to the fact that the biota decomposing meat is essentially aerobic in nature [46, 59].

Although it is possible to decrease the possibility of superficial decomposition in certain food products by storing them in low RH conditions, it should be remembered that the food itself will lose moisture into the atmosphere under such conditions, and thus, it will become undesirable. When selecting appropriate RH conditions, there should be taken into account both the possibility of superficial microbial growth and the quality that the food product needs to have. By altering the gas atmosphere, it is possible to delay superficial decomposition without lowering the relative humidity [46, 60].

2.2.4. *Presence and activities of other microorganisms*

Some food origin organisms produce substances that can inhibit or be lethal for other organisms; these include antibiotics, bacteriocins, hydrogen peroxide, and organic acids. Bacteriocins produced by lactic acid-producing bacteria originated in various food products such as meat, are of high interest. Bacteriocins produced by Gram-positive bacteria are biologically active proteins with bactericidal action. Some bacteriocins produced by these bacteria inhibit a variety of food pathogens including, *B. cereus, C. perfringens, Listeria* spp., *A. hydrophila,* and *S. aureus,* among others [39, 46].

Normally food products can reach the final consumer at home, in community dining rooms, or restaurants. Measures to prevent food poisoning should be implemented at these locations, particularly in areas where large volumes of food are distributed such as cold chain, frozen chain, hot chain, and vacuum cooking. Likewise, in the frozen chain, food temperature is gradually lowered to −18°C and defrosted at temperatures higher than 65°C at the time it will be served to the costumer (not before); while in the hot chain, for example, in a buffet, food is kept at temperatures higher than 65°C and it should be consumed within 12 h maximum [61].

Other important measures are the use of food preservation methods, which can be physical or chemical. Within the physical methods, there are the traditional or industrial pasteurization, dehydration, preservation in modified atmosphere, and irradiation. In order to maintain an adequate quality control and to minimize the risk of food poisoning, microbial markers can be used; these markers do not represent a potential health risk, however, a large number of them indicate deficiencies in hygiene and sanitary quality of food products; it also leads to a decrease in the shelf-life and could be related to the presence of pathogenic microorganisms. The main microbial markers are aerobic mesophilic, total coliforms, fecal coliforms, Enterococci, *E. coli, S. aureus,* and lactic acid bacteria [62].

Once the risk factors are identified, it is necessary to establish a system that allows to prevent and decrease all of them; to do this, a method with scientific basis and systematic profile has been established, this is known as Hazard Analysis and Critical Control Point (HACCP). A microbiological approach should consider the type of microorganism or metabolite (toxins) that threatens human health; the analytical methods for its detection and quantification; the number of samples to be taken and the size of the analytical unit; and the microbiological limits considered to be adequate at specific points in the food chain [63].

3. Foodborne diseases

In food products, we can find different types of toxins such as, bacterial, fungal (mycotoxins), algae or plant toxins, as well as metals, toxic chemicals (zinc, copper, and pesticides), and physical contaminants that can cause diseases in people who eat them; all of these can cause the well-known "foodborne diseases" [64].

Foodborne diseases can be classified into two groups: poisoning and infection.

- Poisoning is caused by the intake of chemical or biological toxins; or toxins produced by pathogens, the latter can be found in food, even if the bacterium is not there.
- Infection is caused by the intake of food containing viable pathogens. Furthermore, a toxic infection (toxicoinfection), formerly known as a toxin-mediated infection, is caused by eating food with bacteria that grow and produce a toxin inside the body [18, 64–66].

To meet the ideal conditions, microorganisms in food grow and produce toxins. By ingesting contaminated food, toxins are absorbed through the intestinal epithelial lining, and it causes local tissue damage. In some cases, toxins can reach organs such as the kidney or the liver, the central nervous system or the peripheral nervous system, where they can cause some damage [18].

The most common clinical symptoms of foodborne diseases are diarrhea, vomit, abdominal cramps, headaches, nausea, pain, fever, vomit, diarrhea with mucus and blood (dysentery), and rectal tenesmus. Some of the microorganisms causing foodborne diseases, either from poisoning, intoxication or toxicoinfection are described in **Tables 2–4**. These diseases are generally diagnosed based on the patient's clinical record or their symptoms [18–20].

Toxins produced by pathogens involved in foodborne diseases have different characteristics, some of them are shown in **Table 5** [9, 11–15, 67].

3.1. Foodborne diseases caused by bacterial toxins

This section will be addressed to some diseases caused by consuming food contaminated with bacterial toxins or microorganisms that produce them. Among some of the most important diseases are the ones transmitted by *V. cholerae, S. aureus, B. cereus C. perfringens, C. botulinum and Listeria monocytogenes.*

3.1.1. Vibrio cholerae

V. cholerae has a free life cycle, it is ubiquitous in aquatic environments; it is able to remain virulent without multiplying in fresh water and sea water for a long time. They are more frequent

Bacteria	Disease/medical complications	Food products involved
Salmonella enterica serovar Typhi and *Salmonella enterica* serovar Paratyphi	Typhoid and paratyphoid fever.	Undercooked pork, beef and poultry, contaminated eggs, and milk.
Salmonella spp.	Salmonellosis (*Salmonella* Typhimurium, *Salmonella* Enteritidis).	Undercooked poultry, cauliflowers, and tomatoes.
Vibrio vulnificus	Septicemia in people with underlying diseases or people who are taking immunosuppressive drugs or steroids.	Seafood, usually oysters.
Mycobacterium bovis	Cervical lymphadenopathy, intestinal lesions, chronic cutaneous tuberculosis.	Contaminated milk.
Mycobacterium avium, subspecies *paratuberculosis*	Crohn's disease.	Pasteurized milk.
Listeria monocytogenes	Meningitis, encephalitis, sepsis in pregnant women, intrauterine or cervical infection that can lead to miscarriage or birth of a dead child.	Raw beef, pork, poultry, vegetables and milk, cheese, ice cream, smoked fish, and raw fish.

Modified from Refs: [18–20].

Table 2. Pathogens that cause infection.

Bacteria	Disease/medical complications	Food products involved
Clostridium botulinum	Paralysis of arms, legs, trunk, and respiratory muscles.	Mixture of oil and nonacid garlic, potatoes cooked at high temperatures, and stews.
Bacillus cereus	Fried rice syndrome.	Rice cooked at high temperatures, sauces, soups, and puddings.
Staphylococcus aureus	Toxic shock syndrome.	Meat and meat products cooked at high temperatures, poultry, and salads with mayonnaise.
Source: Modified from Refs: [18–20].		

Table 3. Pathogens that cause intoxication.

Bacteria	Disease/medical complications	Food products involved
Escherichia coli O157:H7	Hemorrhagic colitis, Hemolytic uremic syndrome in children.	Hamburgers, nonpasteurized milk, contaminated water, spinach, and lettuce.
Shigella spp.	Hemolytic Uremic Syndrome.	Salads, lettuce, raw vegetables, and milk.
Aeromonas spp.	Meningitis, peritonitis, myocarditis, hemolytic uremic syndrome, necrotizing fasciitis in wounds.	Meat (beef, sheep, pork and chicken), vegetables, eggs, fish, seafood, and prepared food.
Cronobacter sakazakii	Permanent neurological or developmental deficits; death.	Powdered infant formula.
Vibrio parahaemolyticus	Gastroenteritis, septicemia and wound infection. Severe infections in immunocompromised people.	Raw or undercooked seafood, usually oysters.
Clostridium perfringens	Clostridial necrotizing enteritis.	Meat juice, stews, cooked beans, meat cooked at high temperatures.
Campylobacter spp.	Campylobacteriosis, arthritis, meningitis, *Campylobacter jejuni* can cause Guillain-Barré Syndrome.	Cheese made with raw milk and chicken meat.
Yersinia enterocolitica	Yersiniosis, enterocolitis, pseudoappendicitis, mesenteric lymphadenitis, infections in wounds, joints and the urinary tract, and Reiter's syndrome.	Nonpasteurized milk, tofu, nonchlorinated water, undercooked meat, oysters and fish.
Vibrio cholerae serogroup O1 or serogroup O139	Cholera.	Contaminated water and raw seafood.
Vibrio cholerae serogroup no-O1	Less severe than Cholera; gastrointestinal infections, sepsis.	Raw, semicooked or recontaminated fish and shellfish after cooking.
Source: Modified from Refs: [18–20].		

Table 4. Pathogens that cause toxico-infection.

Name	Biological effect
Cholera toxin (Ctx) (A-5B)	It activates the adenylyl cyclase; increases the levels of intracellular cAMP promoting fluid and electrolytes secretion in the intestinal epithelium, causing diarrhea. It is a potent exotoxin.
Thermolabile toxin (LT) (A-5B)	Similar effect as the Cholera toxin.
Thermostable toxin (ST)	The binding of ST to the guanylyl cyclase receptor results in an increase of cyclic GMP, affecting the flow of electrolytes. It promotes water and electrolytes secretion from the intestinal epithelium by causing diarrhea.
Shiga toxin (A-5B)	Inactivates the ribosomal subunit 60S and inhibits protein synthesis causing the death of susceptible cells.
Botulinum toxin (A/B)	It is a neurotoxin consisting of a heavy and a light chain linked by a disulfide bond. It is a Zn^{++}-dependent protease. It inhibits the presynaptic release of acetylcholine from peripheral cholinergic neurons, resulting in flaccid paralysis. The neurotoxin exists in seven different serotypes (A-G).
CPE enterotoxin	Lethal, cytotoxic and enterotoxic activity. Stimulates the adenylyl cyclase allowing the increase of cAMP in epithelial cells, which causes diarrhea.
Alpha-toxin	It produces gas gangrene. It has phospholipase (PLC), sphingomyelinase, hemolytic, and dermonecrotic activities. The mature protein is organized into two domains; the amino-terminal, which contains the PLC activity, and the carboxyl-terminal binding that depends on calcium. Depending on the lipid composition of the cell membrane, the Alpha-toxin may be hemolytic in the presence of calcium.
Beta-toxin	It forms selective pores for monovalent cations in lipid bilayers and sensitive cells membranes, so it functions as a neurotoxin capable of producing arterial constriction.
Epsilon-toxin	Produced and secreted by a prototoxin that, when it suffers a specific proteolytic cleavage, it acquires its maximum biological activity. Activation can be catalyzed by proteases such as trypsin, chymotrypsin, and a zinc-dependent metalloproteinase.
Iota-toxin	It has dermonecrotic, cytotoxic, enterotoxic activities, and it causes intestinal histopathological damage. This toxin is binary and consists of a binding peptide (Ib) and an enzymatic peptide (ADP-ribosyltransferase) (Ia). The first one is necessary to internalize the second one. The Iota-toxin requires proteolytic removal of a propeptide fragment, which allows the Ib unit to be inserted into the membrane and to interact with the Ia portion to form a heptameric pore that allows the K^+ and Na^+ ions to escape; in addition to the Ia portion entrance into the cell where it ribosylates the G-actin to depolymerize the actin filaments, with the consequent destruction of the cytoskeleton. The Iota-toxin is generally activated by the effect of the proteases present in the intestinal tract.
Toxin A/Toxin B	It modifies the Rho, a subfamily of GTP-binding proteins that regulate cytoskeletal actin. The deamination of the glutamine residue at position 63 of Rho to a glutamic acid produces a dominant-active Rho protein incapable of hydrolyzing the GTP, resulting in cellular necrosis and bloody diarrhea associated with colitis.
Enterotoxins (A, B, C1, C2, D and E, G, H, I, J)	Enterotoxins are thermostable; they differ in toxicity. Staphylococcal enterotoxins are superantigens that cause massive activation of the immune system, including lymphocytes and macrophages; the exact role in emesis is not known.

Name	Biological effect
Toxic Shock Syndrome Toxin (TSST-1)	Superantigen that acts on the vascular system causing inflammation, fever, and shock.
Cereulide	Thermostable peptide, toxic for the mitochondria when acting as a potassium ionophore.
HBL, NHE, Citotoxin K or CytK	HBL is a three-component hemolysin; two protein subunits, L2 and L1 (cytolytic components), and a B protein (favors binding to the host cell), apart from the hemolytic effect, it is cytotoxic, dermonecrotic and causes vascular permeability. NHE also consists of three components (NheA is a cytolytic component and NhB and NheC favor binding to cells of small intestine). Both toxins are organized into operons (*hbl* and *nhe*), where the genes encoded the NHE components are transcribed together. CytK forms pores in the epithelial cells membrane, and it has necrotizing and cytotoxic activity.

Note: A-5B indicates that the subunits are separately synthesized but associated by noncovalent bonds during secretion and binding to target. 5B indicates that the binding domain of the protein is composed by five identical subunits. A/B denotes a toxin synthesized as a simple polypeptide divided into domains A and B that can be separated by proteolytic cleavage. HBL: hemolysin BL, NHE: nonhemolytic enterotoxin.

Source: Modified from Refs: [9, 11–15, 67].

Table 5. Main toxins produced by pathogens involved in foodborne diseases and their biological effect.

in temperate waters and can be isolated in seafood and fish. The most notable species are *V. cholerae* O1 and O139, causative serogroups of Cholera. Non-O1 strains and the rest of the species cause cholera-like diarrheal syndromes, but they are not as severe, although they frequently produce extraintestinal infections [68–70].

The CTX toxin (Cholera toxin) is the main virulence factor of *V. cholerae* O1 (Ogawa, Inaba, and Hikojima serotypes, Classical and El Tor biotypes) and O139; it contributes to cause profuse diarrhea, after an incubation period from 2 h to 5 days; stools have the appearance of rice water, there is dehydration and electrolyte imbalance, which can lead to death. Approximately 75% of the infected people are asymptomatic, that is, they do not develop the symptoms aforementioned; however, the pathogen is shed in their feces for 7–14 days, which is a very serious source of contamination since it is possible to infect others. The most vulnerable groups are children, adults, and people infected with the HIV virus [68, 69, 71].

This toxin can be identified by the presence of the *ctxAB* gene. *V. cholerae* no-O1 has the *ctx* gene but it is rarely expressed; nevertheless, a faster test is not yet available, although the WHO is currently in the process of validating new rapid diagnoses. The bacteria can be isolated and identified from stool samples by using laboratory procedures [24, 69, 71].

Efficient treatment resides in prompt rehydration through oral solutions or intravenous fluids. The use of antibiotics is suggested only when there is severe dehydration. The supply of safe drinking water, the adequate sanitation, and food security are essential to prevent the emergence of Cholera. Moreover, vaccines administration has emerged because control measures to prevent contamination are insufficient; this is the reason why oral vaccines have been developed as tools to prevent outbreaks. These vaccines are given to more vulnerable populations in areas where the disease is endemic. Experience in different mass vaccination campaigns in countries such as Mozambique, Indonesia, Sudan, and Zanzibar clearly indicates that vaccination requires careful and early planning and preparation, and therefore, it cannot be improvised at the last minute [71].

The lack of toxicity combined with stability and the relative ease to express the Cholera Toxin Subunit B (CTB) has contributed to be an easily manageable adjuvant. The ability to express protein in a wide variety of organisms broadens even further its application potential. CTB is currently being used in vaccines such as Dukoral, a vaccine against *V. cholerae* that consists of dead bacteria and recombinant CTB. It has been approved as adjuvant for vaccines in Europe and in Canada; and given the excellent adjuvant effect, this protein is likely to play an important role in vaccine formulation in the future [72].

3.1.2. Staphylococcus aureus

Staphylococcal foodborne illness is one of the most common diseases acquired by *S. aureus*. It is one of the most concerned diseases by public health programs in the world; it is due to the production of one or more toxins by the bacteria during their growth at permissive temperatures; however, the incubation period of the disease depends on the amount of ingested toxin. Small doses of enterotoxins can cause the disease; for example, a concentration of 0.5 ng/mL in contaminated chocolate milk has been reported to cause large outbreaks [73].

S. aureus produces various toxins. Staphylococcal enterotoxins are a family of nine thermostable enterotoxin serotypes belonging to a large family of pyrogenic toxins (superantigens). Pyrogenic toxins can cause immunosuppression and nonspecific T cell proliferation. Enterotoxins are highly stable and they resist high temperatures (which makes them suitable for industrial use) and environmental conditions of drying and freezing. They are also resistant to proteolytic enzymes (pepsin and trypsin) at low pH, enabling them to be fully functional in the digestive tract after infection [73].

The mechanism by which poisoning is caused is not entirely clear yet. However, enterotoxins have been observed to directly affect the intestinal epithelium and the vagus nerve causing stimulation of the emetic center. It is estimated that 0.1 μg of enterotoxin can cause staphylococcal poisoning in humans. Apart from causing poisoning, *S. aureus* can also cause toxic shock syndrome due to the production of the Toxic Shock Syndrome Toxin 1 (TSST-1) and Enterotoxin Type B [65, 73, 74].

Symptoms include nausea, vomit, abdominal cramps, salivation, diarrhea could be present or absent. The first three symptoms are the most common ones. Usually, it is a self-limiting disease and can be cured in 24–48 h, but it can become severe, especially in children, the elderly, and immunocompromised people. Toxic shock syndrome is characterized by high fever, hypotension, erythematous rash (similar to scarlet fever, peeling of the skin during recovery, flu-like symptoms, vomiting, and diarrhea) [73–75].

The diagnosis of the disease is carried out by detecting the staphylococcal enterotoxin in the food or by recovering at least 10^5 *S. aureus*/g from food leftovers. The enterotoxin can be detected by several methods: bioassays, molecular biology, and immunological techniques. The isolated strains can be genetically characterized by multilocus sequences from the *spa* or *SCCmec* gene, and pulsed-field electrophoresis [73].

The mainly involved food products in outbreaks and where *S. aureus* can grow optimally, since they are stored at room temperature, are meat and its derived products, poultry and eggs, milk and its derived products, salads, and bakery products (cream-filled cakes and stuffed sandwiches) [65, 73].

Other factors that must be taken into account are the emergence of methicillin resistant strains, which may be found in food (mainly in meat and milk). It is important to note that many of the isolates obtained from outbreaks are not tested for antimicrobial susceptibility; due to the various problems that these strains can create, the antimicrobial susceptibility test should be performed. They have been reported to be causative agents of outbreaks in blood infections and wounds in immunocompromised patients in hospitals [65, 73].

Foodborne illness due to *S. aureus* may be preventable. It is known that the permissible temperature for the growth and production of the enzyme is between 6 and 46°C; thus, food products could be cooked above 60°C and refrigerated below 5°C. Therefore, maintaining the cold chain of food can prevent the growth of the microorganism. By using good manufacturing practices and good hygiene practices, the contamination by *S. aureus* can be prevented [73].

3.1.3. *Bacillus cereus*

B. cereus is a ubiquitous microorganism in the environment, and it can easily contaminate any food production and processing system, due to the formation of endospores. The bacterium can survive pasteurization and cooking processes [11, 15].

It has been demonstrated that this microorganism produces, cereulide or emetic toxin; three enterotoxins, hemolysin BL (HBL), nonhemolytic (NHE), cytotoxin K (CytK), which are responsible for the emetic syndrome and diarrhea; and three phospholipases, phosphatidylinositol hydrolase, phosphatidylcholine hydrolase, and hemolytic sphingomyelinase. Cereulide is a thermostable cyclic peptide that causes emesis by stimulating the afferent vagal pathway through its bond to the serotonin receptor. The toxin is produced during the stationary phase of growth of the microorganism and it accumulates in food over time. The structure of the toxin explains its resistance to food processing methods. In contrast, inside the small intestine of the host, the thermolabile enterotoxins, HBL and NHE, produced during the exponential phase of the vegetative growth of the bacterium are the cause of diarrheal syndrome; the proteins that form enterotoxins (binding and lithic factors) are unable to traverse intact the gastric barrier; that is why it is considered that preformed or extracellular enterotoxins in food are not involved in the pathogenesis of the bacterium. It is believed that the spore germination that reaches the small intestine, the growth, and the simultaneous production of the enterotoxin are the ones that cause diarrhea. HBL is a hemolysin formed by three components, two protein subunits (L2 and L1), and one B protein; it has hemolytic, cytotoxic, and dermonecrotic effect, and it induces vascular permeability. NHE also consists of three components: NheA, NheB, and NheC. It has been demonstrated that strains producing emetic toxin do not produce enterotoxin. The cytotoxin K is similar to the Alpha-toxin of *S. aureus* and the Beta-toxin of *C. perfringens* [13, 15, 76].

Furthermore, the enterotoxin FM (EntFM) has been described; it is a 45 kDa polypeptide encoded by the *entFM* gene, located in the bacterial chromosome. It has not been directly involved in food poisoning; however, the presence of the gene in strains that cause diarrheal outbreaks has been detected; in experiments with mice and rabbits, it causes vascular permeability [11].

The emetic syndrome is characterized by nausea and vomit similar to those produced by *S. aureus* poisoning. Symptoms appear soon after consuming food contaminated with the preformed toxin. Generally, poisoning develops with mild symptoms, usually lasting no more than 1 day, but severe cases require hospitalization. The diarrhea that is caused belongs to the secretory type, similar to the one produced by *V. cholerae*. Colic pain occurs similar to that of *C. perfringens* poisoning. Both syndromes are self-limiting [13, 15, 77].

Enterotoxins can be detected by immunoassays or molecular biology (conventional PCR and multiple PCR) by looking for the *ces* gene (nonribosomal production of cereulide); by detecting the *hblD, hblC,* and *hblA* genes encoding the L1, L2, and B protein components of the HBL toxin, respectively; or the *nheA, nheB,* and *nheC* genes of the NHE toxin components. The *16S* ribosomal gene can be looked for by real-time PCR [11, 13, 77].

Apart from causing food poisoning, *B. cereus* can also cause local and systemic infections in immunocompromised patients, neonates, people taking drugs, and patients with surgical or traumatic wounds, or catheters [15].

The most susceptible food products to be contaminated include flours, meats, milk, cheese, vegetables, fish, rice and its derived products; generally, in food with high content of starch. The strains produced by the emetic toxin grow well in rice dishes (fried and cooked) and other starchy products; although, there have been studies where it has been demonstrated that the toxin can be in different types of food products; while strains producing diarrheagenic toxins grow in a wide variety of food products, from vegetables to sauces and stews [15, 77].

Strains isolated from infections have been shown to be sensitive to chloramphenicol, clindamycin, vancomycin, gentamicin, streptomycin, and erythromycin; they are resistant to β-lactam antibiotics, including third-generation cephalosporins [15].

Inadequate cooking temperatures, contaminated equipment, and poor hygiene conditions at the food processing and preparation sites are the major factors that contribute to food poisoning by *B. cereus* and its toxins; that is why, it is suggested to store food at temperatures lower than 4°C or to cook them at temperatures higher than 100°C, and to reheat or cool food rapidly, to avoid prolonged exposure to temperatures that allow spore germination and to diminish the risks of a possible poisoning [11].

3.1.4. *Clostridium perfringens*

C. perfringens is an anaerobic bacterium that creates spores that survive in soil, sediments, and areas subject to both human and animal fecal contamination. It is widely distributed in the environment and is frequently found in the human intestine and in several domestic and wild animals' intestines [78].

C. perfringens is classified into five groups (A, B, C, D, and E), due to the different toxins it produces (alpha, beta, epsilon, and iota). The Alpha-toxin is produced by all the five groups. The Beta-toxin forms selective pores for monovalent ions in the lipid bilayers, functioning as a neurotoxin capable of producing arterial constriction. The Epsilon-toxin is the most potent clostridial toxin after tetanus and botulinum neurotoxins (BoNTs). It is produced and secreted by a prototoxin that acquires its maximum biological activity by undergoing a specific proteolytic cleavage; its activation can be catalyzed by trypsin, chymotrypsin, and a zinc metalloprotease [12].

The toxin receptor is unknown, but it is known to be a surface protein anchored by glycosylphosphatidylinositol. Its main biological activity is the edema generation; it is lethal but not hemolytic. The Iota-toxin is a member of the binary toxin family, since it is formed by a binding peptide (Ib) necessary for the internalization of the enzymatic peptide (Ia; ADP-ribosyltransferase). Proteolytic removal of a propeptide fragment is required to allow Ib to be inserted into the membrane and to interact with Ia. Ib, when inserted into the membrane, forms a heptameric pore that allows the exit of K^+ and Na^+ ions, and the entry of Ia, which once inside the cell, is ribosylated by the G-actin; it depolymerizes the filaments of Actin by destroying the cellular cytoskeleton. The Iota-toxin is dermonecrotic, cytotoxic, enterotoxic, and induces intestinal histopathological damage [12].

However, the virulence of this bacterium is not only due to the presence of these 4 toxins; there have also been described 15 toxins within which the CPE enterotoxin is responsible for causing diarrhea in humans and animals, and it is produced by Type A strains. This toxin is associated with 5 or 15% of gastrointestinal diseases in humans different from food poisoning such as diarrhea produced by antibiotics; the NetB toxin is frequently related to necrotic enteritis in birds and the Beta2-toxin is apparently associated with enteritis. The production of toxins in the digestive tract is associated with sporulation. The disease is foodborne; and only one case has implied the possibility of poisoning caused by the preformed toxin [12, 78, 79].

C. perfringens causes food poisoning characterized by severe abdominal cramps and diarrhea beginning after 8–22 h of food intake, the disease ends 24 h after the intake; although, in some cases the disease may persist for 1–2 weeks. Additionally, there is a more severe but less frequent disease caused by eating a food product contaminated with type C strains; this disease is known as necrotic enteritis or pig-bel disease, and it is often fatal. Deaths caused by necrotic enteritis are due to intestinal infection and necrosis, as well as by septicemia, the elderly people being the most affected population [78].

The disease diagnosis is confirmed by the presence of the toxin in the stools of patients; either by traditional methods (culture from the stools or the food involved) or by molecular methods by looking for the following genes: *cpe* (CPE toxin), *plc* (Alpha-toxin), and *etx* (Epsilon-toxin) [12, 78, 79].

Among the main food products involved are meat and its derived products. The disease can be prevented if the food has been properly cooked; although, there may be a risk of cross-contamination if the cooked food comes in contact with raw and contaminated ingredients, as well as contaminated surfaces [78].

There is no specific treatment or established cure for the infections caused by the toxins of the bacteria. Supportive care includes administration of intravenous fluids, oral rehydration salts solutions, and medication for fever and pain control. The treatment of gas gangrene is based on surgical measures with debridement and removal of the affected tissue and administration of high doses of antibiotics. Necrotizing enterocolitis is treated systemically with penicillin G, metronidazole or chloramphenicol; 50% of the cases require surgical treatment in which a segmental jejunum resection is performed. The antibiotics active against anaerobic bacteria are effective; however, there are strains resistant to penicillin and clindamycin, therefore, it is suggested to perform antimicrobial susceptibility tests, especially in patients with severe disease and those requiring long-term treatments [9, 80].

3.1.5. *Clostridium botulinum*

C. botulinum is a spore-forming microorganism; these spores can remain viable for long periods of time when the environmental conditions are absolutely unfavorable for the development of the microorganism [60].

Four groups are recognized in *C. botulinum*, as well as seven antigenic variants of botulinum neurotoxins (A–G). Groups I and II are primarily responsible for botulism in humans; Group III is responsible for causing botulism in several animal species, and Group IV appears not to be associated with the disease in either humans or animals. Group I is also known as *C. botulinum*-proteolytic (mesophilic microorganisms), while group II is known as *C. botulinum*-non-proteolytic (psychrophilic microorganisms). Group I forms spores that are highly resistant to heat, the "Botulinum cook" (121°C/3 min) given to canned foods with a low content of acid is designed to inactivate them; neurotoxins formed in this group are A, B, F, and H. Group II forms moderately heat-resistant spores, and the neurotoxins formed are B, E, and F. Botulism types A, B, E, and F rarely cause the disease in humans, whereas in animals it is caused by types C and D. Toxins are resistant to proteolytic reactions and to denaturation into the gastric apparatus. Botulinum toxins are metalloproteins with endopeptidase activity that require zinc; the general structure shows two chains with a molecular weight of 150 kDa, the double chain is subdivided into a heavy (H) structure constituted by a nitrogen terminal domain (HN), and a carboxyl-terminal (HC), and a lighter structure (L) that performs the catalytic function of the toxin. HC is responsible for binding to presynaptic receptors for internalization, and HN is called translocation domain [81–83].

C. botulinum, is a bacterial species known simply for producing the botulinum toxin. The number of genes in Group II strains coding for the neurotoxin is variable; there may be one to three genes that encode one to three different neurotoxins; if there are two genes, there can be one active toxin and an inactive toxin, or both toxins can be active. In Group II, the presence of only one gene has been described, that is why there is only one neurotoxin; however, in other studies it has been demonstrated that in Type F strains the toxin has part of Type B and

Type E neurotoxins. Botulinum neurotoxins form complexes with accessory proteins (hemagglutinin and nonhemagglutinin), which protect the neurotoxin and facilitate their adsorption into the host. The hemagglutinin complex of the neurotoxin type A specifically binds the cell adhesion protein, E-cadherin, by binding the epithelial cell and facilitating the adsorption of the neurotoxin complex from the intestinal lumen. Dual toxin-producing strains have been isolated from botulism in humans, the environment, and food; recently there have been found strains that produce three botulinum toxins called F4, F5, and A2. The significance of producing two or more toxins on virulence, as well as the evolutionary consequences are not yet clear. Phylogenetic studies show evidence of horizontal gene transfer; the production of the dual toxin in Group I and the production of a single toxin in Group II is still not clear. Therefore, studies with toxins isolated and purified from the different groups of *C. botulinum* are still being carried out [81–83].

Botulism is a severe disease with a high fatality rate. The typical symptoms are flaccid muscle paralysis, sometimes it starts with blurred vision followed by an acute symmetrical decrease of bilateral paralysis that, if untreated, can lead to paralysis of the respiratory and cardiac muscles. If severe cases are not fatal, the patient may improve his/her condition after months or even years. There are three types of botulism: infant/adult intestinal botulism, wound botulism, and foodborne botulism. The first type (infant/adult intestinal botulism) is an infection associated with the multiplication of the microorganism and neurotoxin formation in the intestine; the second type (wound botulism) is an infection associated with cell multiplication and toxin formation in the wound, often acquired after drug abuse; and the third type (foodborne botulism) is a poisoning caused by the consumption of neurotoxin preformed in food. An amount of 30 ng of toxin is enough to cause the disease and sometimes death. Symptoms appear between 2 h and 8 days after the intake of contaminated food, although they may occasionally appear between 12 and 72 h [81, 82].

Botulism can be diagnosed only by clinical symptoms, but its differentiation from other diseases can be difficult. The most effective and direct way of confirming the disease in the laboratory is by demonstrating the presence of the toxin in the serum, in stools of patients, or in food products consumed by them. One of the most sensitive and widely used methods to detect the toxin is through neutralization in a rodent. This test takes 48 h, and culture of specimens takes from 5 to 7 days. Infant botulism is diagnosed by detecting botulinum toxins and the microorganism in the stools of children [78].

Approximately 90% of the reported cases are related to the consumption of home-made preserved food, especially vegetables; the industrial preparation of meat and fish is rarely associated with botulism. Food products where spores of the bacteria or the botulinum toxin can be found are canned corn, pepper, soups, beets, asparagus, ripe olives, spinach, tuna chicken, chicken liver, ham, sausages, stuffed eggplants, lobster, and honey, just to name a few [78, 82].

To prevent the chances of getting botulism through food, it is necessary to carry out appropriate control measures in food processing and handling, especially when new technologies are introduced or modified. Applying the "Botulinum cook" in the modern industry allows to secure canned foods. The use of chlorine and chlorinated compounds can help sanitize places that handle food industrially. Spores can also be inactivated with ozone and ethylene oxide [81, 82].

3.1.6. *Listeria monocytogenes*

L. monocytogenes is a facultative intracellular microorganism widely distributed in nature, capable of surviving both in the soil and the cytosol of a eukaryotic cell. Considering somatic (O) and flagellar (H) antigens, this bacterium can be classified into 13 serotypes (1/2a, 1/2b, 1/2c, 3a, 3b, 3c, 4a, 4b, 4b, 4c, 4d, 4e, 7), but only the serotypes 1/2a, 1/2b, and 4b are responsible for more than 98% of the cases of human listeriosis. Furthermore, it has also been grouped into four lineages (I, II, III, and IV), where lineage I (serotypes: 1/2b, 3b, and 4b) and lineage II (serotypes: 1/2a, 1/2c, 3a, and 3c) include most strains isolated from clinical cases; lineage I strains have a greater pathogenic potential. Lineages III and IV include strains of serotypes 4a, 4c, and an atypical 4b [84].

L. monocytogenes expresses multiple virulence factors, which allow to enter and survive in several nonphagocytic cells. After cellular internalization, listeriolysin O (LLO) and two phospholipases mediate the escape of the bacterium from the endocytic vesicle into the cytoplasm, where the microorganism divides and submits the F-actin based on mobility to spread from cell to cell. The LLO (coded by the gene *hly*) is a cholesterol-dependent toxin; it is able to form pores in the membrane of phagosomes, allowing *L. monocytogenes* to escape from primary and secondary vacuoles. The cytolytic activity of LLO increases with the action of a phosphatidylinositol phospholipase C (PI-PLC), the substrate of which is phosphatidylinositol; and a phosphatidylcholine phospholipase C (PC-PLC), which is a lecithinase with enzymatic activity over phosphatidylcholine, phosphatidylserine, and phosphatidylethanolamine. PC-PLC is expressed as a protoenzyme and zinc-dependent metalloprotease Mpl is required for its maturation; so once free in the cytosol, the bacterium acquires the necessary nutrients for intracellular multiplication. Some studies have shown that LLO is a critical invasion factor, which perforates the plasma membrane of the host cell to activate the internalization of the bacterium in human hepatocytes. Moreover, other studies have shown that LLO fails to mediate the intracellular survival of *L. monocytogenes* in neutrophils, where early degranulation leads to the release of proteases such as matrix metalloproteinase (MMP)-8, degrading LLO and avoiding the perforation of the membranes [84–86].

L. monocytogenes causes a severe infection known as listeriosis, which is usually acquired after the intake of food contaminated with the microorganism. The disease mainly affects pregnant women, newborns, the elderly, and immunocompromised people, so it is rare for the disease to occur outside the aforementioned groups. Listeriosis is a mild disease in pregnant women, but it is severe in fetus and newborns. People over 65 years of age or immunosuppressed people can develop infection in the bloodstream (sepsis) or in the brain (meningitis or encephalitis). Sometimes the infection can affect bones, joints, thorax, and abdomen. Listeriosis can cause fever and diarrhea similar to that caused by other foodborne microorganisms and is rarely diagnosed. Pregnant women with listeriosis have fever, fatigue, and muscle pain (flu-like symptoms). During pregnancy, the organism can cause miscarriage, stillbirth, premature labor, and infection in the newborn. In the other risk groups, the symptoms are headaches, neck stiffness, confusion, loss of balance, seizures, fever and muscle pain. People with invasive listeriosis usually develop symptoms from 1 to 4 weeks after ingesting food contaminated with the bacterium; although symptoms have been reported after 70 days of exposure or on the same day of the poisoning. The disease is usually diagnosed by culturing the bacterium from tissues or fluids such as blood, cerebrospinal fluid, or placenta. From food products, this microorganism can be detected by various methods such as the use of chromogenic media; immunological methods, although some are nonspecific; molecular methods (hybridization, PCR, and real-time PCR); microarrays or biosensors; and also specific commercial methods. The detection of the *plcA* virulence gene coding for PI-PLC is generally employed to differentiate hemolytic and nonhemolytic strains. Pathogenic and nonpathogenic *Listeria* species can be differentiated by their activities of hemolysin or PI-PLC [87, 88].

L. monocytogenes is a microorganism that can be present in many food products, mainly in dairy products, soft cheeses, cheeses made with unpasteurized milk, celery, cabbage, ice cream, hot dogs, and processed meats [87].

Infection with *L. monocytogenes* can be treated with antibiotics such as ampicillin, although penicillin is more effective. Some experts recommend the use of gentamicin in people with impaired immunity, including neonates, and in cases of meningitis and endocarditis. Ampicillin is only used in pregnant women with isolated listerial bacteremia. Other antibiotics that can be used are trimethoprim-sulfamethoxazole and vancomycin. Cephalosporins should not be used to treat listeriosis because they are ineffective against the microorganism [89, 90].

The general guidelines to prevent listeriosis are similar to those recommended for other food-borne pathogens. For people at high risk, it is recommended not to consume soft cheeses such as Feta, Brie and Camembert, blue cheeses, or Mexican style cheeses (white cheese, fresh cheese, or panela cheese) unless they are made with pasteurized milk; it is also recommended not to consume smoked seafood, *pâté* or refrigerated meat spreads, hot dogs, processed meats or cold cuts, unless they have been reheated at high temperatures; these are just some of the food products that people at high risk should avoid [91].

4. Strategies for disease prevention

Multiple factors associated with the procurement, handling, and food preparation contribute to an increase in the likelihood of contamination, and consequently, consumer's poisoning. Due to the importance of foodborne diseases, the number of cases presented and their severity, it is necessary to know those measures that help preventing or avoiding them; or getting a disease caused by food poisoning related to bacterial toxins [92–94].

Toxigenic microorganisms arrive to food products by cross-contamination; they come from the environment or they belong to the normal microbiota, in the case of animals. Once the contaminated food is ingested and reaches the intestines, the microorganisms get established, colonize, and, if the strain is toxigenic, produce the toxins responsible for the damage. Likewise, an incubation process must occur prior to the first symptoms. To prevent the occurrence of such diseases, health care measures, especially hand hygiene of food handlers, should be carried out; in that way, all food sectors such as restaurants, manufacturing, and distribution companies, pay special attention to hygiene measures for food handling to prevent food handlers from inoculating the bacteria they carry on the skin on their hands. Along with other measures, they must ensure food safety, and for this, food sectors will establish policies and activities to ensure maximum quality and food safety throughout the food chain (from procurement and production to consumption) [92, 95–98].

Some of these standards are described and taken care by the *Codex Alimentarius*, which, together with the World Health Organization and the Food and Agriculture Organization of the United Nations, has the responsibility to develop and standardize the international food standards. Their objective is to ensure the quality of food products and to protect human health, as well as the correct and fair implementation of these standards. The standards of the *Codex Alimentarius* apply to processed, semiprocessed, or raw food products. In addition to all the factors used in food processing, food quality standards seek to ensure that food products are produced in hygienic conditions, and that they preserve their nutritional quality. The main standards include microbiological processes, regarding the use of food additives, pesticide use and pest control, as well as, the permissible limits of drugs or hormones used in animal production [66, 99–103].

For proper handling of food products, facilities, materials, instruments, and equipment must be kept accessible for the cleaning and disinfection process, in order to prevent food contamination by toxigenic bacteria. Cleaning procedures will include the effective removal of food residues or other contaminants; these procedures must be continuous, because some microorganisms have the ability to settle on these surfaces and to survive in adverse conditions by forming biofilm, thus, cleaning with soap and water is not enough. The methods can be chemical, with alkaline and acidic detergents; and physical, with heat, turbulent washes, or vacuum washes. Moreover, brushes or sponges can be used to remove dirt; however, the correct method of use must be considered to ensure efficiency, as well as, not using the same cleaning instrument in areas of processed and unprocessed food. Detergents or disinfectant substances should be used under the conditions proposed by the manufacturer regarding the concentration and time of action, which will depend on the type of surface and the product's presentation (liquid, solid, or semisolid). Such cleaning processes will be subject to regular monitoring and quality control, registering the areas that were cleaned and the person responsible for the cleaning. The cleaning method will be used depending on what is intended to be cleaned; in the case of smooth surfaces, the use of disinfectant and sponges or brushes to remove residues will be enough; this is done *in situ*, contrary to those dismantled equipment that require to be cleaned piece by piece. All of the above related to the establishment's cleaning must be submitted in writing to the personnel responsible for this task for the correct and efficient implementation of cleaning methods [98, 104–106].

Another important aspect in this sector is pest control. A variety of pests lurk at sites where food is produced; special care must be taken because in most cases these pests act as vehicles for toxigenic bacteria and other pathogens, endangering the consumer's health. The most common pests are rodents, flies, and cockroaches. To prevent the presence of pests, food facilities should avoid air vents and cracks; regarding food products, these should be stored in high places, inside sealed containers or bags to prevent rodents from smelling the food. For pest control, insect monitoring should be carried out on a continuous basis, through catch patches that may contain pheromones to attract insects, electric lamps against flying insects, among others. Of all insects, flies are the most common pest in food establishments, and they are an important source of disease transmission to food and other forms of food poisoning. It is important that food establishments eradicate flies pest to avoid any contamination of food products, in restaurants, kitchens, and other establishments where food is prepared; adhesive traps can be employed. Traps are used when managing rodent pests; however, an exhaustive planning must be done to determine the number of traps to be placed, as well as location; pest prevention include specifics such as covering air vents, avoiding cracks, and storage of food in high places, inside sealed containers or in bags to prevent rodents from smelling the food. At this point, the cleaning of the workplaces is of high importance, mainly the kitchen and the surfaces that are in contact with food, to ensure quality and food safety [87, 107, 108].

Food safety is a human right and an obligation of all the governments to ensure it; it refers to the preserved quality of food products without organoleptic alterations, the presence of chemical, physical, or biological pathogens, or other undesirable alterations in the products that may affect the consumer's health. In order to ensure this characteristic, good practices must be put into operation; identification and control of the potential sources of contamination by the establishment, proper storage of food by separating raw food from processed food, and handling of food products depending on their origin (animal or vegetable). Proper waste management and drainage installation need to be taken into account. Regarding the design and equipment distribution, and the areas where the food is prepared, raw food should be separated, and previously processed food should not be exposed in the same surface. Staff restrooms must be distant from food preparation areas to avoid fecal contamination. The use of suitable uniforms and footwear, air quality, ventilation, and temperature control are essential for a working environment that allows a good development of food processing, and reduces, as much as possible, food poisoning by toxigenic bacteria [101, 109].

The Hazard Analysis and Critical Control Point (HACCP) system can be an efficient and systematic alternative to prevent toxico-infection; its function is to identify specific hazards and develop control measures to solve them, guaranteeing food safety by seven basic principles: identifying hazards and preventive measures, identifying critical control points, establishing limits, monitoring critical control points, using corrective measures, verifying processes, and registering the applied processes [63, 110].

As a preventive measure to avoid food contamination and foodborne diseases, World Health Organization (WHO) proposes the five keys for food safety [94].

- Keep clean: It refers to washing hands before and during food preparation; after going to the toilet; washing and sanitizing surfaces and equipment for food preparation, and to keep them away from insects and animals.
- Separate raw and cooked food: Prepare in different surfaces raw and cooked food and use different equipment for each type of food.
- Cook thoroughly: Food cooked thoroughly allow the removal of bacteria and other pathogens; toxins produced by bacteria and pathogens can also be destroyed.

- Keep food at safe temperatures: Do not leave cooked food at room temperature for more than 2 h to avoid bacteria proliferation, and try not to store frozen food for long periods of time.
- Use safe water and raw materials: Safe treated water must be used when preparing food; use fresh food products and wash adequately. Pre-processed products such as pasteurized milk, should be used as directed and not be used beyond their expiry dates.

5. Research

The field of research about bacterial toxins is very wide; the determination of the toxins structure and function has allowed the development of biotechnological applications such as the development of antimicrobial drugs, anti-cancer therapy, and vaccine creation.

Almost all projects focus on the research of vaccines containing portions of attenuated toxin, in order to protect the patient against the effects of the disease. A study carried out by Secore *et al.*, in 2017, showed the efficiency of the tretavalent vaccine against *C. difficile*, which causes nosocomial infections; this vaccine contains TcdA- and TcdB-attenuated toxins and toxin components CDTa and CDTb. This vaccine showed greater effeciency in golden hamsters and in Rhesus monkeys compared to vaccines containing only the TcdA and TcdB antigens. In the case of the botulinum neurotoxin (BoNT), it is known to be of use in the treatment of muscle atrophies, mainly in facial paralysis, muscular hyperactivity, and dystonias. The BoNT has also been used to prevent facial wrinkles. However, it was found to have a preventive effect on headaches, as it is able to lessen it in some diseases such as neuropathic pain, low back pain, myofascial pain, and bladder pain. Studies supporting this statement have been carried out with studies based on human pain, these studies have shown positive and negative results. They are double-blind studies with placebo control. The positive action of the Botulinum toxin (BTX) has been characterized when administered to cells previously exposed to cigarette smoke; this suggests that it is a preventive agent to reduce the risk of necrosis in the respiratory tissue of patients who smoke [111–113].

Another notable example of toxin research is the use of toxins for medical treatments. For example, in studies by Lai et al., they found that the *C. jejuni* distal cytolethal toxin can be incorporated to the lipid rafts on the membrane with the Cj-CdtA/CdtC subunit; the Cj-CdtB subunit goes through the cell membrane, it translocates to the interior of the cell and reaches the nucleus. This is an advantage that can be used to create drugs paired with the attenuated toxin or to a part of it, so that it can be able to reach the nucleus, be separated from the drug, and act as therapy against cancer, without the toxin causing any damage. Several *in vivo* and *in vitro* studies will be needed to establish it as an alternative cancer therapy [114].

The mechanisms that develop in the pathway that creates the pore have been revealed in the study of pore-forming toxins (PFT) in the cell membrane. Nowadays, the mechanism of formation is almost completely known stage by stage. The challenge in the research is to know the process in detail and, from that, design therapies with antibodies, drugs, or other compounds that can inhibit its effects to know how the cell senses the presence of the pore, if it is at a concentration level of ions or by cytoplasmic signals, allowing it to run repair mechanisms of membrane damage [115].

An interesting group of toxins are the immunotoxins, which are formed by a portion of antibody and a portion of toxin; the toxin has an intracellular action to kill the target cells. Most immunotoxins are designed to attack cancer cells; therefore, they are alternative to chemotherapy. The regulation of immunological signals and the treatment against viral and parasite infections are also applications of immunotoxins. Nevertheless, studies should focus on the methods for obtaining the toxin-antibody compounds, because molecular cloning to obtain a hybrid immunotoxin has not been efficient. Therefore, the methods for obtaining and purifying must be improved. The recent results are the creation of smaller immunotoxins with less immunogenicity, leaving only the site of action with the membrane, or the immunogenic site allowing its insertion into the target cell. Related studies are based on the creation and purification of monoclonal antibodies against toxins; for example, the use of an optimized anti-Alpha-toxin antibody of *S. aureus* causing pneumonia. This study showed a decrease in the number of bacteria in lungs and kidneys of the evaluated mice; mice showed minimal swelling and intact lung tissue. Thus, the mice had a higher percentage of survival, even with the combined treatment of the anti-Alpha-toxin antibody plus vancomycin or linezolid [95, 116].

Another alternative is the use of chemicals that inhibit the effect of bacterial toxins. A large number of research papers have been looking for substances that may inhibit the effect of bacterial toxins in human tissue; for example, the use of $Bi3^{+}$ ion to prevent or treat the hemolytic uremic syndrome caused by *E. coli* producing shiga toxin; this ion can be applied to animals and humans. Due to the importance of toxins in the food area, with clinical and pathological consequences, these mechanisms of action and the nature of toxins should be thoroughly investigated, in order to design strategies to prevent and manage effectively toxicoinfections [117].

It should be of particular attention, the use of toxins as an alternative treatment that allows to have tools for treating diseases such as cancer, the use of immunotoxins and pharmacotoxins.

6. Conclusions

Governments should raise food safety as a public health priority, by establishing effective food safety systems to ensure that food producers and suppliers, throughout the food chain, act responsibly and provide safe food to consumers.

Food contamination can occur at any stage of the manufacturing or distribution process, although the responsibility lies primarily with the producers. Nevertheless, a large part of the foodborne diseases are caused by food that has been improperly prepared or handled at home, in food establishments, or in street markets.

It is a joint responsibility for consumers, traders, and governments to work together to implement regulations, enforce laws that support, increase, and sustain food safety.

Acknowledgements

This study was supported by the Grant Secretaría de Investigación y Posgrado del Instituto Politécnico Nacional (SIP 20160609, 20161129, 20172091, 20171254, and 20171099). Andrea Guerrero Mandujano, Luis Uriel Gonzalez Avila, and Ingrid Palma Martinez held a scholarship from CONACyT. The authors are also grateful to Sofia Mulia for her help in preparing the English version of the manuscript of the chapter.

Author details

Cecilia Hernández-Cortez, Ingrid Palma-Martínez, Luis Uriel Gonzalez-Avila, Andrea Guerrero-Mandujano, Raúl Colmenero Solís and Graciela Castro-Escarpulli*

*Address all correspondence to: chelacastro@hotmail.com

Departamento de Microbiología, Escuela Nacional de Ciencias Biológicas, Instituto Politécnico Nacional, Ciudad de Mexico, Mexico

References

[1] Ospina MML, Martínez DME, Pacheco GOE, Quijada BH. Vigilancia y análisis de riesgo en salud pública. Protocolo de Vigilancia en Salud Pública. Intoxicaciones por sustancias químicas. Instituto Nacional de Salud. 2016;**PRO-R02.006**(Versión 02):1-75

[2] World Health Organization. Informe Estimación de la carga mundial de las enfermedades de transmisión alimentaria. Ginebra [Internet]. 2015 [Updated: 2017]. Available from: http://www.who.int/mediacentre/news/releases/2015/foodborne-disease-estimates/es/ [Accessed: February 2017]

[3] Ramírez-Peña EO. Etiology of acute diarrheal disease: An improved system for monitoring outbreaks of foodborne diseases in Peru. Revista Cuerpo Médico. HNAAA. 2014;**7**(1):54

[4] Kirk MD, Pires SM, Black RE, Caipo M, Crump JA, Devleesschauwer B, Döpfer D, Fazil A, Fischer-Walker CL, Hald T, Hall AJ, Keddy KH, Lake RJ, Lanata CF, Torgerson PR, Havelaar AH, Angulo FJ. World Health Organization estimates of the global and regional disease burden of 22 foodborne bacterial, protozoal, and viral diseases, 2010: A data synthesis. PLoS Med. 2015;**12**:e1001921. DOI: 10.1371/journal.pmed.1001921

[5] Iriarte MJ, Ugarte JC, Salazar L. Utility of the airbone endotoxins assay in different occupational environments as a risk indicator by biological agents. Mapfre Medicina. 2001;**12**(4):234-240

[6] Ramachandran G. Gram-positive and Gram-negative bacterial toxins in sepsis. A brief review. Virulence. 2014;**5**(1):213-218

[7] Romero HS, Iregui CA. El Lipopolisacárido. Revista de Medicina Veterinaria. 2010; **19**:37-45

[8] Sears CL, Kaper JB. Enteric bacterial toxins: Mechanisms of actions and linkage to intestinal secretion. Microbiology and Molecular Biology Reviews. 1996;**60**:167-215

[9] Todar K. Todar's Online Textbook of Bacteriology. Bacterial Protein Toxins 2008-2012 [Internet]. Available from: http://textbookofbacteriology.net/proteintoxins.html [Accessed: February 2017]

[10] Fraser A. Clemson Food Safety Education Program. Section 2: Foodborne Bacterial Pathogens [Internet]. 2012. Available from: www.foodsafetysite.com [Accessed: February 2017]

[11] Sánchez J, Correa M, Castañeda-Sandoval LM. *Bacillus cereus* un patógeno importante en el control microbiológico de los alimentos. Revista Facultad Nacional de Salud Pública. 2016;**34**(2):230-242. DOI: 10.17533/udea.rfnsp.v34n2a12

[12] Morris WE, Fernández-Miyakawa ME. Toxinas de *Clostridium perfringens*. Revista Argentina de Microbiología. 2009;**41**(4):251-260. DOI: S0325-75412009000400010

[13] Ehling-Schulz M, Guinebretiere MH, Monthán A, Berge O, Fricker M, Svensson B. Toxin gene profiling of enterotoxic and emetic *Bacillus cereus*. FEMS Microbiology Letters. 2006;**260**(2):232-240. DOI: 10.1111/j.1574-6968.2006. 00320.X

[14] Dressler D, Adib Saberi F, Reis Barbosa E. Botulinum toxin. Mechanisms of action. Arquivos de Neuro-Psiquiatria. 2005;**63**(1):180-185. DOI: S0004-282X2005000100035

[15] Lindbäck T, Granum PE. Detection and purification of *B. cereus* enterotoxins. In: Adley C, editor. Methods in Biotechnology. Vol. 21. Food-Borne Pathogens: Methods and Protocols. Totowa, NJ: Humana Press Inc; 2006. pp. 15-26. DOI: 9781588294654-c2

[16] Crerar SK, Dalton CB, Longbottom HM. Foodborne disease: Current trends and future surveillance needs in Australia. Medical Journal of Australia. 1996;**165**(11-12):672-675

[17] Pires SM, Fischer-Walker CL, Lanata CF, Devleesschauwer B, Hall AJ, Kirk MD, Duarte ASR, Black RE, Angulo FJ. Aetiology-specific estimates of the global and regional incidence and mortality of diarrhoeal diseases commonly transmitted through food. Plos One. 2015;**10**(12):e0142927. DOI: 10.1371/journal.pone.0142927

[18] Addis M, Sisay D. A review on major food borne bacterial illnesses. Journal of Tropical Diseases & Public Health. 2015;**3**(176):1-7. DOI: 10.4176/2329-891X.1000176

[19] Lopez-Garcia R, Douglas LP, Ayala CE, Guzmán-Pérez SE, López-García R, Trujillo S. Microbial toxins in foods: Algal, fungal and bacterial. In: Helferich WG, Winter CK, editors. Food Toxicology. U.S.A: CRC Press; 2000. DOI: 0.1201/9781420038316.ch5

[20] Lima GC, Loiko MR, Casarin LS, Tondo EC. Assessing the epidemiological data of *Staphylococcus aureus* food poisoning occurred in the State of Rio Grande do Sul, southern Brazil. Brazilian Journal of Microbiology. 2013;**44**(3):759-763. DOI: 0.1590/S1517-83822013005000063. eCollection 2013

[21] Kotiranta A, lounatmaa K, Haapasalo M. Epidemiology and pathogenesis of *Bacillus cereus* infections. Microbes and Infection. 2000;**2**(2):189-198. DOI: 10.1016/S1286-4579(00)00269-0

[22] Tewari A, Abdullah S. *Bacillus cereus* food poisoning: International and Indian perspective. Journal of Food Science and Technology. 2015;**52**(5):2500-2511. DOI: 10.1007/s13197-014-1344-4

[23] Feng L, Chen X, Liu S, Zhou Z, Yang R. Two family outbreak of botulism associated with the consumption of smoked ribs in Sichuan Province, China. International Journal of Infectious Diseases. 2015;**30**:74-77. DOI: 10.1016/j.ijid.2014.10.008

[24] Böhme K, Fernández-No IC, Barros-Velázquez J, Gallardo JM, Cañas B, Calo-Mata P. Species identification of food spoilage and pathogenic Bacteria by MALDI-TOF mass fingerprinting. In: Kapiris K, editor. Food Quality. Croatia: InTech; 2012. pp. 27-47. DOI: 10.5772/33884

[25] Grass JE, Gould LH, Mahon BE. Epidemiology of foodborne disease outbreaks caused by *Clostridium perfringens*, Unites States, 1998-2010. Foodborne Pathogens and Disease. 2013;**10**(2):131-136. DOI: 10.1089/fpd.2012.1316

[26] World Health Organization. WHO Estimates of the Global Burden of Foodborne Diseases: Foodborne Disease Burden Epidemiology Reference Group 2007-2015. Switzerland: WHO Library Cataloguing-in-Publication Data; 2015. pp.61-89

[27] Valero A, Magdevis-Yanet R, Posada-Izquierdo GD, Pérez-Rodríguez F, Carrasco E, García-Gimeno RM. Risk factors influencing microbial contamination in food service centres. In: Makun HA, editor. Significance, Prevention and Control of Food Related Diseases. Croatia: Intech; 2016. pp. 27-58. DOI: 10.5772/63029

[28] Jay JM, Loesner NJ, Golden DA. In: Heldman DR, editor. Modern Food Microbiology. 7th ed. Maryland, Aspen: Springer; 1998. p. 790

[29] Malangu N. Risk factors and outcomes of food poisoning in Africa. In: Makun HA, editor. Significance, Prevention and Control of Food Related Diseases. Croatia: Intech; 2016. pp. 59-97. DOI: 10.5772/62274

[30] Fukuda K. Food safety in a globalized world. Bulletin of the World Health Organization. 2015;**93**:212. DOI: 10.2471/BLT.15.154831

[31] World Health Organization and Food and Agriculture Organization of the United Nations. *Codex Alimentarius*. 4th ed. Rome: 2009. p. 125

[32] Raspor P. Total food chain safety: How good practices can contribute? Trends in Food Science & Technology. 2008;**19**:405-412

[33] Nevin S. The knowledge and practice of food safety by young and adult consumers. Food Control. 2009;**20**(6):538-542. DOI: 10.1016/j.foodcont.2008.08.006

[34] Jevšnik M, Hlebec V, Raspor P. Consumers' awareness of food safety from shopping to eating. Food Control. 2007;**19**(8):737-745

[35] Scallan E, Hoekstra RM, Frederick JA, Robert VT, Marc-Alain W, Roy SL, Jones JL, Griffi PM. Foodborne illness acquired in the United States – Major pathogens. Emerging Infectious Diseases. 2011;**17**(1):7-15. DOI: 10.3201/eid1701.P11101

[36] Blackburn CW, Blackburn CdW, McClure P, Mcclure PJ. Foodborne Pathogens-Hazards, Risk Analysis and Control. Cambridge, England: CRC Press, Woodhead Publishing Limited; 2002. p. 571

[37] Robertson G. Food Packaging Principles and Practices. 2nd ed. U.S.A: CRC Press, Taylor and Francis; 2006. p. 568

[38] Caswell J, Mojduszka E. Using informational labeling to influence the market for quality in food products. American Journal of Agricultural Economics. 1996;**78**(5):1248-1253

[39] Madigan MT, Martinko JM, Stahl D, Clark DP. Brock Biology of Microorganisms. 13th ed. U.K: Pearson Benjamin Cummings; 2010

[40] McSwane D, Salfinger Y, Nummer B, Winslow A. Microbiology (of the Food Code). In: Bradsher J, Wojtala G, Kaml C, Weiss C, Read D, editors. Regulatory Foundations for the Food Protection Professional. New York: Springer; 2015. pp. 77-89

[41] Tyrewala A. What restaurants should do during power or water emergencies. In: Almanza B, Ghiselli R, editors. Hazardous Foods: Food Safety. Canada: Apple Academic Press;2014. pp. 213-232

[42] Prescott LM, Harley JP, Klein DA. Microbiología. 3rd ed. Mexico: Mc GrawHill-Interamericana; 2009. p. 1220

[43] Valero A, Carrasco E, García-Gimeno RM. Principles and methodologies for the determination of shelf-life in foods. In: Eissa AHA, editor. Trends in Vital Food and Control Engineering. Croatia: InTech; 2012. pp. 3-42. DOI: 10.5772/35353

[44] Banwart GJ. Basic Food Microbiology. 2nd ed. New York: Chapman and Hall/Van Nostrand Reinhold; 1989. p. 772

[45] Dashdorj D, Amna T, Hwang I. Influence of specific taste-active components on meat flavor as affected by intrinsic and extrinsic factors: an overview. European Food Research and Technology. 2015;**241**(2):157-171. DOI: 10.1007/s00217-015-2449-3

[46] Adams MR, Moss MO. Food Microbiology. Guildford, UK: The Royal Society of Chemistry; 1995

[47] Akhtar S, Sarker MR, Hossain A. Microbiological food safety: A dilemma of developing societies. Critical Reviews in Microbiology. 2014;**40**(4):348-359. DOI: 10.3109/1040841X.2012.742036

[48] Carrasco E, Valero A, Pérez-Rodríguez F, García-Gimeno RM, Zurera G. Risk management in environment, production and economy. In: Savino M, editor. Food Safety Risk Management. Croatia: Intech; 2011. pp. 77-102. DOI: 10.5772/17757

[49] Huang H, Liu L, Ngadi MO. Recent developments in hyperspectral imaging for assessment of food quality and safety. Sensors. 2014;**14**(4):7248-7276. DOI: 10.3390/s140407248

[50] Wildman RE. Handbook of Nutraceuticals and Functional Foods. U.S.A: CRC Press; 2016. p.543

[51] Gracias KS, McKillip JL. A review of conventional detection and enumeration methods for pathogenic bacteria in food. Canadian Journal of Microbiology. 2004;**50**(11): 883-890. DOI: 10.1139/w04-080

[52] Tilg H, Moschen AR. Food, immunity, and the microbiome. Gastroenterology. 2015;**148**(6):1107-1119. DOI: 10.1053/j.gastro.2014.12.036

[53] Blackburn C de W, McClure PJ. Foodborne Pathogens: Hazards, Risk Analysis and Control. The Netherlands: Elsevier; 2009. p. 1193

[54] Lee SJ, Si J, Yun HS, Ko G. Effect of temperature and relative humidity on the survival of foodborne viruses during food storage. Applied and Environmental Microbiology. 2015;**81**(6):2075-2081. DOI: 10.1128/AEM.04093-14.

[55] Aung MM, Chang YS. Temperature management for the quality assurance of a perishable food supply chain. Food Control. 2014;**40**:198-207. DOI: 10.1016/j.foodcont.2013.11.016

[56] Peelman N, Ragaert P, Vandemoortele A, Verguldt E, De Meulenaer B, Devlieghere F. Use of biobased materials for modified atmosphere packaging of short and medium shelf-life food products. Innovative Food Science & Emerging Technologies. 2014;**26**:319-329. DOI: 10.1016/j.ifset.2014.06.007

[57] Cheng T, Li R, Kou X, Wang S. Influence of controlled atmosphere on thermal inactivation of *Escherichia coli* ATCC 25922 in almond powder. Food Microbiology. 2017;**64**:186-194. DOI: 10.1016/j.fm.2017.01.007

[58] Pu H, Li Z, Hui J, Raghavan GV. Effect of relative humidity on microwave drying of carrot. Journal of Food Engineering. 2016;**190**:167-175. DOI: 10.1016/j.jfoodeng.2016.06.027

[59] Choi S, Jun H, Bang J, Chung SH, Kim Y, Kim BS, Kim H, Beuchat LR, Ryu JH. Behaviour of *Aspergillus flavus* and *Fusarium graminearum* on rice as affected by degree of milling, temperature, and relative humidity during storage. Food Microbiology. 2015;**46**:307-313. DOI: 10.1016/j.fm.2013.08.016

[60] Likotrafiti E, Smirniotis P, Nastou A, Rhoades J. Effect of relative humidity and storage temperature on the behavior of *Listeria monocytogenes* on fresh vegetables. Journal of Food Safety. 2013;**33**(4):545-551. DOI: 10.1111/jfs.12087

[61] Arévalo CA. Novel technologies associated to hospital foodservice Spain. In: Glosa SL, editor. Update in Hospital Food Science. Spain. 2009. ISBN: 978-84-7429-429-3.pp. 95-117

[62] Silva Jr EA. Manual of Hygienic Control in Food Service Systems. Vol. 623. 6th ed. São Paulo: Varela; 2007. ISBN: 8585519533

[63] Kafetzopoulos DP, Psomas EL, Kafetzopoulos PD. Measuring the effectiveness of the HACCP food safety management system. Food Control. 2013;**33**(2):505-513. DOI: 10.1016/j.foodcont.2013.03.044

[64] Center for Disease Control and Prevention. Health Practices on Cruise Ships: Training for Employees [Internet]. Available from: https://www.cdc.gov/nceh/vsp/training/videos/environadd.htm

[65] Nyenje ME, Ndip RN. The challenges of foodborne pathogens and antimicrobial chemotherapy: A global perspective. African Journal Microbiology Research. 2013;**7**(14):1158-1172. DOI: 10.5897/AJMRx12.014

[66] World Health Organization. Inocuidad de los alimentos [Internet]. 2016 [Updated: March 2017]. Available from: http://www.who.int/foodsafety/areas_work/food-standard/es/ [Accessed: March 2017]

[67] Pal P. Role of cholera toxin in *Vibrio cholerae* infection in humans – A review. International Letters of Natural Sciences. 2014;**22**:22-32. DOI: 10.18052/www. scipress. com/ILNS.22.22

[68] Jahan S. Cholera – Epidemiology, prevention and control. In: Makun HA, editor. Significance, Prevention and Control of Food Related Diseases. Croatia: InTech; 2016. pp. 145- 157. DOI: 10.5772/63358

[69] García-Lázaro M, Almodóvar Pulido MC, Rivero A, Torre-Cisneros J. Cólera y otras infecciones del género *Vibrio*. Medicine. 2010;**10**(52):3489-3496. DOI: 10.1016/S0304-5412 (14)70776-0

[70] World Health Organization. World Health Organization [Internet]. 2015 [Updated: 2017]. Available from: http://www.who.int/cholera/en/ [Accessed: March 2017]

[71] Stratmann T. Cholera toxin subunit B as adjuvant – An accelerator in protective immunity and a break in autoimmunity. Vaccines. 2015;**3**(3):579-596. DOI: 10.3390/vaccines3030579

[72] Kadariya J, Smith TC, Thapaliya D. *Staphylococcus aureus* and staphylococcal food-borne disease: An ongoing challenge in public health. Hindawi Publishing Corporation. BioMed Research International, vol. 2014, Article ID 827965; pp.1-9. DOI: 10.1155/2014/827965

[73] Zaghloul MZ. *Staphylococcus aureus* toxic shock syndrome. Tropical Medicine & Surgery. 2015;**3**(2):1-2. DOI: 10.4172/2329-9088.1000e125

[74] Spaulding AR, Salgado-Pabón W, Kohler PL, Horswill AR, Leung DYM, Schlieverta PM. Staphylococcal and streptococcal superantigen exotoxins. Clinical Microbiology Reviews. 2013;**26**(3):422-447. DOI: 10.1128/CMR.00104-12

[75] Pérez PI. *Bacillus cereus* y su papel en las intoxicaciones alimentarias. Revista Cubana de Salud Pública. 2012;**38**(1):98-108. DOI: 10.1590/S0864-34662012000100010

[76] Messelhäusser U, Frenzel E, Blöchinger C, Zucker R, Kämpf P, Ehling-Schulz M. Emetic *Bacillus cereus* are more volatile than thought: Recent foodborne outbreaks and prevalence studies in Bavaria (2007-2013). BioMed Research International, vol. 2014, Article ID 465603, pp. 1-9. DOI:10.1155/2014/465603

[77] Wageningen University, Food-Info Foundation. Food-Info [Internet]. 2014 [Updated: August 14, 2014]. Available from: http://www.food-info.net/es/bact/intro.htm/ [Accessed: February 2017]

[78] Ahsani MR, Mohammadabadi MR, Shamsaddini MB. *Clostridium perfringens* isolate typing by multiplex PCR. The Journal of Venomous Animals and Toxins including Tropical Diseases. 2010;**16**(4):573-578. DOI: 10.1590/S1678-91992010000400006

[79] Miranda C, Rojo MD. *Clostridium perfringens*: Infecciones de piel y tejidos blandos [Internet]. Granada: Hospital Universitario Virgen de las Nieves. 2010. Available from: http://www.seimc.org/contenidos/ccs/revisionestematicas/bacteriologia/clostper.pdf

[80] Illinois Poison Center. Toxinas de *Clostridium perfringens* [Internet]. 2016 [Updated: March 2017]. Available from: https://illinoispoisoncenter. org/ipc_media/pdf/CPTs_Spa.pdf [Accessed: March 2017]

[81] Carter AT, Peck MW. Genomes neurotoxins and biology of *Clostridium botulinum* group I and Group II. Research in Microbiology. 2015;**166**(4):303-317. DOI: 10.1016/j.resmic.2014.10.010

[82] Micali M. *Clostridium Botulinum* and C. *perfringens* in vegetable foods: Chemistry of related toxins. In: Foods of Non-Animal Origin. Switzerland: Springer International Publishing; 2016.pp. 19-39

[83] Pellett S, Tepp WH, Bradshaw M, Kalb SR, Dykes JK, Lin G, Nawrocki EM, Pier CL, Barr JR, Maslanka SE, Johnson EA. Purification and characterization of botulinum neurotoxin FA from a genetically modified *Clostridium botulinum* strain. mSphere. 2016;**1**(1):1-18. DOI: 10.1128/mSphere.00100-15

[84] Vera A, González G, Domínguez M, Bello H. Principales factores de virulencia de *Listeria monocytogenes* y su regulación. Revista Chilena de Infectología. 2013;**30**(4):407-416. DOI: 10.4067/S0716-10182013000400010

[85] Arnett E, Vadia S, Nackerman CC, Oghumu S, Satoskar AR, McLeish KR, Uriarte SM, Seveau S. The pore-forming toxin listeriolysin O is degraded by neutrophil metalloproteinase-8 and fails to mediate *Listeria monocytogenes* intracellular survival in neutrophils. Journal of Immunology. 2014;**192**:234-244. DOI: 10.4049/jimmunol.1301302

[86] Vadia S, Arnett E, Haghighat A-C, Wilson-Kubalek EM, Tweten RK, Seveau S. The pore-forming toxin listeriolysin O mediates a novel entry pathway of *L. monocytogenes* into human hepatocytes. PLoS Pathogens. 2011;**7**(11):e1002356:1-e1002356:19. DOI: 10.1371/journal.ppat.1002356

[87] Centers for Disease Control and Prevention. *Listeria* (Listeriosis) [Internet]. 2016 [Updated: March 2017]. Available from: https://www.cdc.gov/listeria/index.html [Accessed: March 2017]

[88] Janzten MM, Navas J, Corujo A, Moreno R, López V, Martínez-Suárez JV. Review. Specific detection of *Listeria monocytogenes* in foods using commercial methods: from chromogenic media to real-time PCR. Spanish Journal of Agricultural Research. 2006;**4**(3):235-247. DOI: 10.5424/sjar/2006043-198

[89] Agency for Health Protection and Promotion. *Listeria Monocytogenes* a Clinical Practice Guideline [Internet]. 2016 [Updated: March 2017]. Available from: http://www.infectologia.edu.uy/images/stories/pdf/4_guias_clinicas/agente_causal/bacterias/Ontario_AHPP_Listeria_Monocytogenes_A_Clinical_Practical_Guideline.pdf [Accessed: March 2017]

[90] Morobe IC, Obi CL, Nyila MA, Matsheka MI, Gashe BA. Molecular characterization and serotyping of *Listeria monocytogenes* with a focus on food safety and disease prevention. In: Jimenez-Lopez JC, editor. Biochemical Testing. Croatia: Intech; 2012. pp. 197-216. DOI: 10.5772/33009

[91] Centers for Disease Control and Prevention. *Listeria* (Listeriosis) Prevention [Internet]. 2016 [Updated: March 2017]. Available from: https://www.cdc.gov/listeria/prevention.html [Accessed: March 2017]

[92] Moreno GM, Alejandra A. Higiene alimentaria para la prevención de trastornos digestivos infecciosos y por toxinas. Revista Médica Clínica Las Condes. 2010;**21**(5):749-755. DOI: 10.1016/S0716-8640(10)70596-4

[93] Havelaar AH, Kirk MD, Torgerson PR, Gibb HJ, Hald T, Lake RJ, Praet N, Bellinger DC, de Silva NR, Gargouri N, Speybroeck N, Cawthorne A, Mathers C, Stein C, Angulo FJ, Devleesschauwer B. World Health Organization global estimates and regional comparisons of the burden of foodborne disease in 2010. PLoS Medicine. 2015;**12**(12):e1001923. DOI: 10.1371/journal.pmed.1001923

[94] World Health Organization. WHO Estimates of the Global Burden of Foodborne Diseases: Foodborne Disease Burden Epidemiology Reference Group 2007-2015 [Internet]. 2017. [Updated: March 2017]. Available from: http://apps. who. Int/iris/bitstream/10665/199350/1/9789241565165_eng.pdf [Accessed: March 2017]

[95] Oliver MA, Gregory PJ. Soil, food security and human health: A review. European Journal of Soil Science. 2015;**66**(2):257-276. DOI: 10.1111/ejss.12216

[96] Scharff RL, Besser J, Sharp DJ, Jones TF, Peter GS, Hedberg CW. An economic evaluation of PulseNet: A network for foodborne disease surveillance. American Journal of Preventive Medicine. 2016;**50**(5):S66-S73. DOI: 10.1016/j.amepre.2015.09.018

[97] Sadilek A, Kaut HA, DiPrete L, Labus B, Portman E, Teitel J, Silenzio V. Deploying nEmesis: Preventing foodborne illness by data mining social media. In: Proceedings of the 28th AAAI Conference on Innovative Applications (IAAI-16); U.S.A:AAAI. 2016. pp.3982-3990

[98] Uçar A, Yilmaz MV, Çakıroğlu FP. Food Safety – Problems and Solutions. In: Makun HA, editor. Significance, Prevention and Control of Food Related Diseases. Croatia: InTech; 2016. p. 2-25. DOI: 10.5772/63176

[99] Masson-Matthee MD. The codex alimentarius commission and its standards. Netherlands: Springer T.M.C. ASSER PRESS; 2007. p. 370

[100] Tritscher A, Miyagishima K, Nishida C, Branca F. Ensuring food safety and nutrition security to protect consumer health: 50 years of the *Codex Alimentarius* Commission. Bulletin of the World Health Organization. 2013;**91**(7):468-468. DOI: 10.2471/BLT.13.125518

[101] da Cunha DT, Braga ARC, de Camargo PE, Stedefeldt E, de Rosso VV. The existence of optimistic bias about foodborne disease by food handlers and its association with training participation and food safety performance. Food Research International. 2015;**75**:27-33. DOI: 10.1016/j.foodres.2015.05.035

[102] Devleesschauwer B, Haagsma JA, Angulo FJ, Bellinger DC, Cole D, Döpfer D,Fazil A, Fèbre ME, Gibb HJ, Hald T, Kirk MD, Lake RJ, de Noordhout CM, Mathers CD, McDonald SA, Pires SM, Speybroeck N, Thomas MK, Torgerson PR, Wu F, Havelaar HA, Praet N. Methodological framework for World Health Organization estimates of the global burden of foodborne disease. PLoS One. 2015;**10**(12):e0142498. DOI: 10.1371/journal.pone.0142498

[103] World Health Organization and Food and Agriculture Organization of the United Nations. *Codex Alimentarius*. Normas Internacionales de Alimentos [Internet]. 2017 [Updated: 15 march 2017]. Available from: http://www.fao.org/fao-who-codexalimentarius/codex-home/es/ [Accessed: February 2017]

[104] Capita R, Alonso-Calleja C. Antibiotic-resistant bacteria: A challenge for the food industry. Critical Reviews in Food Science and Nutrition. 2013;**53**(1):11-48. DOI: 10.1080/10408398.2010.519837

[105] Lelieveld HL, Holah J, Napper D. Hygiene in Food Processing: Principles and Practice. 2nd ed. Woodhead Publishing, U.K: Elsevier; 2014. p. 640

[106] Lelieveld HL, Holah J, Gabric D. Handbook of Hygiene Control in the Food Industry. Cambridge England: Woodhead Publishing; 2016. p. 619

[107] Stejskal V, Aulicky R, Kucerova Z. Pest control strategies and damage potential of seed-infesting pests in the Czech stores. Plant Protect Science. 2014;**50**(4):165-173

[108] Trematerra P. Aspects related to decision support tools and integrated pest management in food chains. Food Control. 2013;**34**(2):733-742. DOI: 10.1016/j.foodcont.2013.06.020

[109] Mainuddin M, Kirby M. National food security in Bangladesh to 2050. Food Security. 2015;**7**(3):633-646. DOI: 10.1007/s12571-015-0465-6

[110] Trafiałek J, Kolanowski W. Implementation and functioning of HACCP principles in certified and non-certified food business: A preliminary study. British Food Journal. 2017;**19**(4):1-30. DOI: 10.1108/BFJ-07-2016-0313

[111] Luvisetto S, Gazerani P, Cianchetti C, Pavone F. Botulinum toxin type a as a therapeutic agent against headache and related disorders. Toxins. 2015;**7**(9):3818-3844. DOI: 10.3390/toxins7093818

[112] Karayel H, Kaya B, Caydere M, Terzioğlu A, Aslan G. Prevention of unfavourable effects of cigarette smoke on flap viability using botulinum toxin in random pattern flaps: An experimental study. Plastic Surgery. 2015;**23**(3):177-182

[113] Secore S, Wang S, Doughtry J, Xie J, Miezeiewski M, Rustandi RR, Horton M, Xoconostle R, Wang B, Lancaster C, Kristopeit A, Wang SC, Christanti S, Vitelli S, Gentile MP, Goerke A, Skinner J, Strable E, Thiriot DS, Bodmer JL, Heinrichs JH. Development of a novel vaccine containing binary toxin for the prevention of *Clostridium difficile* disease with enhanced efficacy against NAP1 strains. PloS One. 2017;**12**(1):e0170640. DOI: 10.1371/journal.pone.0170640

[114] Lai CK, Chen YA, Lin CJ, Lin HJ, Kao MC, Huang MZ, Lin YH, Chiang-Ni C, Chen CJ, Lo UG, Lin LC, Lin H, Hsieh JT, Lai CH. Molecular mechanisms and potential clinical applications of *Campylobacter jejuni* cytolethal distending toxin. Frontiers in Cellular and Infection Microbiology. 2016;**6**(9):1-8. DOI: 10.3389/fcimb.2016.00009

[115] Dal Peraro M, Van Der Goot FG. Pore-forming toxins: Ancient, but never really out of fashion. Nature Reviews Microbiology. 2016;**14**(2):77-92. DOI: 10.1038/nrmicro.2015.3

[116] Hua L, Hilliard JJ, Shi Y, Tkaczyk C, Cheng LI, Yu X, Datta V, Ren S, Feng H, Zinsou R, Keller A, O'Day T, Du Q, Cheng L, Damschroder M, Robbie G, Suzich J, Stover CK, Sellman BR. Assessment of an anti-alpha-toxin monoclonal antibody for prevention and treatment of *Staphylococcus aureus*-induced pneumonia. Antimicrobial Agents and Chemotherapy. 2014;**58**(2):1108-1117. DOI: 10.1128/AAC.02190-13

[117] Subils T, Casabonne, C, Balagué C. The inhibitory effect of colloidal bismuth hydroxide gel on *Escherichia coli* O157:H7 and on the activity of Shiga toxins. BMC Research Notes. 2014;**7**(1):875. DOI: 10.1186/1756-0500-7-875

Chapter 4

Carbon Monoxide Intoxication: Experiences from Hungary

Edit Gara

Additional information is available at the end of the chapter

http://dx.doi.org/10.5772/intechopen.70010

Abstract

Carbon monoxide (CO) is odorless, colorless, tasteless, and nonirritating gas. Hence, mild CO poisoning often remains unrecognized and appears lethally. Carbon and gas systems, unfavorable architectural designs and machines may also cause intoxications. The prevalence rates in Hungary ranged from 2.37 to 3.80 cases per 100,000 people per year between 2013 and 2015; fatality rates have been decreased from 5.96 in 2013 to 3.38 in 2015. Given the vagueness and the broad spectrum of complaints, misdiagnosis of CO toxicity is common. The gold standard diagnosis is detecting the level of circulating carboxyhemoglobin (CO-Hgb). The measurement of CO-Hgb can be performed via blood-gas analyses or by spectrophotometry. Treatment protocol should follow the ACBDE rule. Administration of 100% oxygen should be performed as soon as possible. Later in-hospital management includes evaluation, treatment and prevention of further peripheral organ damage and long-term neurological complications. Fetuses and children are prone to suffer more severe intoxication due to higher oxygen demand. Though hyperbaric oxygen is the mainstay therapy, a prompt cesarean section is effective in preventing further intoxication. In conclusion, fatal CO intoxication can occur due to plain early signs and symptoms. Hyperbaric oxygen therapy should be considered in severe intoxication, in fetal and children.

Keywords: carbon monoxide poisoning, pathophysiology, differential diagnose, intoxication in pregnancy, treatment options, prevalence in Hungary

1. Introduction

Carbon monoxide (CO) is an odorless, colorless, tasteless, and nonirritating gas product of carbon and gas combustion. CO is also present in cigarette smoke and vehicle combustion gas. CO diffuses through general building constructions (brick and wood). Generally, atmospheric concentration of CO is low, however, in urban and industrial regions it may be elevated. Poisoning usually occurs via impaired operating heating and mechanical systems and fire emergencies.

CO enters human body via breathing and gas exchange, furthermore CO is also generated endogenously in small amounts during oxygen consumption in healthy subjects. The hemoxidase enzyme, responsible for the catabolism of hemoglobin into biliverdine, is responsible for endogenous CO production.

CO has higher affinity in binding to hemoglobin then oxygen, thus development of carboxyhemoglobin (CO-Hgb) is responsible for the major signs and symptoms, and late complications associated with CO intoxication such as cardiovascular and neurological complications due to hypoxia which are often lethal.

The aim of this chapter is to summarize the toxicokinetics, epidemiology, pathophysiology, signs and symptoms, diagnosis, differential diagnosis and treatment options of carbon monoxide poisoning. In doing so, a case report involving a whole family that suffered severe carbon monoxide intoxication will be presented including the story of a successful management of a pregnant woman (one of the family members) who underwent an urgent cesarean section to protect the baby from carbon monoxide intoxication. This will help to elaborate on treatment options to be carried out pre- and during hospitalization; and discuss the merits of hyperbaric oxygen therapy.

2. Toxicokinetics of carbon monoxide

CO is formed as a by-product of burning organic compounds; that is why poisoning by CO is common during power outages due to storms, as a result of the improper use of gasoline-powered portable generators to provide electricity and indoor use of charcoal briquettes for cooking and heating. Other sources of CO include improperly vented gas water heaters, kerosene space heaters, charcoal grills, malfunctioning or obstructed exhaust systems stoves, portable heaters, fires, cigarette smoke, and automobile exhausts.

In a healthy adult alveolar CO concentration, during one cigarette smoke is increased to 400–500 ppm. Nonsmoker individual in the same room is also exposed to CO, resulting 25–100 ppm alveolar concentration [1].

CO is absorbed and eliminated through the lungs. The amounts inhaled and exhaled are dependent on the alveolar-capillary pressure gradient of oxygen and alveolar diffusion. CO intoxication also occurs by inhalation of methylene chloride vapors, a volatile liquid found in degreasers, solvents, and paint removers. The liver metabolizes as much as one-third of inhaled methylene chloride to CO. A significant percentage of methylene chloride is stored in the tissues, and continued release results in elevated CO levels for at least twice as long as with direct CO inhalation. The half-time of CO in a healthy adult takes 4 hours breathing on air, 1.5 hours breathing on 100% oxygen, and 20 minutes in hyperbaric oxygen circumstances [2].

3. Prevalence of carbon monoxide poisoning in Hungary

Carbon monoxide intoxication cases have been documented in Hungary from 2012. Hence, as shown in **Figure 1**, the total number of cases was, respectively, 235 in 2013, 375 in 2014, and 355 in 2015.

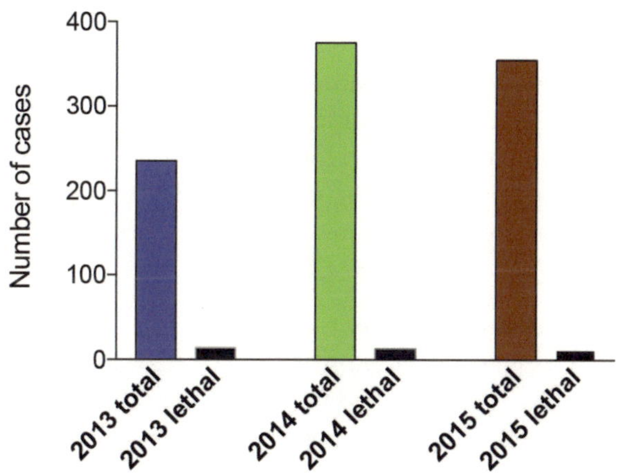

Figure 1. Prevalence of carbon monoxide poisoning in Hungary. Figure shows total number of cases and lethal cases in 2013, 2014, and 2015.

Parameters	2013	2014	2015
# Cases	235	375	355
# Population	9,910,000	9,880,000	9,860,000*
# Cases/100,000 people	2.37	3.80	3.60
# Deaths due to CO	14	13	12
Case fatality rate	5.96	3.47	3.38

*Source: Hungarian Central Statistics Office.

Table 1. Rates of CO poisoning and deaths from 2013 to 2015.

These figures translate to 2.37–3.80 cases per 100,000 people per year. Since, the number of deaths from CO poisoning were, respectively, 14 in 2013, 13 in 2014, and 12 in 2015, the case fatality rates have been decreasing from 5.96 in 2013 to 3.38 in 2015 (**Table 1**). These figures when compared to other countries such the USA, they appear to below [3].

The decrease in the case of fatality rates can be explained not only by the decreasing population, but also by the efforts of the Hungarian National Ambulance that successfully initiated a widespread campaign to increase awareness of CO intoxication. In this project, education focuses on safe handling of household heating systems, importance of regular, controlled, and authorized servicing of equipment and the use of CO level detector devices.

4. Pathophysiology

Carbon monoxide poisoning leads to impaired oxygen delivery and utilization at the cellular level. In doing so, it affects several organs including the brain, heart, and other organs with the highest oxygen requirement. It causes cellular hypoxia by impedance of oxygen delivery as it reversibly binds hemoglobin, resulting in relative functional anemia. Because it binds hemoglobin 230–270 times more avidly than oxygen, even small concentrations can result in significant levels of carboxyhemoglobin (HbCO).

Several studies have indicated that CO may cause brain lipid peroxidation and leukocyte-mediated inflammatory changes in the brain, a process that may be stopped by hyperbaric oxygen therapy. Studies have demonstrated release of nitric oxide free radicals from platelet and vascular endothelium, following exposure to CO concentrations of 100 ppm. One study suggests a direct toxicity of CO on myocardium that is separate from the effect of hypoxia [4].

It should be noted that the severity of CO poisoning depends on Ref. [5]:

- The time of the exposure.
- The concentration of inhaled CO gas.
- Alveolar-capillary diffusion parameters (e.g., general pulmonology status).
- Accompanied illnesses and general condition of the patient.

Exogenous CO intake is regulated via alveolar-capillary diffusion rate. Alveolar-capillary diffusion is dependent on the permeability of the alveolar membrane and from the hemoglobin concentration of alveolar capillaries. Diffusion efficacy of CO in the alveoli is 80%, similarly as for oxygen. The hemoglobin binding efficacy of CO is 200–250 times greater than those of oxygen. Thus, in the presence of CO, oxygen-hemoglobin binding is impaired, however partial oxygen pressures are normal. Main pathological step behind CO intoxication and the related organ dysfunction is the severe tissue hypoxia, caused by elevated levels of CO-Hgb. The hemoglobin-oxygen dissociation curves are shifted to the left, meaning that less oxygen can bind to Hgb at the same partial oxygen pressure levels and CO-Hgb cannot deliver oxygen to the peripheral tissues effectively (**Figure 2**). Furthermore, CO also has higher binding efficacy

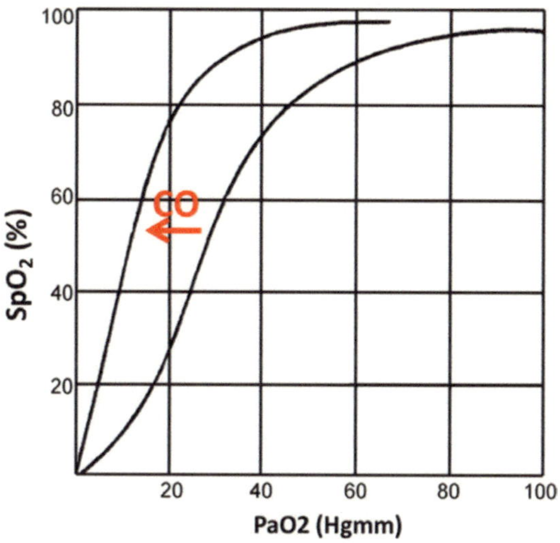

Figure 2. Effects of CO poisoning on hemoglobin-oxygen dissociation curve. In response to CO intoxication the Hgb-O_2 dissociation curve is shifted to the left, physiological sigmoid shape of the curve is impaired, and tissue O_2 delivery is decreased. CO: carbon monoxide, SpO_2%: oxygen saturation, PaO_2: partial oxygen pressure.

to myoglobin than oxygen. This results in more severe peripheral myogenic ischemia and also myocardial ischemia. Partial O_2 pressure is normal, thus forced respiratory responses to compensate tissue hypoxia are lacking. CO also binds to the cytochrome oxidase and NADPH systems at high concentration or long time exposure poisoning. This causes impaired mitochondrial activity and cellular energy development.

5. Signs and symptoms

Signs and symptoms of CO intoxication depend on the CO concentration, thus the CO-Hgb levels. **Table 2** provides a list of general symptoms depending on gas concentration and CO-Hgb levels. Generally, tissue hypoxemia dominates and causes the most severe complications in the cardiovascular and central nervous system. Physical signs of CO intoxication lack unique features. CO-Hgb may cause cherry-pink color on skin, however it only occurs in high levels of CO-Hgb, when the accompanied cyanosis usually lighten cherry-pink sign. Further organ specific signs and symptoms are discussed below.

5.1. Cardiovascular signs and symptoms

Co-Hgb and CO-myoglobin impair myocardial oxygen delivery. Ischemic myocardium is a severe complication in CO poisoning. Clinical features include decreased inotrope function of the left ventricle, accompanied by hypotension and hemodynamic instability. Furthermore, arrhythmogenic complication occurs in one-third of CO-intoxicated patients. Myocardial tissue hypoxia can trigger atrial and ventricular arrhythmias. Malignant ventricular arrhythmia (ventricular tachycardia or ventricular fibrillation) may occur at high CO-Hgb levels, which

CO concentration	Symptoms	CO-Hgb level
35 ppm	Mild headache, vertigo	5–20%
100 ppm	Headache, vertigo, fatigue	
200 ppm	Previous listed above + altered reflexes and cognitive alert	
400 ppm	Previous listed above + nausea, vomiting, tachycardia, tachypnea, palpitation, angina pectoris	30–50%
800 ppm	Previous listed above + arrhythmia, convulsion, respiratory insufficiency, loss of consciousness	
1600 ppm	Convulsions, loss of consciousness, lethal in 2 hours	50–66%
3200 ppm	Convulsions, loss of consciousness, lethal in 30 minutes	
6400 ppm	Loss of consciousness, lethal in 20 minutes	>66%
12,800 ppm	Loss of consciousness after 2–3 breaths, lethal in minutes	

Table 2. Symptoms of CO intoxication in relation with CO concentration and CO-Hgb levels.

may be lethal. Myocardial ischemia may also cause chest pain, angina pectoris and can trigger vegetative reflexes (nausea, vomiting, sweating, and vertigo).

5.2. Neurological signs and symptoms

Loss of consciousness and acute neurological symptoms are due to neuronal hypoxemia. However, after surviving acute intoxication, major studies reported late-onset neuropsychiatric syndrome related to CO poising [6, 7]. This includes change in personality, depressive disorders, cognitive deficits, and psychomotor imbalance. Exact signaling pathways are not yet detailed, general brain hypoxemia/anoxia tends to be responsible for long-term neurological complications.

6. CO poisoning in pregnancy

CO poisoning is rare condition in pregnancy. When occurs, it is a critical condition, the mother and the fetus may suffer severe long-term complications. Due to fetal hemoglobin transport system, the intoxication of the fetus is usually more severe than it is in the mother [8]. Fetal hemoglobin desaturation has higher levels in tissue transport, than adult hemoglobin, even more the fetal gas exchange via the placenta eliminates CO slowly [9]. CO poisoning in pregnancy can cause severe hypoxic/anoxic damage in all fetal organs and tissues. Prenatal injury of the central nervous system may lead to life-long mental and somatic dysfunction, attention deficit disorder or behavioral disorders, due to high sensitivity for hypoxic attacks. Mainly, fetal cortical region and basal ganglions suffer in case of tissue hypoxia [10].

Pathophysiology of CO intoxication of the fetus includes:

1. Maternal O_2 transport via the placenta is impaired in correlation with the elevated CO-Hgb level of the mother

2. CO enters fetal circulation via passive diffusion or facilitated diffusion through the placenta and forms fetal-CO-Hgb, further worsening fetal hypoxemia. Placental CO diffusion is dependent on gestation age and weight of the fetus. In later stage pregnancy, placental diffusion capacity increases and CO intoxication are more severe on the fetus. Many cases presented in the literature lethal, in utero CO intoxication in pregnancies close to terminus [11].

3. Fetal-Hgb binds CO 172 times more than O_2 (lower affinity than adult Hgb), albeit CO binding capacity is longer in time than in adult Hgb. Usually fetal CO-Hgb levels are 10–15% higher than maternal CO-Hgb.

7. Diagnosis and differential diagnosis

Given the vagueness and the broad spectrum of complaints, misdiagnosis of carbon monoxide (CO) toxicity is common. Hence, it is necessary to specifically inquire about possible exposures when considering the diagnosis. In some nonfire-related incidents, the most common symptoms were headaches (37%) followed by dizziness (18%), and nausea (17%) [10]. When a patient has a history compatible with CO exposure and when more than one patient in a group or household presents with similar complaints, the following symptoms have been noted: malaise, flu-like symptoms, fatigue, dyspnoea on exertion, chest pain, palpitations, lethargy, confusion, hallucination, agitation, visual disturbance, syncope, seizure, and neurological symptoms [5].

It should be noted that chronic exposure to CO may produce the above symptoms; but what is more common is the gradual-onset neuropsychiatric symptoms such as memory disturbance including retrograde and anterograde amnesia, impaired judgment and psychosis. Some patients may develop delayed neuropsychiatric symptoms, often after severe intoxications associated with coma. After recovery from the initial incident, patients present several days to weeks later with neuropsychiatric symptoms such as those just described. Two-third of patients eventually recover completely.

The gold standard diagnosis of CO poisoning can be accomplished only by detecting the level of circulating carboxyhemoglobin (CO-Hgb). The measurement of CO-Hgb can be performed via blood-gas analyses or by spectrophotometry by performing SpO_2 measurements. However, general SpO_2 sensors are not able to detect CO-Hgb, a special equipment is required. Either arterial or venous blood can be used for testing. The analysis of CO-Hgb requires direct spectrophotometric measurement in specific blood-gas analyzers. It is noteworthy that the latest emergency defibrillator-monitor systems are equipped with CO-Hgb sensors. Equally, it is important to underline that even in case of severe CO-Hgb intoxication, normal SpO_2 levels can be sensed, due to similar spectrophotometry waveform of oxy- and CO-Hgb. Thus, diagnosis in emergency pre-hospital care may be challenging. Even more, differential diagnose of CO poisoning includes wide range of acute and chronic medical conditions. Early signs and symptoms are atypical, thus it is extremely important to be aware and keep in mind the possibility of CO intoxication, when the circumstances of the scenario suggest. In severe cases, every medical condition that may cause loss of consciousness should be ruled out.

The main differential diagnoses considerations include ruling out:

- other intoxications such as by ethyl- or methyl-alcohol, cyanide, drugs of abuse, or medications;
- infective neurological disorders such as encephalitis or meningitis;
- metabolic disorders such as hypoglycemia, hepatic coma, hypothyroid coma, diabetic ketoacidosis, and lactic acidosis;
- psychiatric conditions.

During in-hospital diagnostics several nonspecific tests can be performed, which help clinicians to determine and quantify the severity of organ specific tissue damage. In this concept, cardiac biomarkers can estimate myocardial ischemia: for example, troponin I, T, and creatine kinase. Peripheral myogenic injury may be estimated via myoglobin urine levels. NT-pro-BNP is able to mirror elevated left ventricular filling pressure and heart failure, especially in the case of severe myocardial ischemia and related acute heart decompensation. Further laboratory tests are able to estimate renal (BUN, creatinine) and hepatic function (liver transaminase). Blood count, ion levels, and glucose levels are also measured routinely. To follow-up metabolic status, blood-lactate should be investigated. Elevated lactate levels suggest more severe CO poisoning and are the predictor of worse outcome [8].

In the most severe cases, radiology scanning of the central nervous system is required to estimate damages. Hence computer tomography (CT), magnetic resonance imaging (MRI), or positron emission tomography (PET) scans are advisable to detect organic neurological complications, mainly bilateral ischemic focus in basal ganglions and subcortical white matter damages. Rarely, haemorrhagic complication can also occur if there is a severe central nervous hypoxia/anoxia in high metabolic demand areas of the brain.

8. Treatment options

Treatment protocol should follow the ACBDE rule, as for every emergency scenario. Airway, breathing, circulation, disability, and exposure should be assessed and treated in respective order. In short, it means that the clinical team whether first responders or people first attending to the patient, must ensure that the airways are clear from any obstruction, that the breathing is present or is restored and efficient, that blood circulation is assured; that further complications and disability are prevented, and that the victim is removed or shielded from further exposure. In sequence, the treatment options include pre-hospital care and hospital care in emergency departments.

8.1. Pre-hospital care

Pre-hospital care includes the following:

- Promptly removing the patient from continued exposure and immediately institute oxygen therapy with a nonrebreather mask.
- Performing intubation for the comatose patient for airway protection, or if necessary, for ventilatory support and provide 100% oxygen therapy.
- Instituting cardiac monitoring.
- Alerting the emergency department of the up-coming comatose or unstable patients because rapid or direct transfer to a hyperbaric center may be indicated.
- Drawing early blood samples for accurate correlation between CO-Hgb measurements and clinical status.
- Obtaining an estimate of exposure time, if possible.
- Avoid exertion to limit tissue oxygen demand.

In CO intoxication, the most important approach is to remove the patient from CO-intoxicated gas area as soon as safely possible and provide high flow 100% oxygen inhale by nonrebreathing masks. The respiratory, hemodynamic status, and consciousness level defines whether the patient needs further respiratory (mechanical ventilation) or hemodynamic support. Controlled hyperventilation provides faster CO elimination. These should be administered as soon as possible, even in pre-hospital first medical contact. For those patients, who suffered CO intoxication in fire event, care should be taken on burns and burn-syndrome-related secondary SIRS (systemic inflammatory response syndrome).

First medical contact

- Detecting CO
- Assessing all possible intoxicated patients
- 100% oxygen ASAP to all poisoned
- Assessing the severity of signs and symptoms
- Assessing special needs: children, pregnancy

In-hospital treatment

- Evaluating CO-Hgb levels and severity
- Assessing peripheral organ dysfunction
- Assessing central nervous complication
- Preventing further hypoxic tissue damage
- Considering special treatment options
- Neuropsychiatric follow-up

Textbox 1. Summarizes key elements of first medical contact and in-hospital treatment.

8.2. Hospital care

In-hospital management requires thorough assessment and support of all damaged organs. Pre- and intra-hospital care should take careful consideration on myocardial ischemia. ECG recording should be carefully analyzed and actions should be taken to decrease myocardial injury and prevent further myocardial ischemia. High-flow oxygen therapy, is needed to prevent myocardial and central nervous ischemic injury, to support renal function, and to compensate metabolic disturbances. The administration of hyperbaric oxygen therapy is the mainstay therapy for CO intoxication. Hyperbaric oxygen therapy initiates CO-Hgb elimination from the human body, and increase partial oxygen pressure and oxygen delivery of circulating blood. During hyperbaric oxygen therapy, the Hgb–oxygen dissociation curve is shifted to the right, thus oxygen binding of Hgb and tissue oxygen delivery is increased. Myoglobin and cytochrome systems bind CO in lower rate. Every patient with CO intoxication may benefit from hyperbaric oxygen therapy, however availability and costs tailor patient population for this treatment. Patients should be selected via the following criteria [9, 12]:

- CO-Hgb level above 25%.
- Loss of consciousness.
- Evidence of organ ischemic function (e.g., renal or myocardial injury).
- Severe metabolic imbalance (lactatemia).
- Pregnancy.

Hyperbaric oxygen therapy is proven to decrease late neurological complications and deficit in CO intoxication. Neuropsychiatric tests are able to estimate loss of function, these may help finding those patients who benefit the most from rarely available and expensive therapy [13, 14]. Hyperbaric oxygen therapy should be administered as soon as possible, but at least in 6 hours to exposure time. It is cautioned here that, although some studies have reported major reductions in delayed neurologic sequelae, cerebral oedema, pathologic central nervous system (CNS) changes, and reduced cytochrome oxidase impairment as a result of hyperbaric oxygen therapy, some systematic reviews have not revealed a clear benefit of HBO, so no clear guidelines for its use have been determined. [15, 16].

8.3. CO intoxication treatment in pregnancy

The major cornerstone of treating a pregnant woman with CO intoxication is to decrease fetal CO-Hgb level. Fetal oxygenation must be provided; noting that in pregnancy, hyperbaric oxygen therapy is superior to urgent cesarian section [15]. However, hyperbaric oxygen therapy is rarely available, thus in many cases, urgent cesarean section is the only option to support fetal oxygenation. Fetal CO-Hgb levels cannot be directly measured but can be estimated. Moreover, fetal ultrasound or MRI scan, if available, can be used to check for central nervous system damage and guide further therapy for the new-born if a cesarian section was performed [16].

9. Case report

This case report is provided from the Hungarian National Pediatric Ambulance Service. The ambulance got a call from a family member who said that their 6-year-old child suffered from convulsions while in the bathroom; but regained consciousness spontaneously, though he still had impaired mental function and could not answer simple questions. It is important to note that convulsion in a 6-year-old child may result from several conditions; hence a skillful questioning is necessary to establish the most likely cause.

Fortunately, the Hungarian pediatric ambulance services are equipped with the latest emergency care machines including CO detectors. When the ambulance arrived at the scene, the CO detectors alarmed a high concentration of CO (335 ppm). Beside the 6-year-old child, there were also five adults in the flat. The child was conscious, with altered mental status. All people were immediately evacuated from the flat to fresh air and the fire service was called on scene, to detect source of CO. The pediatric ambulance with its LifePak®15 ECG-defibrillator system could measure SpCO via spectrophotometry detectors. The SpCO measurements showed more than 30% CO-Hgb levels in all people who were in the flat. Hence, high-flow oxygen therapy using nonrebreathing oxygen masks was provided to all victims. All of them were in a stable condition based on the vital signs (heart rate, blood pressure, ECG monitor, Neurological evaluation (Glasgow Come Scale)), though adults had moderate symptoms of fatigue, dizziness, and vertigo. With the use of the removal from further exposure and the administration of oxygen, the mental status of the child also improved and he did not experience any longer convulsions.

With regard to the pregnant woman among the victims, it should be noted that she was one of the adult patients was pregnant woman. She was 26-year old and in the 39th week of her pregnancy. Her initial SpCO assessment showed a 28% CO-Hgb level, a severe CO intoxication. Her management was continued in the hospital, her CO-Hgb levels had decreased to 14.5% at the time of hospital admission. Given the high level of CO-Hgb levels, an emergency cesarean section was carried out in order to maintain fetal oxygenation. This was performed within 1 hour after hospital admission. This procedure was needed because there was only one hyperbaric oxygen chamber available in Hungary, so organizing an emergency hyperbaric oxygen therapy would have been difficult and time-consuming lost time. The fetal CO-Hgb level was 5% at the time of birth, which is the level of a smoking adult. The new-born was otherwise healthy and received high-flow oxygen support until total elimination of CO-Hgb. The mother also eliminated her remaining CO-Hgb in the following 1.5 hours. The mother and the baby were discharged from the hospital being in good health.

The lessons learnt from the above case were that ambulance services with latest diagnosis equipment and devices are critical in recognizing a diagnosis of CO quickly and facilitation medical care secondly, the administration of oxygen must be performed as soon as possible; thirdly, that an efficient triage should be performed by the providers who first see the victims in order to identify those who are in critical situations and who should be prioritized such as children and pregnant women; finally, the performance of an urgent cesarean section has been effective in preventing accumulation of CO in fetal and thus saved the life of the baby.

10. Concluding remarks

The key learning points from this chapter include that CO is silent killer; fatal CO intoxication can occur and present with plain, nonspecific signs and symptoms. Prevention is a key to avoid severe intoxication: education, safe heating systems, and use of CO detectors. Furthermore, the first medical contact has an important role in recognizing CO intoxication with the use of diagnosing devices and sometimes, based on the signs and symptoms. It is important to perform a differential diagnosis based on information gathered from patients and relatives. With regard to actual management of CO intoxication, the administration of high flow, 100% oxygen therapy must be administered as soon as possible in pre-hospital care. Later in-hospital management should include the evaluation, treatment, and prevention of further organ damage and the neurological deficits. More importantly, prompt care and interventions are required for pregnant women because children and fetus are prone to suffer more severe CO intoxication. Therefore, hyperbaric oxygen therapy should be initiated as soon as possible when available or an emergency cesarean section should be performed to save the fetus from CO intoxication.

Acknowledgements

Eva Gesztes Dr, Gabor Zacher Dr and Richard Doroszlai for the management of the child and the pregnant woman in the case report and providing their clinical data for this chapter.

Author details

Edit Gara

Address all correspondence to: gara.editgara@gmail.com

Semmelweis University, Budapest, Hungary

References

[1] Aubard Y. Carbon monoxide poisoning in pregnancy. British Journal of Obstetrics and Gynecology. 2000;**107**:833-838

[2] Prockop LD, Chichkova RI. Carbon monoxide intoxication: An updated review. Journal of Neurological Sciences. 2007;**262**:122-130

[3] Hungarian Central Statistical Office Database. Available from: www.ksh.hu/engstadat

[4] Damlapinar R, Arikan FI, Sahin S, Dallar Y. Lactate level is more significant than carboxyhemoglobin level in determining prognosis of carbon monoxide intoxication of childhood. Pediatric Emergency Care. 2015 Jul 14;**37**(1):1-7

[5] Ernst A, Zibrak JD. Carbon monoxide poisoning. New England Journal of Medicine. 1998;**339**(22):1603

[6] Thom SR, Taber RL, Mendiguren II, Clark JM, Hardy KR, Fisher AB. Delayed neuropsychologic sequelae after carbon monoxide poisoning: Prevention by treatment with hyperbaric oxygen. Annals of Emergency Medicine. 1995;**25**(4):474

[7] Kwon OY, Chung SP, Ha YR, Yoo IS, Kim SW. Delayed postanoxic encephalopathy after carbon monoxide poisoning. Emergency Medicine Journal. 2004;**21**(2):250

[8] Hutter CD, Blair ME. Carbon monoxide – Does foetal exposure cause sudden infant death syndrome? Medical Hypotheses. 1996;**46**:1-4

[9] Greginor JL, Tosi JM, Ruhlmann és mtsai S. Acute carbon monoxide intoxication during pregnancy. One case report and review of the literature. Emergency Medicine Journal. 2001;**18**(5):399-401

[10] Wu L, Wang R. Carbon monoxide, endogenous production, physiological functions, and pharmacological applications. Pharmacological Reviews. 2005;**57**(4):585-630

[11] Farrow JR, Davis GJ, Roy és mtsai TM. Fetal death due to nonlethal maternal carbon monoxide poisoning. Journal of Forensic Sciences. 1990;**35**:1448-1452

[12] Brown DB, Mueller GL, Golich FC. Hyperbaric oxygen treatment for carbon monoxide poisoning in pregnancy: A case report. Aviation, Space, and Environmental Medicine. 1992;**63**(11):1011-1014

[13] Devine SA, Kirkley SM, Palumbo CL. MRI and neuropsychological correlates of carbon monoxide exposure: A case report. Environmental Health Perspectives. 2002;**110**(10):1051-1055

[14] Pepe G, Castelli M, Nazerian és mtsai P. Delayed neuropsychological sequelae after carbon monoxide poisoning: Predictive risk factor in the emergency department. Scandinavian Journal of Trauma, Resuscitation and Emergency Medicine. 2011 Mar 17; **19**:16

[15] Gabrielli A, Layon AJ. Carbon monoxide intoxication during pregnancy: A case presentation and pathophysiologic discussion, with emphasis on molecular mechanisms. Journal of Clinical Anesthesia. 1995;**7**(1):82-87

[16] Koren G, Sharav T, Pastuszak és mtsai A. A multicenter, prospective study of fetal outcome following accidental carbon monoxide poisoning in pregnancy. Reproductive Toxicology. 1991;**5**:397-403

Toxicity of β-Lactam Antibiotics: Pathophysiology, Molecular Biology and Possible Recovery Strategies

Elif Bozcal and Melih Dagdeviren

Additional information is available at the end of the chapter

http://dx.doi.org/10.5772/intechopen.70199

Abstract

Beta (β)-lactam antibiotics are wide-spectrum antibiotics used for various bacterial infections. The aim of this chapter is to summarize the knowledge about the toxicity of β-lactam antibiotics and issues associated to their inappropriate use. This review has highlighted that β-lactam antibiotics are a group of products that have a chemical structure characterized by a β-lactam ring and are one of the most common antibacterial agents. However, due to the inappropriate use including abuse and misuse, resistance to the β-lactam antibiotics is currently a global crisis. Moreover, even when used appropriately, they have been linked to triggering allergic reactions like urticaria, bronchoconstriction, also severe conditions like immune-mediated haemolytic anaemia and intravascular haemolysis. It is known that some β-lactam antibiotics are neurotoxic, some are nephrotoxic, some are genotoxic and some are toxic to urogenital system. Several factors are involved in the occurrence of toxic effects including the dosage and renal status. Several strategies are possible to overcome β-lactam antibiotics-triggered toxicity, including rational prescribing, substitution combination and phage therapy which seems promising. Public health education for clinical teams and patients is essential in ensuring that this group of antibiotics are retained in therapeutics.

Keywords: β-lactam antibiotics, β-lactamase, toxicity, side effects, treatment strategies

1. Introduction

Beta (β)-lactam antibiotics are one of most commonly used class of antimicrobial agents around the world. β-lactam or β-lactamase inhibitor antibiotics are substances that disrupt bacterial cell-wall formation via penicillin-binding proteins (PBPs) where they bind covalently at the terminal step of peptidoglycan cross-linking in bacteria [1]. The first generation of β-lactam antibiotics were penicillins, followed by cephalosporins; later carbapenems and monocyclic β-lactams that have been recently introduced and are currently in service for the treatment of infectious disease caused by pathogenic bacteria [2]. However, following the occurrence of resistance to the penicillin, new β-lactam antibiotics are being researched for enhancing the spectrum efficiency against the β-lactam-resistant bacteria [3]. In terms of life-threatening infections, β-lactam antibiotics are almost indispensable for therapies in intensive care units (ICUs). However, the therapy with β-lactam antibiotics remains unresolved since β-lactamase resistance is disseminating rapidly among pathogenic bacteria. The most serious types of β-lactamase resistance today are extended-spectrum β-lactamases (ESBLs), carbapenemases and metallo-β-lactamases (MBLs) [1, 4, 5].

The large amount of use and misuse of β-lactam antibiotics has been inducing the β-lactam resistance for decades; besides β-lactam antibiotics have many side or adverse effects including allergy and toxicity [6, 7]. Since beta-lactam rings are different in their structure, they can be recognized by the immune system and this leads to hypersensitivity in some patients [8]. For example, cephalosporin can induce a range of hypersensitivity reaction and anaphylaxis in patients with IgE-mediated allergy [9]. Also, β-lactams are the most known causes of drug-induced fevers [10]. β-lactam antibiotics are neurotoxic, nephrotoxic, genotoxic and some are reproductive toxic. The nephrotoxic effects of β-lactams lead to proximal tubular necrosis [11]. Some are toxic to reproductive system; tazobactam/piperacillin has a toxic effect on reproductive systems and also developmental toxicity reported that tazobactam has an influence on maternal toxicity [12]. Another significant point for the side effects of β-lactams is the toxicity on central nervous system. It can be observed after the administration of β-lactam antibiotics such as penicillin; hence, clinical data have reported disorientation, twitching, somnolence and myoclonus [7]. β-lactam antibiotics such as imipenem and cephaloridine have been reported to cause an irreversible injury to the renal anionic substrate uptake and respiration [13]. Since this effect is dose-dependent, it can be resolved through dosing reduction based on renal function test results [6].

To overcome the resistance and toxicity of β-lactam antibiotics, many attempts have been reported. Developing more stable and more effective strategies is the key factor. For instance, ampicillin/sulbactam, amoxicillin/clavulanate, ticarcillin/clavulanate and piperacillin/tazobactam are the most used β-lactamase inhibitor combinations for clinicians [2]. Moreover, the selection of right β-lactam antibiotics for patients who have an antibiotic allergy is important. To overcome this issue, some of allergy tests are available, for example, penicillin skin testing [14]. Fighting with bacteria via the phage therapy is another option to overcome toxicity/allergy of β-lactams and it reduces the resistance risk of β-lactams. A unique and effective phage against metallo-β-lactamase producing *Pseudomonas aeruginosa* (*P. aeruginosa*) has been used to treat a catfish infection. However, this phage is not useful for the treatment of infections in human [15]. By the way, combination of phages and antibiotics is possible; it is called phage–antibiotic synergy (PAS) and has been proven successful in some bacteria normally resistant to β-lactam antibiotics such as cefotaxime [16]. Interestingly, some studies have reported that phages were not toxic on mammalian cells [17, 18]. Thus, the aim of this chapter is to summarize the knowledge about the toxicity

http://dx.doi.org/10.5772/intechopen.70199

of β-lactam antibiotics and issues associated to their inappropriate use. It is hoped that a good understanding of the structures, mechanisms of action and risk factors leading to resistance to β-lactam antibiotics will assist both clinicians and researchers in the design of anti-resistance interventions.

2. Classes of beta (β)-lactam antibiotics

Beta (β)-lactam antibiotics are a class of antibiotics that contain a β-lactam ring in their molecular structures. Generally, β-lactam antibiotics have a common function: inhibition on cell-wall biosynthesis of the peptidoglycan layer in the bacteria. And this makes β-lactams the most extensively used antibiotics [19]. For over 70 years, penicillin and related antibiotics have been used extensively for the control and treatment of bacterial infections. Improving the efficiency of these antibiotics is still important, and it captivates increasing attention of researchers to overcome the infections depending on highly resistant bacteria. Development of new β-lactam group of antibiotics generally depends on enhancing the spectrum efficiency against the pathogenic bacteria. Besides, resistance mechanisms with special features may be targeted [1].

Over the years, countless penicillin derivatives have been produced including penicillins, cephalosporins, carbapenems, oxapenems, oxacephams as well as monocyclic, spirocyclic and multicyclic ring systems [2]. The first β-lactam antibiotic was 'penicillin G' in the beginning of 1940s [1]. Afterwards, naturally occurring penicillin was 'penicillin V' which was an oral formulation, still in use for the therapeutic purposes. Followed by the occurring resistance to the penicillin, semi-synthetic penicillins were developed such as methicillin [20]. Moreover, some of the significant penicillins from the beginning up to date are the following: oxacillin, cloxacillin, ampicillin, nafcillin, amoxicillin, carbenicillin, ticarcillin, piperacillin, termocillin and mecillinam [20].

Cephalosporins are another subgroup of β-lactam antibiotics, and the first penicillinase-stable cephalosporin was discovered during 1950s [21]. It was efficient for the treatment of infectious diseases mainly caused by penicillinase-producing pathogenic bacteria [22]. Numerous cephalosporins are in use nowadays including cefotaxime, ceftriaxone, cefepime, ceftazidime and cefuroxime [23]. A new addition has been made to the cephalosporin family with a siderophore-substituted cephalosporin (S-649266) that contains a catechol segment which facilitates entry into bacterial cells through iron transportation system. Moreover, this cephalosporin is stable against several carbapenemases [24].

Furthermore, carbapenems are also members of the β-lactam antibiotics which act by binding to penicillin-binding proteins and lead to the inhibition of bacterial cell-wall synthesis. However, they have broader spectrum than other cephalosporins and have been proven successful against *Enterobacteriaceae* including ESBLs [25]. Carbapenem-related agents and other carbapenems that have extended-spectrum activity include meropenem, imipenem, ertapenem and doripenem which have been used widely [1].

Finally, at molecular level, it is worth noting that there is a peptidoglycan layer which is critical for bacterial cell-wall structural wholeness and stability, particularly in Gram-positive organisms, being the outermost and primary component of the wall [26]. During the final stage formation of the peptidoglycan, there is a transpeptidation step catalysed by DD-transpeptidases which are PBPs. β-lactam antibiotics inhibit these PBPs and ultimately lead to cell lysis [27]. It should be noted that PBPs are classified according to their molecular mass: the first category is low-molecular-mass PBPs that are monofunctional, for example, D-Ala-D-Ala carboxypeptidases; the second category is high-molecular-mass PBPs that are bifunctional enzymes containing a transpeptidase (D-Ala-D-Ala-dependent) and a transglycosylase [1, 28, 29].

3. Specific cases of resistance to β-lactam antibiotics

In most instances, particularly in case of life-threatening bacterial infections, antibiotics are the core of treatment [19]. Two of the main goals of β-lactam antibiotics are prevention and treatment of bacterial infections occasioned by susceptible bacteria [1]. Antimicrobial resistance has a greater risk for critically ill patients. For example, it is well known that ICUs are facing a major problem with β-lactam antibiotics [30]. Moreover, many case studies have been reported issues intensively with regard to resistance to the β-lactam antibiotics. A recent case was reported about extensively drug-resistant (particularly β-lactams) *Escherichia coli (E. coli),* which was isolated from the urine of a 63-year-old man from Phetchabun, Thailand. A craniotomy resulted that it is also difficult to treat infections like this via β-lactam antibiotics [31]. Another case was reported from an 87-year-old woman, who had clinical signs, for example, fever, dysuria and suprapubic pain. Urine culture produces a positive result for *Klebsiella pneumoniae* and *E. coli,* both resistant to multiple antibiotics including β-lactams [32]. β-lactam resistance can be seen in serious infections such as cystic fibrosis. Pollini and coworkers reported that a metallo-β-lactamase-producing *P. aeruginosa* identified in a cystic fibrosis patient was resistant to carbapenems [33]. Furthermore, New Delhi β-lactamase-1 (NDM-1) producing *Enterobacteriaceae* infections have been found in patients suffering from type 2 diabetes mellitus infections [34]. Bacteria that produce NDM-1 have been dealt with resistance also in other classes of antimicrobials and virulently restrict treatment options [34].

It is important to note that the clinical outcomes in patients with *P. aeruginosa* infection are poor, with a case fatality rate being higher in patients with MBL-producing *P. aeruginosa* [35]. A recently approved antibiotic is ceftolozane (cephalosporin), which is a combination with tazobactam, has shown a potent activity and has been used successfully for treatment of the urinary tract and intra-abdominal infections [36]. Furthermore, there was a report from an organ transplant unit where a 61-year-old lung transplant patient in Chicago had *Serratia marcescens (S. marcescens)* infection with imipenem resistance. Since beta-lactam antibiotics could not be used, several antibiotics were prescribed instead such as trimethoprim-sulfamethoxazole, itraconazole, ceftriaxone, cefepime and levofloxacin; this is clearly a costly exercise [37].

There is an observation that patients at a high risk for developing colonization with β-lactam resistance include both the severely ill and well-on patients. Likewise, patients with medical devices like urinary catheters are also prone to antibiotic-resistant bacteria [38]. Moreover, the length of hospital stay is another risk factor; patients who have stayed more than 3 days in hospitals and who have been previously treated with β-lactam antibiotics might be considered as a risk factor for the acquisition of β-lactamase resistance [39]. Furthermore, it has been reported in Italy that the risk factors for ESBL-producing *S. marcescens* and *K. pneumoniae* acquisition in neonatal ICU include low birthweight, gestational period and the use of invasive devices [40].

Further observations have noted that clinical isolates that have ESBL-produced *E. coli* strains occur generally in hospitalized patients exposed to invasive procedures [41]. It is also noted that when antibiotics are cheap and accessible, this encourages their overuse and subsequent resistance [42]. It has been reported that there is a positive relationship between antibiotic consumption and the emergence and spreading of resistant bacterial strains. One of the most significant reasons of this is the lack of enforcement of legislation which result in the sale of antibiotics without a prescription in many countries [43].

4. Factors and mechanisms involved in resistance to β-lactam antibiotics

Clinicians can prescribe beta-lactams without a real need; yet the health condition could have been treated by diet or rest. Sometimes, the consumers can take drugs without a medical advice or can take more doses than prescribed doses because of mental illnesses like Alzheimer's disease or dementia. Though some people know that antibiotics are used against bacterial infections, few are aware that antibiotics are not useful for viral infections [44]. When antibiotics are used in viral infections, they can trigger bacterial resistance while infections are not cured because of their viral background. Clinicians, surgeons, patients, consumers and caretakers as well require up-to-date information about the appropriate usage of β-lactam antibiotics because their misuse can cause severe conditions including bacterial resistance or allergic/toxic side effects [45].

It should be remembered that resistance to penicillin was noted in early 1940s; this finding has no clinical significance until the 1970s [20]. However, β-lactam resistance became a global crisis nowadays [46]. Resistance to the β-lactams usually occurs by three different mechanisms: decreased access of antimicrobials to the target PBPs (efflux pumps), altered PBPs (affinity of binding decreased) and β-lactamase production [1].

Although efflux pumps are found in almost all bacterial species, the β-lactamase production is the most efficient of the three mechanisms. This resistance mechanism generally depends on plasmids that include various virulence genes consisting of multiple β-lactamases of different classes in this way. This is why β-lactamase resistance can sprawl among various bacterial species. There are two types of β-lactamases: (a) serine-β-lactamases and (b) MBLs. Serine-β-lactamases comprise ESBLs and carbapenemases that hydrolyse carbapenem antibiotics and cephalosporins [2, 20]. We can suffice to say that the most common mechanism for drug resistance to β-lactam antibiotics is bacterial synthesis of β-lactamases. Many bacteria synthesize beta-lactamases that degrade beta-lactam antibiotics before they reach the cell wall. Gram-positive bacteria that produce beta-lactamase excrete the enzyme into the extracellular space. Gram-negative bacteria excrete beta-lactamase into the periplasmic space located between the cytoplasmic membrane and the outer membrane, where the cell wall is located; while the genes that encode beta-lactamases can be located on either (a) the bacterial chromosome; (b) plasmids; or (c) transposable elements which enhance the spread of beta-lactamases among different bacterial species [47].

Carbapenemases are distinct among the β-lactamases; they are able to hydrolyse most of the penicillins, cephalosporins and carbapenems. In 1980s and 1990s, carbapenems were considered as the 'last resort antibiotics' which used primarily against ESBL- or AmpC-producing bacteria. Molecular classes of A, B and D β-lactamases are known as carbapenemases. The carbapenemase resistance generally occurs in bacteria involving OprD porin loss, overexpression of efflux systems, overproduction of AmpC-type β-lactamase and acquisition of carbapenemase-encoding genes [46]. A and D enzymes are the group of carbapenemases having serine-based hydrolytic mechanisms; however, the group of B carbapenemases are known as MBLs [48]. Also, MBLs are inhibited by chelate-divalent cations like EDTA. The group A carbapenemases include members of the *S. marcescens enzyme* (SME), imipenem-hydrolysing-β-lactamase (IMI), not metallo-enzyme carbapenemase (NMC), Guiana-extended-spectrum (GES) and *K. pneumoniae* carbapenemases (KPC) families and their hydrolytic mechanism requires their active serine site at position 70 [37]. This feature gives them the ability to hydrolyse many β-lactam antibiotics like carbapenems, cephalosporins, penicillins and aztreonam, and all are inhibited by clavulanate and tazobactam [37]. SME-1 was first reported in England from two *S. marcescens* isolates. SME-1 has identical features with SME-2 and SME-3. SME-3 β-lactamases differentiate from SME-1 gene by a single amino acid substitution of tyrosine for histidine at position 105 [49], and SME-1 is encoded by chromosome in bla_{SME-1} gene [37]. Since chromosomally encoded bla_{SME-1} gene was not detected in any plasmids, mobile genetic elements can be concluded that there is a limitation of SME-1 enzyme distribution [50]. The IMI and NMC-A enzymes have been found in clinical isolates of *Enterobacter cloacae* from the United States, Croatia, Finland and France. Most bla_{IMI-1} genes are located on chromosome and it is related to *imi-R* gene that limits their dissemination and their expression at a high level [51]. NMC-A and IMI-1 have 97% amino acid similarity and they are similar to the SME-1, with approximately 70% of amino acid identity encoded by bacterial genome B [52]. The GES family enzymes consist of 26 variants of GES. For example, GES-1 was reported from *K. pneumoniae* strain in year 2000. The other GES enzymes are the following: GES-2, GES-4, GES-5, GES-6, GES-11, GES-14 and GES-18 are able to hydrolyse imipenem. Among these enzymes, GES-2 and GES-5 have carbapenemase activity. *K. pneumoniae* carbapenemases are another carbepenemases, identified in *K. pneumoniae.* These enzymes are known as one of the most significant enzymes due to their effectiveness to the carbapenems [53].

OXA-type β-lactamases include Group D carbapenemases and OXA referred to oxacillinases since they hydrolyse isoxazolyl penicillin oxacillin [51]. Nowadays, OXA-type enzymes contain over 400 enzymes. With regard to their amino acid sequences, OXA-type enzymes have 12 subgroups accommodating OXA-23, OXA-24/40, OXA-48, OXA-51, OXA-58, OXA-134a, OXA-143, OXA-211, OXA-213, OXA-214, OXA-229 and OXA-235 [54]. In spite of OXA enzymes that were generally detected in *Acinetobacter* species, these enzymes were started to be reported in other *Enterobacteriaceae* members such as *Salmonella* spp. and *P. aeruginosa;* this showed that OXA-type β-lactamases can spread to the *Enterobacteriaceae* members [54–56].

ESBLs are implicated in serine β-lactamases [48]. ESBLs are able to hydrolyse extended-spectrum cephalosporin; thereof they are active against the β-lactam antibiotics such as ceftazidime, ceftriaxone and oxyimino-monobactams. ESBLs are generally produced by Gram-negative bacteria including *Enterobacteriaceae* such as *E. coli* and *K. pneumoniae* [57]. The types of ESBLs are TEM- β-lactamases, SHV-β-lactamases and CTX-M-type β-lactamases. TEM-type ESBLs are originated from TEM-1 and TEM-2; however, the number of TEM-type ESBLs is over 100. The most prevalent TEM-type ESBLs were detected in *E. coli* and *K. pneumoniae* [58]. SHV-type ESBLs are more widespread according to the TEM-type ESBLs and more than 100 SHV-type ESBLs are known around the world mainly reported from *Enterobacteriaceae*, *P. aeruginosa* and *Acinetobacter* spp. CTX-M-type ESBLs have the ability to hydrolyse cefotaxime and cefepime. In contrast to TEM and SHV enzymes, CXT-M-type ESBLs have no point mutations in their structures [58]. Until today, 128 different types of CTX-M were reported such as CTX-M-1, CTX-M-2, CTX-M-8, CTX-M-9 and CTX-M-25. Likewise, the type of CTX-M-15 is the most prevalent in *E. coli* strains [59].

The class B MBLs can be divided into four subclasses according to their structure: (a) B1aVIM, imipenemase (IMP), DIM, SPM; (b) B1b: NDM, (c) B2: cphA, (d) B3: LI and AIM [37, 60]. Moreover, Tripoli metallo-β-lactamase (TBM-1) was also included in MBLs [58, 61]. The earlier MBLs were reported in Japan in 1980s called imipenemase in *P. aeruginosa* [62]. After that, several varieties of IMP were reported such as Verona integron-encoded metallo-β-lactamase (VIM) and SPM-type enzymes and it was reported that VIM-producing bacteria are distributed intensely [63]. The New Delhi metallo-β-lactamase is a globally distributed enzyme discovered of late. NDM was reported for the first time in year 2009 and referred to as NDM-1. NDM-1 can bind and hydrolyse all beta-lactams with the exception of aztreonam. There are 13 different NDMs reported: NDM-1 to 14. The variation of these NDM types results from mutation within the gene encoding the β-lactamase [64]. #NDM-1 has drawn attention since the gene encoding these MBLs is located in a mobile genetic element and the pattern of spread proves to be more complex [65]. NDM can coexist with other antibiotic-resistant genes. Recently, plasmid-mediated NDM was reported in Thailand and coexisted with colistin resistance [31]. Co-carriage of ESBL, AmpC and NDM-1 genes among carbapenem-resistant *Enterobacteriaceae* in India [66] was reported. There are several MBL types reported occasionally. For instance, GIM-1 MBL was reported in a clinical isolate (*P. aeruginosa*) in Germany in year 2002, firstly. In recent years, GIM-1 was started to be reported in other bacterial species such as *S. marcescens*, *E. cloacae* and *Acinetobacter pittii* [60, 67]. Similarly, SIM-1 was obtained uncommonly and an integron-encoded blaSIM-1 was reported from *Acinetobacter baumannii* in Korea firstly [68]. Moreover, TMB-1 was reported in an *Achromobacter xylosoxidans* strain isolated from a hospital environment sample in Tripoli, Libya [69].

5. Toxicity of β-lactam antibiotics

There are several β-lactam antibiotics, and they have various side effects (**Table 1**). Although it is very hard to gather data on all the adverse effects and present them in this section, a description of toxic side effects known to be associated with the use of this category of antibiotics is subsequently presented.

Antibiotic	Adverse/side effects	Toxicity grade	Populations-circumstances	Type of study	References
Cephaloglycin	Nephrotoxicity	Moderate	Rabbit kidney extracts	Experimental	[13]
Imipenem	Nephrotoxicity	Severe	Rabbit kidney extracts	Experimental	[13]
L-695,256 is a novel 2-fluorenonyl carbapenem	Haemolytic anaemia	Moderate	Rhesus monkeys	Experimental	[70]
L-695,256 is a novel 2-fluorenonyl carbapenem	Regenerative anaemia	Mild	Squirrel monkeys	Experimental	[70]
Penicillin	Epileptic seizures	Moderate	Rats	Experimental	[71]
	Hemorrhagic cystitis	Moderate	Infection patient adult	Case	[88]
Piperacillin	Nephrotoxicity	Moderate	1200 patients	Randomized control trial	[83]
	Convulsion	Mild	Schizophrenic adult, ECT taken	Case	[72]
Cefotiam	Convulsion	Mild	Schizophrenic adult, ECT taken	Case	[72]
Cefuroxime	Retinal toxicity	Mild	Cataract patient adult	Case	[73]
Cefazolin	Nephrotoxicity	Mild	Hospitalized adult infectious patients	Case-control	[81]
Ceftriaxone	Nephrotoxicity	Mild	Hospitalized adult infectious patients	Case-control	[81]
	Genotoxicity	Moderate	Human lymphocytes	Experimental	[85]
Amoxicillin	Genotoxicity	Severe	Human gastric cells	Experimental	[86]
FCE 22891 a penem antibiotic	Urotoxicity	Severe	Rats	Experimental	[87]

Table 1. Illustrative adverse effects of β-lactam antibiotics.

The use of β-lactam antibiotics has been linked to triggering allergic reactions like urticaria, bronchoconstriction, also severe conditions like immune-mediated haemolytic anaemia and intravascular haemolysis [70]. It is known that some β-lactam antibiotics are neurotoxic, some are nephrotoxic, some are genotoxic and some are toxic to urogenital system.

Neurotoxic side effects of β-lactam antibiotics are well-known conditions for decades. The administration route and the dose of antibiotic are important factors that determine whether a neurological dysfunction would occur. β-lactam antibiotics can trigger epilepsy or seizures because of their chemical structures of β-lactams that make them capable of binding to the gamma-aminobutyric acid (GABA) receptors in the brain. Some of the β-lactams are GABA receptor antagonists [7]. This is the reason why penicillin injection can be used as an epilepsy model in rats [71]. In a case report, it was proposed that β-lactams triggered a tardive seizure in a patient after an electroconvulsive therapy [72]. It has been noted also that the retina is a target for neurotoxic pathologies. In a case report after the cataract surgery, cefuroxime

http://dx.doi.org/10.5772/intechopen.70199

was given in normal dosing ranges but it induced a retinal toxicity; fortunately, the resulting visual loss was recovered after a week [73]. Neurotoxicity induced by β-lactams can be a result of renal failure, which increases the amount of the antibiotic in the circulating blood. Hence, even in normal dosing ranges, β-lactam antibiotics pose risks in case of renal failure [74]. The relationship between the nervous system and β-lactams is not just the toxicity, but the molecular interaction may also have positive consequences. β-lactams may have neuroprotective roles in some instances [75]. The molecular glutamate mechanism takes place for that protection [76]. Also, β-lactams can help in treating ischaemic rat brain during the acute phase [77]. The effect of β-lactams on the glutamate receptors affects the lab animals' behaviour. Rats' dependence on alcohol and morphine may be decreased with the β-lactam application [78–80].

Nephrotoxicity is a very serious side effect of antibiotics generally. β-lactam antibiotics are both dangerous as a mono therapy or as a combination therapy agent [81]. These chemicals induce toxicity in kidneys via a couple of molecular mechanisms. Tubular cells are under threat because of the excess active transport from blood to these cells; however, less efflux and accumulation happens. The other mechanism is acylation of target proteins, which cause respiratory arrest by inactivation of mitochondrial anionic substrate carriers in cells. The other nephrotoxic side effects occur via lipid peroxidation of renal cortex [11, 82]. For critically ill patients, it is very dangerous to use antibiotics such as tazobactam with piperacillin because of the toxic effect on renal tubule [83].

Genotoxic effects of some β-lactams have been shown in some studies done in vitro. Ceftazidime is toxic to bone marrow stromal cells via DNA polymerase inhibition [84]. Ceftriaxone genotoxicity was shown in human peripheral blood lymphocytes, while amoxicillin genotoxicity was studied with both human lymphocytes and gastric mucosa cells resulting in β-lactams having genotoxicity risk [85, 86].

Also, β-lactam antibiotics have toxic effects on the urogenital system. A synthetic β-lactam caused urothelial hyperplasia in rats but scientist suggested that chemical is not toxic to human [87]. In a case study, it has been reported that penicillin-G induced haemorrhagic cystitis, but the patient recovered in 8 days [88]. Some of the β-lactams toxicity grades and possible adverse effects were shown in **Table 1**.

6. Strategies to overcome β-lactam antibiotic-triggered toxicity

After any toxic reaction in an organism, the resulting defects could be very severe and cannot be reversed; hence, there is a need for special care for recovery. When it is established that there is no recovery, substituting the toxic chemical or product can help reduce the risk of side effects.

The potential strategies to overcome β-lactam antibiotic-triggered toxicity are as follows:

1. Replacing the toxic β-lactam with a non-allergic/toxic one,
2. Using phage therapy instead of chemicals,

3. Using β-lactamase inhibitors,
4. Using other chemicals in combination with β-lactams,
5. Performing a dialysis (for very severe cases),
6. Rational drug prescribing and treatment monitoring.

In implementing the substitution strategy, one way is to use other available β-lactam antibiotics for clinical use called ESBLs such as cephalosporins, carbapenem, imipenem, monobactam and aztreonam [2]. Another strategy is designing/choosing a β-lactamase inhibitor which makes it possible to use a smaller dose of or a mild β-lactam. Clavulanic acid, tazobactam and sulbactam are known inhibitors that are used for this purpose [2, 89].

With regard to phage therapy, it has always been an alternative to the antibiotics; however, the concerns about the production cost have made it difficult. The phage therapy has been kept on the shelves for decades: a less toxic option which was as effective as antibiotics [90]. But it is nowadays on the table as a potential replacement for β-lactam antibiotics in the near future. It has been successfully applied to cultured African catfish, which were infected by *P. aeruginosa* and positive results have evaluated, while there was a resistance for β-lactam antibiotics [15], and phage therapy may be a logical substitute for β-lactam antibiotics in the near future.

With regard to combination strategy, β-lactam antibiotics have been used with aminoglycosides and they created a synergistic effect, which helped to reduce the doses required for both groups. This strategy has been able to increase the efficiency of the β-lactam antibiotics [91–94]. But clinicians should be aware that, because of a possibility of unexpected adverse effects, dialysis facilities should be available [95].

With regard to rational prescribing, clinical teams including doctors, nurses and pharmacists need to work hand in hand in order to select, purchase, control, restrict and ensure that patients are prescribed β-lactam antibiotics only when needed and that the patients must be counselled on the appropriate use thereof. Considering preventive medicine perspective, it is cheaper trying to limit the misuse/abuse of β-lactam antibiotics.

7. Concluding remarks

The above review has highlighted that β-lactam antibiotics are a group of products that have a chemical structure characterized by a β-lactam ring and are one of the most common antibacterial agents. However, due to inappropriate use including abuse and misuse, resistance to the β-lactam antibiotics is currently a global crisis. It usually occurs by three different mechanisms: decreased access of antimicrobials to the target PBPs (efflux pumps), altered PBPs (affinity of binding decreased) and β-lactamase production.

Moreover, even when used appropriately, they have been linked to triggering allergic reactions like urticaria, bronchoconstriction, also severe conditions like immune-mediated haemolytic anaemia and intravascular haemolysis [70]. It is known that some β-lactam antibiotics are neurotoxic, some are nephrotoxic, some are genotoxic and some are toxic to urogenital system. Several factors are involved in the occurrence of toxic effects including the dosage and the renal status. Several strategies to overcome β-lactam antibiotics triggered toxicity include rational prescribing, substitution combination and phage therapy which seems promising. Public health education for clinical teams and patients is essential in ensuring that this group of antibiotics are retained in therapeutics.

Author details

Elif Bozcal[1]* and Melih Dagdeviren[2]

*Address all correspondence to: elif.bozcal@istanbul.edu.tr

1 Department of Biology, Faculty of Science, Basic and Industrial Microbiology Section, Istanbul University, Istanbul, Turkey

2 Department of Biology, Faculty of Science, General Biology Section, Ege University, Izmir, Turkey

References

[1] Bush K, Bradford PA. Beta-lactams and beta-lactamase inhibitors: An overview. Cold Spring Harbor Perspectives in Medicine. 2016;**6**: pii: a025247. DOI: 10.1101/cshperspect.a025247

[2] Konaklieva MI. Molecular targets of beta-lactam-based antimicrobials: Beyond the usual suspects. Antibiotics. 2014;**3**:128. DOI: 10.3390/antibiotics3020128

[3] Watkins RR, Papp-Wallace KM, Drawz SM, Bonomo RA. Novel beta-lactamase inhibitors: A therapeutic hope against the scourge of multidrug resistance. Frontiers in Microbiology. 2013;**4**:392. DOI: 10.3389/fmicb.2013.00392

[4] Cai XF, Sun JM, Bao LS, Li WB. Risk factors and antibiotic resistance of pneumonia caused by multidrug resistant *Acinetobacter baumannii* in pediatric intensive care unit. World Journal of Emergency Medicine. 2012;**3**(3):202-207. DOI: 10.5847/wjem.j.issn.1920-8642.2012.03008

[5] Mereuta AI, Tuchilus C, Badescu AC, Iancu LS. Metallo-beta-lactamase-mediated resistance among carbapenem-resistant *Pseudomonas aeruginosa* clinical isolates. Revista medico-chirurgicala a Societatii de Medici si Naturalisti din Iasi. 2011;**115**(4):1208-1213

[6] Lagace-Wiens P, Rubinstein E. Adverse reactions to beta-lactam antimicrobials. Expert Opinion on Drug Safety. 2012;**11**(3):381-399. DOI: 10.1517/14740338.2012.643866

[7] Chow KM, Hui AC, Szeto CC. Neurotoxicity induced by beta-lactam antibiotics: From bench to bedside. European Journal of Clinical Microbiology & Infectious Diseases. 2005;**24**(10):649-653. DOI: 10.1007/s10096-005-0021-y

[8] Ariza A, Mayorga C, Fernández TD, Barbero N, Martín-Serrano A, Pérez-Sala D. Hypersensitivity reactions to β-lactams: Relevance of hapten-protein conjugates. Journal of Investigational Allergology and Clinical Immunology. 2015;**25**(1):12-25

[9] Dickson SD, Kimberly CS. Diagnosis and management of immediate hypersensitivity reactions to cephalosporins. Clinical Reviews in Allergy & Immunology. 2013;**45**(1):131-142. DOI: 10.1007/s12016-013-8367-x

[10] Cunha BA. Antibiotic side effects. The Medical Clinics of North America. 2001;**85**(1): 149-185

[11] Tune BM. Nephrotoxicity of beta-lactam antibiotics: Mechanisms and strategies for prevention. Pediatric Nephrology. 1997;**11**(6):768-772

[12] Michael PT. Management of complications associated with cancer or antineoplastic treatment during pregnancy. In: Lishner M, Koren G, editor. Cancer in Pregnancy and Lactation. Section 3: Cambridge University Press; UK. 2011. pp. 117-128

[13] Tune BM, Hsu CY. The renal mitochondrial toxicity of beta-lactam antibiotics: In vitro effects of cephaloglycin and imipenem. Journal of the American Society of Nephrology. 1990;**1**(5):815-821

[14] Robinson JL, Hameed T, Carr S. Practical aspects of choosing an antibiotic for patients with a reported allergy to an antibiotic. Clinical Infectious Diseases. 2002;**35**(1):26-31. DOI: 10.1086/340740

[15] Khairnar K, Raut MP, Chandekar RH, Sanmukh SG, Paunikar WN. Novel bacteriophage therapy for controlling metallo-beta-lactamase producing *Pseudomonas aeruginosa* infection in catfish. BMC Veterinary Research. 2013;**9**:264. DOI: 10.1186/1746-6148-9-264

[16] Viertel TM, Ritter K, Horz HP. Viruses versus bacteria-novel approaches to phage therapy as a tool against multidrug- resistant pathogens. The Journal of Antimicrobial Chemotherapy. 2014;**69**(9):2326-2336. DOI: 10.1093/jac/dku173

[17] Skurnik M, Pajunen M, Kiljunen S. Biotechnological challenges of phage therapy. Biotechnology Letters. 2007;**29**(7):995-1003. DOI: 10.1007/s10529-007-9346-1

[18] Carlton RM, Noordman WH, Biswas B, de Meeste ED, Loessner MJ. Bacteriophage P100 for control of *Listeria monocytogenes* in foods: genome sequence, bioinformatic analyses, oral toxicity study, and application. Regulatory Toxicology and Pharmacology. 2005;**43**(3):301-312. DOI: 10.1016/j.yrtph.2005.08.005

[19] Cho H, Uehara T, Bernhardt TG. Beta-lactam antibiotics induce a lethal malfunctioning of the bacterial cell wall synthesis machinery. Cell. 2014;**159**(6):1300-1311. DOI: 10.1016/j.cell.2014.11.017

[20] Worthington RJ, Melander C. Overcoming resistance to beta-lactam antibiotics. Journal of Organic Chemistry. 2013;**78**(9):4207-4213. DOI: 10.1021/jo400236f

[21] Newton GG, Abraham EP. Isolation of cephalosporin C, a penicillin-like antibiotic containing D-alpha-aminoadipic acid. The Biochemical Journal. 1956;**62**(4):651-658

[22] Lin JK, Huang TS, Luh KT. Penicillinase-type of beta-lactamase responsible for the ampicillin resistance in *Escherichia coli* NTUH 9501-1. Taiwan yi xue hui za zhi. Journal of the Formosan Medical Association. 1989;**88**(1):1-7

[23] Egorov AM, Sazykin IuO. Cephalosporin antibiotics: The first ones by their significance and complexity of their discovery. Antibiotiki i khimioterapiia=Antibiotics and Chemotherapy. 2001;**46**:3-6

[24] Kohira N, West J, Ito A, Ito-Horiyama T, Nakamura R, Sato T, Rittenhouse S, Tsuji M, Yamano Y. In vitro antimicrobial activity of siderophore cephalosporin S- 649266 against *Enterobacteriaceae* clinical isolates including carbapenem-resistant strains. Antimicrobial Agents Chemotherapy. 2015;**60**(2):729-734. DOI: 10.1128/AAC.01695-15

[25] Falagas ME, Lourida P, Poulikakos P, Rafailidis PI, Tansarli GS. Antibiotic treatment of infections due to carbapenem-resistant *Enterobacteriaceae*: Systematic evaluation of the available evidence. Antimicrobial Agents and Chemotherapy. 2014;**58**(2):654-666. DOI: 10.1128/AAC.01222-13

[26] Uehara T, Park JT. Growth of *Escherichia coli:* Significance of peptidoglycan degradation during elongation and septation. Journal of Bacteriology. 2008;**190**(11):3914-3922. DOI: 10.1128/JB.00207-08

[27] Fernandez A, Perez A, Ayala JA, Mallo S, Rumbo-Feal S, Tomas M, et al. Expression of OXA-type and SFO-1 beta-lactamases induces changes in peptidoglycan composition and affects bacterial fitness. Antimicrobial Agents and Chemotherapy. 2012;**56**(4):1877-1884. DOI: 10.1128/AAC.05402-11

[28] Goffin C, Ghuysen JM. Multimodular penicillin binding proteins: An enigmatic family of orthologs and paralogs. Microbiology and Molecular Biology Reviews. 1988;**62:**1079-1093

[29] Massova I, Mobashery S. Kinship and diversification of bacterial penicillin-binding proteins and beta-lactamases. Antimicrobial Agents and Chemotherapy. 1998;**42**:1-17

[30] Shorr AF, Zilberberg MD. Continuous infusion of beta-lactams: A blissful option for the intensive care unit. Journal of Thoracic Disease. 2016;**8**(12)**:**E1637-E1640. DOI: 10.21037/jtd.2016.12.47

[31] Paveenkittiporn W, Kerdsin A, Chokngam S, Bunthi C, Sangkitporn S, Gregory CJ. Emergence of plasmid-mediated colistin resistance and New Delhi metallo-beta-lactamase genes in extensively drug-resistant *Escherichia coli* isolated from a patient in Thailand. Diagnostic Microbiology and Infectious Disease. 2017;**87**(2):157-159. DOI: 10.1016/j.diagmicrobio.2016.11.005

[32] Sidjabat H, Nimmo GR, Walsh TR, Binotto E, Htin A, Hayashi Y, et al. Carbapenem resistance in *Klebsiella pneumoniae* due to the New Delhi Metallo-beta-lactamase. Clinical Infectious Diseases: An Official Publication of the Infectious Diseases Society of America. 2011;**52**(4):481-484. DOI: 10.1093/cid/ciq178

[33] Pollini S, Fiscarelli E, Mugnaioli C, Di Pilato V, Ricciotti G, Neri AS et al. *Pseudomonas aeruginosa* infection in cystic fibrosis caused by an epidemic metallo-beta-lactamase-producing

clone with a heterogeneous carbapenem resistance phenotype. Clinical Microbiology and Infection. 2011;**17**(8):1272-1275. DOI: 10.1111/j.1469-0691.2011.03466.x

[34] Pillai DR, McGeer A, Low DE. New Delhi metallo-beta-lactamase-1 in *Enterobacteriaceae:* Emerging resistance. Canadian Medical Association Journal. 2011;**183**(1):59-64. DOI: 10.1503/cmaj.101487

[35] Willmann M, Kuebart I, Marschal M, Schroppel K, Vogel W, Flesch I, et al. Effect of metallo-beta-lactamase production and multidrug resistance on clinical outcomes in patients with *Pseudomonas aeruginosa* bloodstream infection: A retrospective cohort study. BMC Infectious Diseases. 2013;**13**:515. DOI: 10.1186/1471-2334-13-515

[36] Huntington JA, Sakoulas G, Umeh O, Cloutier DJ, Steenbergen JN, Bliss C, Goldstein EJ. Efficacy of ceftolozane/tazobactam versus levofloxacin in the treatment of complicated urinary tract infections (cUTIs) caused by levofloxacin-resistant pathogens: Results from the ASPECT-cUTI trial. The Journal of Antimicrobial Chemotherapy. 2016;**71**(7):2014-2021. DOI: 10.1093/jac/dkw053

[37] Queenan AM, Bush K. Carbapenemases: The versatile beta-lactamases. Clinical Microbiology Reviews. 2007;**20**(3):440-458. DOI: 10.1128/CMR.00001-07

[38] Jacobsen SM, Stickler DJ, Mobley HL, Shirtliff ME. Complicated catheter-associated urinary tract infections due to *Escherichia coli* and *Proteus mirabilis*. Clinical Microbiology Reviews. 2008;**21**(1):26-59. DOI: 10.1128/CMR.00019-07

[39] Shaikh S, Fatima J, Shakil S, Rizvi SM, Kamal MA. Risk factors for acquisition of extended spectrum beta lactamase producing *Escherichia coli* and *Klebsiella pneumoniae* in North-Indian hospitals. Saudi Journal of Biological Sciences. 2015;**22**(1):37-41. DOI: 10.1016/j.sjbs.2014.05.006

[40] Crivaro V, Bagattini M, Salza MF, Raimondi F, Rossano F, Triassi M, et al. Risk factors for extended-spectrum beta-lactamase-producing *Serratia marcescens* and *Klebsiella pneumoniae* acquisition in a neonatal intensive care unit. The Journal of Hospital Infection. 2007;**67**(2):135-141. DOI: 10.1016/j.jhin.2007.07.026

[41] Pena C, Gudiol C, Tubau F, Saballs M, Pujol M, Dominguez MA. Risk-factors for acquisition of extended-spectrum beta-lactamase-producing *Escherichia coli* among hospitalised patients. Clinical Microbiology and Infection. 2006;**12**(3):279-284. DOI: 10.1111/j.1469-0691.2005.01358.x

[42] Ventola CL. The antibiotic resistance crisis: Part 2: Management strategies and new agents. P &T: A Peer-Reviewed Journal for Formulary Management. 2015;**40**(5):344-335

[43] Malangu N. Chapter 3: Risks associated with international trading of medicines by non-licensed entities and non-professionals. In: Macek A, editor. International Trade - On the Brink of Change. 2017. InTech, DOI: 10.5772/66471

[44] Mouhieddine TH, Olleik Z, Itani MM, Kawtharani S, Nassar H, Hassoun R, et al. Assessing the Lebanese population for their knowledge, attitudes and practices of

antibiotic usage. Journal of Infection and Public Health. 2015;**8**(1):20-31. DOI: 10.1016/j.jiph.2014.07.010

[45] Brink AJ, Feldman C, Grolman DC, Muckart D, Pretorius J, Richards GA, et al. Appropriate use of the carbapenems. South African Medical Journal. 2004;**94**(10 Pt 2): 857-886

[46] Cacci LC, Chuster SG, Martins N, Carmo PR, Girao VB, Nouer SA, Moreira BM. Mechanisms of carbapenem resistance in endemic *Pseudomonas aeruginosa* isolates after an SPM-1 metallo-beta-lactamase producing strain subsided in an intensive care unit of a teaching hospital in Brazil. Memórias do Instituto Oswaldo Cruz. 2016;**111**(9):551-558. DOI: 10.1590/0074-02760160116

[47] Hall BG et al. Independent origins of subgroup Bl+B2 and subgroup B3 metallo-β-lactamases. Journal of Molecular Evolution. 2003;**59**:133-141. DOI: 10.1007/s00239-003-2572-9

[48] Horsfall LE, Izougarhane Y, Lassaux P, Selevsek N, Lienard BM, Poirel L et al. Broad antibiotic resistance profile of the subclass B3 metallo-beta-lactamase GOB-1, a di-zinc enzyme. The FEBS Journal. 2011;**278**(8):1252-1263. DOI: 10.1111/j.1742-4658.2011.08046.x

[49] Queenan AM, Shang W, Schreckenberger P, Lolans K, Bush K, Quinn J. SME-3, a novel member of the *Serratia marcescens* SME family of carbapenem-hydrolyzing beta-lactamases. Antimicrobial Agents and Chemotherapy. 2006;**50**(10):3485-3487. DOI: 10.1128/AAC.00363-06

[50] Marciano DC, Karkouti OY, Palzkill TA. Fitness cost associated with the antibiotic resistance enzyme SME-1 beta-lactamase. Genetics. 2007;**176**(4):2381-2392. DOI: 10.1534/genetics.106.069443

[51] Jeon JH, Lee JH, Lee JJ, Park KS, Karim AM, Lee CR, et al. Structural basis for carbapenem-hydrolyzing mechanisms of carbapenemases conferring antibiotic resistance. International Journal of Molecular Sciences. 2015;**16**(5):9654-9692. DOI: 10.3390/ijms16059654

[52] Kocsis B, Szabó D. Antibiotic resistance mechanisms in *Enterobacteriaceae.* Microbial pathogens and strategies for combating them: Science, technology and education. In: Méndez-Vilas A, editor. FORMATEX; Spain. 2013. pp. 251-257

[53] Jaskulski MR, Medeiros BC, Borges JV, Zalewsky R, Fonseca MF, Marinowic DR. Assessment of extended-spectrum beta-lactamase, KPC carbapenemase and porin resistance mechanisms in clinical samples of *Klebsiella pneumoniae* and *Enterobacter* spp. International Journal of Antimicrobial Agents. 2013;**42**(1):76-79. DOI: 10.1016/j.ijantimicag.2013.03.009

[54] Evans BA, Amyes SG. OXA beta-lactamases. Clinical Microbiology Reviews. 2014; **27**(2):241-263. DOI: 10.1128/CMR.00117-13

[55] Koh TH, Sng LH, Wang GC, Hsu LY, Zhao Y. IMP-4 and OXA beta-lactamases in *Acinetobacter baumannii* from Singapore. The Journal of Antimicrobial Chemotherapy. 2007;**59**(4):627-632. DOI: 10.1093/jac/dkl544

[56] Bert F, Branger C, Lambert-Zechovsky N. Comparative activity of beta-lactam agents (carbapenem excepted) against *Pseudomonas aeruginosa* strains with CARB or OXA beta-lactamases. Chemotherapy. 2004;**50**(1):31-34. DOI: 10.1159/000077282

[57] Kotapati S, Kuti JL, Nightingale CH, Nicolau DP. Clinical implications of extended spectrum beta-lactamase (ESBL) producing *Klebsiella* species and *Escherichia coli* on cefepime effectiveness. The Journal of Infection. 2005;**51**:211-217

[58] Ghafourian S, Sadeghifard N, Soheili S, Sekawi Z. Extended spectrum beta-lactamases: Definition, classification and epidemiology. Current Issues in Molecular Biology. 2015; **17**:11-21

[59] Paterson DL, Bonomo RA. Extended-spectrum β-lactamases: A clinical update. Clinical Microbiology Reviews. 2005;**18**(4):657-686. DOI: 10.1128/CMR.18.4.657-686.2005

[60] Skagseth S, Carlsen TJ, Bjerga GE, Spencer J, Samuelsen O, Leiros HK. Role of residues W228 and Y233 in the structure and activity of metallo-beta-lactamase GIM-1. Antimicrobial Agents and Chemotherapy. 2016;**60**(2):990-1002. DOI: 10.1128/AAC.02017-15

[61] Kayama S, Shigemoto N, Shimizu W, Kuwahara R, Ikeda M, Ikebe K, et al. Tripoli metallo-beta-lactamase-1 (TMB-1)-producing Acinetobacter spp. with decreased resistance to imipenem in Japan. Antimicrobial Agents and Chemotherapy. 2014;**58**(4):2477-2478. DOI: 10.1128/AAC.01790-13

[62] Watanabe M, Iyobe S, Inoue M, Mitsuhashi S. Transferable imipenem resistance in *Pseudomonas aeruginosa*. Antimicrobial Agents and Chemotherapy. 1991;**35**:147-151

[63] Castanheira M, Bell JM, Turnidge JD, Mathai D, Jones RN. Carbapenem resistance among *Pseudomonas aeruginosa* strains from India: Evidence for nationwide endemicity of multiple metallo-beta-lactamase clones (VIM-2, -5, -6, and -11 and the newly characterized VIM-18). Antimicrobial Agents and Chemotherapy. 2009;**53**(3):1225-1227. DOI: 10.1128/AAC.01011-08

[64] Zmarlicka MT, Nailor MD, Nicolau DP. Impact of the New Delhi metallo-beta-lactamase on beta-lactam antibiotics. Infection and Drug Resistance. 2015;**8**:297-309. DOI: 10.2147/IDR.S3918

[65] Bonomo RA. New Delhi metallo-beta-lactamase and multidrug resistance: A global SOS? Clinical Infectious Diseases: An Official Publication of the Infectious Diseases Society of America. 2011;**52**(4):485-487. DOI: 10.1093/cid/ciq179

[66] Manoharan A, Barla GS, Peter R, Sugumar M, Mathai D. Multidrug resistance mediated by co-carriage of extended-spectrum beta-lactamases, AmpC and New Delhi metallo-beta-lactamase-1 genes among carbapenem-resistant *Enterobacteriaceae* at five Indian medical centres. Indian Journal of Medical Microbiology. 2016;**34**(3):359-361. DOI: 10.4103/0255-0857.188350

[67] Kaase M, Szabados F, Pfennigwerth N, Anders A, Geis G, Pranada AB, et al. Description of the metallo-beta-lactamase GIM-1 in *Acinetobacter pittii*. The Journal of Antimicrobial Chemotherapy. 2014;**69**(1):81-84. DOI: 10.1093/jac/dkt325

[68] Lee K, Yum JH, Yong D, Lee HM, Kim HD, Docquier JD, Rossolini GM, Chong Y. Novel acquired metallo-beta-lactamase gene, bla(SIM-1), in a class 1 integron from *Acinetobacter baumannii* clinical isolates from Korea. Antimicrobial Agents and Chemotherapy. 2005;**49**(11):4485-4491. DOI: 10.1128/AAC.49.11.4485-4491.2005

[69] El Salabi A, Borra PS, Toleman MA, Samuelsen O, Walsh TR. Genetic and biochemical characterization of a novel metallo-beta-lactamase, TMB-1, from an *Achromobacter xylosoxidans* strain isolated in Tripoli, Libya. Antimicrobial Agents and Chemotherapy. 2012;**56**(5):2241-2245. DOI: 10.1128/AAC.05640-11

[70] Lankas GR, Coleman JB, Klein HJ, Bailly Y. Species specificity of 2-aryl carbapenem-induced immune-mediated hemolytic anemia in primates. Toxicology. 1996;**108**(3): 207-215

[71] Culic M, Pekovic S, Stojiljkovic M, Saponjic J, Jankovic B, Rakic L. The effect of cortical lesion on systemic penicillin epilepsy in rats. Neuroscience. 1992;**51**(2):439-444

[72] Saito T, Nakamura M, Watari M, Isse K. Tardive seizure and antibiotics: Case reports and review of the literature. The Journal of ECT. 2008;**24**(4):275-276. DOI: 10.1097/YCT.0b013e31816ba986

[73] Faure C, Perreira D, Audo I. Retinal toxicity after intracameral use of a standard dose of cefuroxime during cataract surgery. Documenta Ophthalmologica. 2015;**130**(1):57-63. DOI: 10.1007/s10633-014-9465-7

[74] Chow KM, Szeto CC, Hui AC, Li PK. Mechanisms of antibiotic neurotoxicity in renal failure. International Journal of Antimicrobial Agents. 2004;**23**(3):213-217

[75] Mao J. Glutamate transporter: An unexpected target for some antibiotics. Molecular Pain. 2005;**1**:5. DOI: 10.1186/1744-8069-1-5

[76] Rothstein JD, Patel S, Regan MR, Haenggeli C, Huang YH, Bergles DE, et al. Beta-lactam antibiotics offer neuroprotection by increasing glutamate transporter expression. Nature. 2005;**433**(7021):73-77. DOI: 10.1038/nature03180

[77] Kim SY, Jones TA. The effects of ceftriaxone on skill learning and motor functional outcome after ischemic cortical damage in rats. Restorative Neurology and Neuroscience. 2013;**31**(1):87-97. DOI: 10.3233/RNN-2012-120245

[78] Goodwani S, Rao PS, Bell RL, Sari Y. Amoxicillin and amoxicillin/clavulanate reduce ethanol intake and increase GLT-1 expression as well as AKT phosphorylation in mesocorticolimbic regions. Brain Research. 2015;**1622**:397-408. DOI: 10.1016/j.brainres.2015.07.008

[79] Rao PS, Goodwani S, Bell RL, Wei Y, Boddu SH, Sari Y. Effects of ampicillin, cefazolin and cefoperazone treatments on GLT-1 expressions in the mesocorticolimbic system and ethanol intake in alcohol-preferring rats. Neuroscience. 2015;**295**:164-174. DOI: 10.1016/j.neuroscience.2015.03.038

[80] Rawls SM, Baron DA, Kim J. Beta-lactam antibiotic inhibits development of morphine physical dependence in rats. Behavioural Pharmacology. 2010;**21**(2):161-164. DOI: 10.1097/FBP.0b013e328337be10

[81] Khalili H, Bairami S, Kargar M. Antibiotics induced acute kidney injury: Incidence, risk factors, onset time and outcome. Acta Medica Iranica. 2013;**51**(12):871-878

[82] Dekant W, Vamvakas S. Biotransformation and membrane transport in nephrotoxicity. Critical Reviews in Toxicology. 1996;**26**(3):309-334. DOI: 10.3109/10408449609012526

[83] Jensen JU, Hein L, Lundgren B, Bestle MH, Mohr T, Andersen MH, et al. Kidney failure related to broad-spectrum antibiotics in critically ill patients: Secondary end point results from a 1200 patient randomised trial. BMJ Open. 2012;**2**(2):e000635. DOI: 10.1136/bmjopen-2011-000635

[84] Guest I, Uetrecht J. Drugs toxic to the bone marrow that target the stromal cells. Immunopharmacology. 2000;**46**(2):103-112

[85] Metovic A, Mackic-Djurovic M, Ibrulj S. Analysis of chromosome aberrations contained in vitro human peripheral blood lymphocytes after treatment with ceftriaxone. Medical Archives. 2013;**67**(4):228-232

[86] Arabski M, Kazmierczak P, Wisniewska-Jarosinska M, Poplawski T, Klupinska G, Chojnacki J, et al. Interaction of amoxicillin with DNA in human lymphocytes and H. pylori-infected and non-infected gastric mucosa cells. Chemico-Biological Interactions. 2005;**152**(1):13-24. DOI: 10.1016/j.cbi.2005.01.004

[87] Iatropoulos MJ, Newman AJ, Dayan AD, Brughera M, Scampini G, Mazue G. Urinary bladder hyperplasia in the rat: Non-specific pathogenetic considerations using a beta-lactam antibiotic. Experimental and Toxicologic Pathology. 1994;**46**(4-5):265-274. DOI: 10.1016/S0940-2993(11)80098-9

[88] Kim MK, Kang CK, Kim MJ, Jun KI, Lee YK, Jeong SJ, et al. Penicillin G-induced hemorrhagic cystitis: A case and review of the literature. Korean Journal of Internal Medicine. 2013;**28**(6):743-745. DOI: 10.3904/kjim.2013.28.6.743

[89] Koch AL. Bacterial wall as target for attack: Past, present, and future research. Clinical Microbiology Reviews. 2003;**16**(4):673-687

[90] Cisek AA, Dabrowska I, Gregorczyk KP, Wyzewski Z. Phage therapy in bacterial infections treatment: One hundred years after the discovery of bacteriophages. Current Microbiology. 2017;**74**(2):277-283. DOI: 10.1007/s00284-016-1166-x

[91] Nageeb W, Metwally L, Kamel M, Zakaria S. In vitro antimicrobial synergy studies of carbapenem-resistant *Acinetobacter baumannii* isolated from intensive care units of a tertiary care hospital in Egypt. Journal of Infection and Public Health. 2015;**8**(6):593-602. DOI: 10.1016/j.jiph.2015.05.007

[92] Hopefl AW. Overview of synergy with reference to double beta-lactam combinations. DICP. 1991;**25**(9):972-977

[93] Drusano GL, Ambrose PG, Bhavnani SM, Bertino JS, Nafziger AN, Louie A. Back to the future: Using aminoglycosides again and how to dose them optimally. Clinical Infectious Diseases. 2007;**45**(6):753-760. DOI: 10.1086/520991

[94] Gomez L, Estrada C, Gomez I, Marquez M, Estany C, Marti JM, et al. Low-dose beta-lactam plus amikacin in febrile neutropenia: Cefepime vs. piperacillin/tazobactam, a randomized trial. European Journal of Clinical Microbiology & Infectious Diseases. 2010;**29**(4):417-427. DOI: 10.1007/s10096-010-0879-1

[95] Tune BM. The renal toxicity of beta-lactam antibiotics: Mechanisms and clinical implications. In: De Broe ME, Porter GA, Bennett WM, Verpooten GA, editors. Clinical Nephrotoxins. Springer; USA. 1998. pp. 121-134. DOI: 10.1007/978-94-015-9088-4

Chapter 6

Acute Poisoning with Neonicotinoid Insecticide

Nicolai Nistor, Otilia Elena Frăsinariu and
Violeta Ştreangă

Additional information is available at the end of the chapter

http://dx.doi.org/10.5772/intechopen.72004

Abstract

Neonicotinoids are a class of insecticides considered less toxic to humans than organophosphates, carbamates, organochloride and pyrethroids. The purpose of this chapter was to systematize existing data in the literature on acute intoxication with neonicotinoids to help practitioners. Clinical manifestations vary across different human systems. Gastrointestinal symptoms consist of nausea, vomiting, abdominal pain and corrosive lesions. In the central nervous system, headaches, agitation, confusion, fasciculations, seizures or coma may occur, while tachycardia or bradycardia, hypertension, hypotension and palpitations occur in the cardiovascular system. Respiratory effects are dyspnea, aspiration pneumonia or respiratory failure. Solvents that drive the insecticide also have an important role in the toxic effects. There are no specific biological tests of neonicotinoid intoxication, and their dosing is not routinely available. Treatment is symptomatic. Mortality is less than 3%, well below the poisoning with anticholinesterase insecticides, like organophosphates and carbamates.

Keywords: neonicotinoids, insecticides, poisoning, cardiovascular symptoms

1. Introduction

Poisoning with insecticides is a public health problem in many countries [1]. Organophosphates and carbamates are the principal cause of serious poisonings, sometimes leading to death. Due to the high toxicity of these compounds, new insecticides called neonicotinoids (synthetic analogs of nicotine) have been created [2].

The term "neonicotinoid" was initially used by Izuru Yamamoto for imidacloprid and related insecticides to differentiate the new insecticidal active compounds of n-AChRs from older nicotine insecticides [3].

Neonicotinoids are used in agriculture, horticulture and forestry to combat various pests. They are also used to combat fleas in domestic animals, as well as against household pests. After spraying, they act by direct contact with the insects, or by ingestion, when the insects pierce or consume the vegetative parts of plants [4]. Neonicotinoids are developed and continue to be launched on the market, often in the absence of direct human toxicity data. The human toxicity of these insecticides is often extrapolated from studies on animals, whose relevance is unclear. Therefore, more studies on acute intoxications with this class of insecticides are needed. The information resulting from these studies can contribute to the risk assessment and management of patients with neonicotinoid intoxications and support the decisions of the regulatory agencies for these substances [5]. The insecticidal activity of neonicotinoids results mainly from the agonist effect on the insects' postsynaptic nicotinic receptors for acetylcholine. They are attached to the nicotinic receptors of the postsynaptic membranes from both nerve and muscle cells and thus disrupt the transmission of the nervous influx into the central and peripheral nervous system. Additionally, this interaction with the nicotinic receptors determines their desensitization, leading to a loss of synaptic transmission of the nervous impulse [6, 7]. In recent years, some studies have suggested that neonicotinoids have a negative impact on bees near crops exposed to neonicotinoids. It is known that exposure to thiamethoxam may cause bees to be disoriented [8, 9]. In 2013, the European Food Safety Agency published a report confirming that neonicotinoids pose a risk to bees and pollinators. For this reason, under the precautionary principle, the European Commission has decided to temporarily suspend the use of three neonicotinoid substances (imidacloprid, clothianidin and thiamethoxam) for seed treatment in the agriculture of all EU member States [10]. However, in some countries, based on derogations from the ministry, they are still used.

In a large study conducted recently in three countries in Europe (the United Kingdom, Germany and Hungary), the results were contradictory: in the United Kingdom and Hungary, neonicotinoids had a negative impact on bees, while in Germany they did not seem to have affected their health status [11]. The findings of another recent Canadian study, conducted in Ontario and Quebec, are that neonicotinoids have negative effects on bees, including a 23% decrease in their life span [12]. It is therefore necessary to continue the studies on this subject in order to reach a clear and definitive scientific conclusion. Neonicotinoid insecticides are considered to have low toxicity in humans because they interact much less with nicotinic receptors in vertebrates than in insects and penetrate less the blood-brain barrier. Provided that they are less toxic in humans, neonicotinoid insecticides have become increasingly used throughout the world. However, the ingestion of large amounts of these insecticides has been associated with the occurrence of severe poisoning [13].

Hence, this review was performed in order to clarify some aspects of the diagnosis and treatment of poisonings with neonicotinoids, useful for practitioners who face such cases and maybe helping improve management of these intoxications. The physicochemical properties, toxicokinetics, experimental data and mechanism of action of neonicotinoids, clinical symptoms, diagnosis, treatment and prognosis of acute intoxication with this relatively new class of insecticides are discussed below.

http://dx.doi.org/10.5772/intechopen.72004

2. Physicochemical properties of neonicotinoids

Neonicotinoids are classified by the EPA as both Class II and Class III agents and are labeled with the signal word "Warning" or "Caution." Imidacloprid, the first neonicotinoid insecticide discovered in 1994 in Japan, is a structural analogue of nicotine derived from N-nitroguanidine

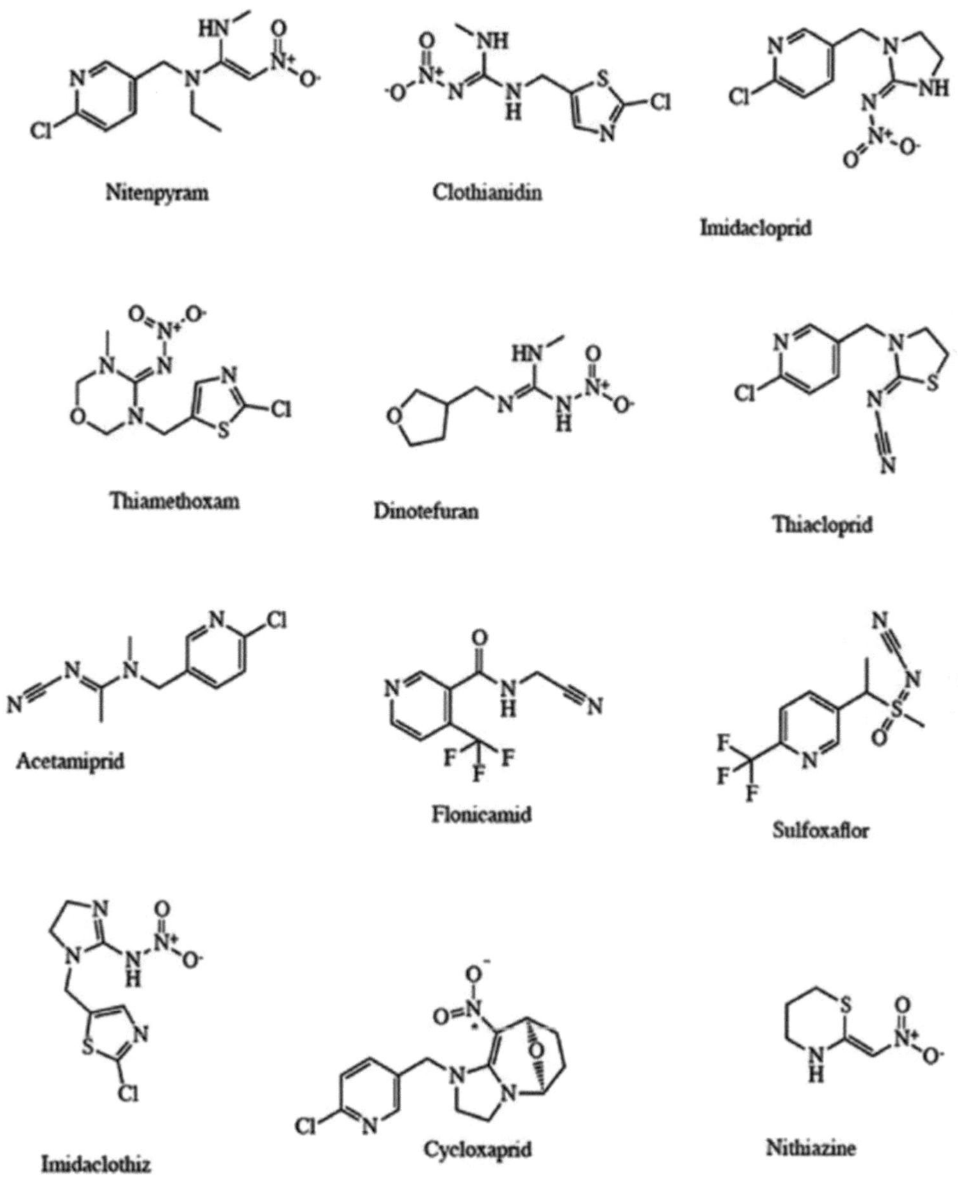

Figure 1. Common names and molecular structures of the neonicotinoids [14].

Generation of neonicotinoids	Type of neonicotinoid	Physical state
First-generation neonicotinoids	Imidacloprid	Clear crystals or beige powder
	Nitenpyram	Pale yellow crystals
	Acetamiprid	White crystals, white fine powder, odorless
	Thiacloprid	Yellow crystalline powder, odorless
Second-generation neonicotinoids	Thiamethoxam	Slightly creamy crystalline powder, odorless
	Clothianidin	Clear colorless solid powder, odorless
Third-generation neonicotinoids	Dinotefuran	White crystalline solid, odorless
	Sulfoxaflor	White solid
	Cycloxaprid	Wettable powder

Table 1. The physical state of neonicotinoids.

and is the best sold worldwide. Currently, besides imidacloprid, the neonicotinoid family includes thiamethoxam, clothianidin, thiacloprid, acetamiprid, dinotefuran, nitenpyram, nitiazine, imidaclothiz, flonicamid, sulfoxaflor and cycloxaprid, the chemical structure of which is shown in **Figure 1** [14]. Currently, neonicotinoids are homologated in agriculture in more than 120 countries, being sold under various commercial names [14] (**Table 1**).

3. Toxicokinetics

Most human toxicity data available are about imidacloprid. Penetration through the skin (predominantly in the agricultural environment) of neonicotinoid insecticides is not quantified in humans. Intoxication through the respiratory tract is negligible given that these molecules are nonvolatile. However, there may be a secondary swallowing of the inhaled aerosol microparticles. The first prospective study conducted in Sri Lanka by Mohamed F. et al. on 68 patients (61 with voluntary ingestion and 7 with cutaneous exposure) showed that the mean plasma concentration of imidacloprid was 10.58 ng/l, IQR: 3.84–15.58 ng/l, range: 0.02–51.25 ng/l. In seven patients, the plasma concentration remained elevated for 10–15 h postingestion, suggesting that absorption and/or elimination may be prolonged at high doses. The time-concentration profiles have demonstrated a rapid initial absorption [5]. The plasma peak is reached within 2 h. There is no preferential distribution in fat-rich tissues [15]. In insects, mammals and plants, neonicotinoids undergo phase I and phase II biotransformation (**Figure 2**).

In vitro studies on the metabolism of neonicotinoids have indicated the importance of cytochrome P450s (CYP) in their oxidation and reduction. Through a variety of human CYP isoenzymes, imidacloprid is oxidized to 5-hydroxyimidacloprid and imidacloprid olefin and reduced to nitrosoguanidine, aminoguanidine and urea imidacloprid. The most active CYP isoenzyme for oxidation of the imidacloprid residue is CYP 3A4 (CYP most abundant in humans), followed by CYP 2C19, 2A6 and 2C9. For nitroreduction, the most active CYP are: CYP 1A2, 2B6, 2D6 and 2E1 [16, 17].

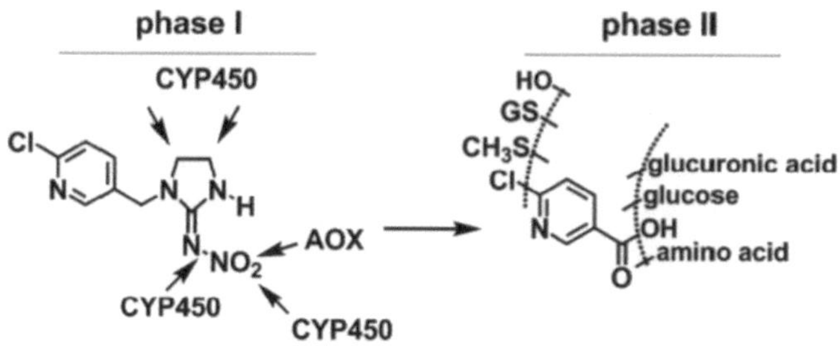

Figure 2. Sites of metabolite attack on IMI and 6-chloronicotinic acid (CNA) for phase I and phase II reactions [16].

Thiamethoxam is converted to clothianidin, which is more active than the parent molecule, mostly by CYP 3A4 and to a lesser extent by CYP 2C19 and 2B6, and is demethylated by 2C19. Clothianidin is demethylated by CYP 3A4, 2C19 and 2A6 [18]. There is no accumulation of neonicotinoids in the body: over 90% are eliminated in less than 24 h and totally in 48 h [15, 19].

4. Experimental data and mechanisms of action

Neonicotinoids are neither irritating to eyes and skin (rabbit) nor sensitizing (guinea pigs) [15]. Their acute toxicity to mammals is variable depending on the type of neonicotinoid. The amount of toxic product that kills 50% of the experimental animals, called the lethal dose (LD 50), is illustrated in **Table 2** for the main neonicotinoids.

With an LD 50 of 425–475 mg/kg administered orally in rats, the toxicity of imidacloprid is mild to moderate. A single 42 mg/kg dose has no effect. After 2–6 h, poisoned animals present with apathy, trembling with ataxia, hypothermia and respiratory arrest [19, 20].

Neonicotinoids have been designed to be effective as insecticides by contact or ingestion [21]. In both insects and humans, neonicotinoids behave as postsynaptic acetylcholine receptor agonists, which are neurotransmitters of the central nervous system, the parasympathetic nervous system and some of the sympathetic system. Their irreversible linkages with these receptors initially stimulate, then rapidly block the Na^{+}/K^{+} channels and inhibit the transmission of the nervous influx. Their high insect toxicity is explained by the predominance of nicotinic receptors in the central nervous system of these species, by

Common name	Local effects	Rat oral LD50	Rabbit dermal LD50
Acetamiprid	Absent	450	>2000
Clothianidin	Absent	>5000	>2000
Dinotefuran	Absent	2000	>2000
Imidacloprid	Absent	4870	>2000
Thiamethoxam	Absent	>5000	>2000

Table 2. Neonicotinoid pesticides mammalian toxicities (mg/kg of body weight) [7].

the absence of the blood-brain barrier and by their affinity for some insect-specific receptor subtypes, in particular α4β2 [19]. In mammals, the predominant receptor subtype is α4p2, which is found to have the highest density in the thalamus. In the developing brain, this subtype is involved in proliferation, apoptosis, migration, differentiation, synapse formation and neuronal circuits [22]. Given that in mammals nicotinic receptors have a wider distribution (neuromuscular junction), the neonicotinoid affinity for these receptors is lower and the central action is reduced because of poor intracerebral penetration [17]. The toxicity of imidacloprid is very low in dermal exposure and is moderate in case of ingestion. In case of inhalation, the toxicity is variable: as dust it is considered to be slightly toxic, but as aerosols it is very toxic [23].

5. Epidemiology of acute poisoning with neonicotinoids in humans

Despite the widespread use of neonicotinoids, there are few reports in the literature on human toxicity. The first case report was made in 2001 by Wu IW et al. Clinical manifestation included drowsiness, disorientation, dizziness, oral and gastroesophageal erosions, hemorrhagic gastritis, productive cough, fever, leukocytosis and hyperglycemia. The patient recovered without complications with supportive treatment and was discharged 4 days after ingestion [24]. Most cases were reported in USA (Texas), France, China and Sri Lanka [25, 26, 13]. The epidemiological aspects resulting from these studies are summarized in **Table 3**.

Studies	Cohort of the study	Country of study	Epidemiological findings
Forrester M et al., 2014 [25]	1142 cases of acute intoxication reported by Texas Intoxication Control Centers over the period 2000–2012 (retrospective study)	USA	• 77% with imidacloprid • 17% with dinotefuran • 64% female • 32 serious cases (2.9%) • Intoxication mode: ingestion (51%), cutaneous (44%) and ocular (11%) • 28% children aged <5 years and 9% aged 6–19 years • 97% accidental
Boels D, Chataigner D, 2014 [26]	482 cases of acute poisoning with imidacloprid between January 1999 and December 2012 (retrospective study)	France	• Increase from 8 cases in 1999 to 34 cases in 2012 • 120 cases (28%) were children <5 years • 37 cases (8.6%) children aged 5–14 years • 389 poisonings were accidental, 24 voluntary, and in 15 cases it was not possible to specify the circumstances of intoxication • Seven cases were serious, requiring intensive care

Studies	Cohort of the study	Country of study	Epidemiological findings
Phua DH et al, 2009 [13]	70 cases of acute intoxication reported by the Taiwan National Poison Center between 1987 and 2007 (retrospective study)	China	• Dramatic increase in the number of cases between 2003 and 2007: 58 cases out of the total of 70 • Two children with accidental poisoning • 67 males • 48 cases were suicidal attempts, of which eight consumed ethanol • Toxic: imidacloprid (64 cases), acetamiprid (4) and clothianidin (2). • Two deaths (mortality rate 2.9%)
Mohamed F et al., 2009 [5]	68 cases of acute poisoning with imidacloprid between March 2002 and March 2007 (prospective study)	Sri Lanka The dosing was done in laboratories in Australia	• 61 out of 68 patients (91%) were intoxicated by ingestion • 82% were voluntary poisonings

Table 3. The main epidemiological aspects of neonicotinoid intoxication studies.

The prevalence of voluntary intoxication was different from one study to another: only 2% in the study in Texas and 4.9% in the study in France, as opposed to the studies in China and Sri Lanka, where 81% and 82%, respectively, were classified as an attempt of suicide [25, 26, 13].

There are also differences in childhood poisoning frequency: in the study conducted in Texas, 37% were patients under the age of 19, and in France 36.6% were children under the age of 14, whereas the study in China recorded only two children with accidental poisoning. The study in Sri Lanka does not specify the age of the patients.

Regarding the manner of intoxication, in the US study only 51% of poisoning occurred through ingestion, compared to 91% (61/68 cases) in Sri Lanka and 81% (57/70) in China.

In addition to these studies, several sporadic cases have been reported. Thus, eight cases were reported in India [27–33], two in Turkey [34, 35], two in Portugal [36], two in Colombia [37], two in Japan [38], one case in Saudi Arabia [39], Iran [40], Poland [41] and four cases in Taiwan [41–45].

6. Clinical symptoms of poisoning by neonicotinoids

Symptoms of neonicotinoid poisoning appear to be less severe in humans than in insects, because their affinity for human nicotinic receptors is lower and they do not cross the blood-brain barrier. Clinical picture is better known for intoxication with imidacloprid, which is the oldest neonicotinoid used as an insecticide. A large study conducted in Texas between 2000 and 2012 on 1142 patients with neonicotinoid exposure found that the main symptoms are: eye irritation and dermatitis, nausea, vomiting, corrosive oral mucosal lesions,

Symptomatology	Benign forms Minor, mild symptoms that spontaneously regress	Moderate forms Pronounced or prolonged symptoms or signs	Severe forms Severe symptoms that threaten vital prognosis
Neurological	• Sleepiness, vertigo, ataxia, tinnitus • Glasgow score 12–14 • Slight agitation • Minor extrapyramidal symptoms • Minor cholinergic/anticholinergic symptoms • Paresthesia • Minor visual and hearing impairments	• Disturbances of consciousness with delayed response to pain • Glasgow score 8–11 • Apnea, bradypnea • Confusion, agitation, hallucinations, delirium • Localized or generalized seizures (rarely) • Marked extrapyramidal symptoms • Noticeable cholinergic/anticholinergic symptoms • Isolated paralysis without affecting vital functions • Visual and auditory disturbances	• Deep coma with inappropriate or absent response to pain • Glasgow score 3–7 • Depression or respiratory failure • Extreme agitation • Generalized seizures • Convulsive state, opisthotonus • Generalized paralysis or paralysis that affects vital functions • Blindness, deafness
Eye	• Irritation, conjunctival hyperemia, tears • Minor eyelid edema	• Marked irritation • Limited, circumscribed corneal involvement • Punctual keratitis	• Corneal ulcer • Corneal perforations • Definitive sequelae
Skin	• Irritation, first-degree burns • Second-degree burns and <10% body surface area (BSA)	• Second-degree burns with 10–50% BSA to adult and 10–30% BSA to child • Third-degree marks <2% BSA	• Second-degree burns >50% BSA to adult and >30% BSA to child • Third-degree burns >2% BSA
Bites/stinging	• Edema, localized pruritus • Discrete pain	• Localized edema involving the entire member • Localized necrosis • Moderate pain	• Extensive edema comprising the adjacent member and the adjacent parts • Critical location of edema with danger to the integrity of the upper airways

http://dx.doi.org/10.5772/intechopen.72004

Symptomatology	Benign forms Minor, mild symptoms that spontaneously regress	Moderate forms Pronounced or prolonged symptoms or signs	Severe forms Severe symptoms that threaten vital prognosis
Muscle	• Slight or moderate pain • Sensitivity to palpation • Rhabdomyolysis • CPK: 250–1500 ui/l	• Pain, stiffness, cramps • Fasciculations • Rhabdomyolysis • CPK: 1500–10,000 ui/l	• Intense pain, extreme rigidity • Extensive cramps • Extended, diffuse fasciculations • Rhabdomyolysis with complications • CPK > 10,000 ui/l • Compartment syndrome
Kidney	• Proteinuria and/or minimal hematuria	• Proteinuria and/or massive hematuria • Oliguria, polyuria • Serum creatinine: 200–500 mmol/l	• Kidney failure, anuria • Serum creatinine >500 μmol/l
Blood	• Minor hemolysis • Methemoglobinemia ranging from 10 to 30%	• Hemolysis • Methemoglobinemia ranging from 30 to 50% • Coagulation disorders without bleeding • Anemia, leukopenia, thrombocytopenia	• Massive hemolysis • Methemoglobinemia >50% • Coagulation disorders with bleeding • Anemia, leukopenia, severe thrombocytopenia
Liver	• ASAT, ALT: 2–5 times normal	• ASAT, ALAT: 5–50 times normal • Without obvious clinical signs of liver dysfunction	• ASAT, ALT >50 times normal • Affecting clotting factors • Clinical signs of liver failure

Table 4. The symptomatology of imidacloprid poisoning depending on severity [26].

dizziness, hypertension and tachycardia [25]. The French Toxicity Co-ordination Committee analyzed 428 cases of exposure to imidacloprid between 1999 and 2012, of which over 27% were children under 5 years of age. As a result of this study, the symptomatology was better outlined according to the severity of the intoxication (mild, moderate or severe), as illustrated in **Table 4** [26].

There was reported a case with concomitant intoxication with imidacloprid and alcohol ingestion, resulting in multiple organ failure [45]. Another case was reported by Agarwal and Srinivas, manifesting severe neuropsychiatric disorders and rhabdomyolysis [31]. In Colombia, Estrada et al. signaled two cases admitted with digestive manifestations, coma (Glasgow score 6 and 3, respectively) and respiratory failure with 70–75% Sa O_2. One of the patients also presented dormant miosis and was thus given atropine [37]. In Saudi Arabia, there was a case with generalized erythematous maculopapular rash typical of leukoclastic vasculitis, which was confirmed by biopsy. It also associated hepatic and renal dysfunction, requiring dialysis [40]. Another case reported in Taiwan presented fatal ventricular fibrillation [45].

The main symptoms of acetamiprid poisoning are severe nausea, vomiting, muscle weakness, hypothermia and convulsions [46]. Clinical manifestations include tachycardia, hypotension, electrocardiogram changes, hypoxia and thirst in the case of the highest serum concentration of acetamiprid. The symptoms were partly similar to acute organophosphate intoxication [30]. In one case, ventricular fibrillation that lasted 11 h after ingestion was described [45]. Similar to imidacloprid poisonings, there was reported a case of severe multiple organic dysfunction [43]. Another case of acetamiprid intoxication was by suicidal ingestion, where symptoms included prolonged muscle weakness, similar to the intermediate syndrome in organophosphorus intoxication. The case resolved in about 3 weeks [35].

Symptoms of thiamethoxam intoxication are less known, and cases are rarely reported. Vinod et al. noted a case manifesting nausea, vomiting, agitation and multiple episodes of generalized tonic-clonic seizures within the first 2 h of ingestion of thiamethoxam. Subsequently, coma, hypotension, renal failure, metabolic acidosis and rhabdomyolysis occurred, with fatal outcome 36 h after ingestion [29].

Solvents used in neonicotinoid insecticide solutions can also play an important part in poisoning symptoms. Although not all solvents contained by neonicotinoid insecticides are known, most of them use N-methylpyrrolidone. Ingestion of a large amount of this substance irritates the upper gastrointestinal tract and causes oral ulceration, nausea, vomiting, dysphagia, odynophagia and abdominal pain [24].

7. Diagnosis of poisoning incidents

The diagnosis is based on anamnesis and clinical symptoms. There are no specific abnormalities of acute poisoning with neonicotinoids [5]. There may be metabolic disturbances (**Table 5**). Dosage of neonicotinoids is not routinely available, its interest being purely medicolegal. Depending on the symptomatology of each case, additional investigations may be necessary.

Clinical forms	Mild	Moderate	Severe
Acidobasic disorders	• HCO_3: 15–20 or 30–40 mmol/l • pH: 7.25–7.32 or 7.50–7.59	• HCO_3: 10–14 sau > 40 mmol/l • pH: 7.16–7.24 sau 7.60–7.69	• HCO_3 < 10 mmol/l • pH < 7.15 or >7.7
Electrolytic disorders	• K: 3–3.4 or 5.2–5.9 mmol/l • Moderate hypoglycemia: 0.5–0.7 g/l or 2.8–3.9 mmol/l • Short-term hyperthermia	• K: 2.5–2.9 or 6–6.9 mmol/l • Severe hypoglycemia: 0.3–0.5 g/l or 1.7–2.8 mmol/l • Prolonged hyperthermia	• K: <2.5 or >7 mmol/l • Severe hypoglycemia <0.3 g/l or <1.7 mmol/l • Malignant hyperthermia/hypothermia

Table 5. Metabolic disorders depending on the severity of intoxication [26].

Depending on the intensity and duration of cardiovascular, respiratory and digestive symptoms, three degrees of severity can be distinguished (**Table 6**):

1. Benign: mild symptoms that spontaneously regress;
2. Moderate: pronounced or prolonged symptoms/signs;
3. Severe: severe symptoms that may influence the vital prognosis.

Forms	Cardiovascular symptoms	Respiratory symptoms	Digestive symptoms
Benign	• Isolated extrasystoles • Discrete, transient hypotension • Transient, discrete hypertension	• Airways irritation • Coughing, breathlessness • Slight dyspnea • Slight bronchospasm • Abnormal thoracic radiography with or without minor symptoms	• Vomiting • Diarrhea • Abdominal pain • Minor oral ulceration • Endoscopy: erythema, stage I edema
Moderate	• Sinus bradycardia: ○ Adults 40–50 b/min ○ Children 60–80 b/min ○ New born 80–90 b/min • Frequent premature beats • Atrial flutter/fibrillation • AVB grade I or II • Prolonged QRS and QTc • Repolarization modifications • Myocardial ischemia • Hypo/hypertension	• Prolonged cough • Stridor, bronchospasm • Dyspnea • Hypoxia requiring oxygen administration • Abnormal pulmonary radiography with moderate symptoms	• Pronounced or prolonged vomiting • Diarrhea • Abdominal pain • First-grade burns of a critical area or II and III grade burns on limited areas • Dysphagia • Endoscopy: stage IIa transient ulcerative lesions

Forms	Cardiovascular symptoms	Respiratory symptoms	Digestive symptoms
Severe	• Severe sinus bradycardia: ○ Adults <40 b/min ○ Children <60 b/min ○ New born <80 b/min • Severe sinus tachycardia ○ Adults >180 b/min ○ Children >190 b/min ○ New born >200 b/min • Ventricular dysrhythmia with vital prognosis • AVB grade III • Asystole • Myocardial infarction • Shock • Malignant hypertensive disorder	• Respiratory failure: severe bronchospasm, dyspnea, airway obstruction, ARDS, pulmonary edema, glottis edema, bronchopneumonia, pneumopathy, pneumothorax • Abnormal pulmonary radiography with severe symptoms	• Severe digestive hemorrhage • Digestive perforation • Enlarged II and III grade burns • Severe dysphagia • Endoscopy: transmural ulcer lesions, circumferential lesions, perforations stage IIB, III and IV

Table 6. Degrees of severity according to intensity and duration of cardiovascular, respiratory and digestive symptoms [26].

Differential diagnosis should take into account intoxications with other pesticides. This poisonings can mimic light forms of organophosphorus or carbamates intoxications. Also, many cases reported involved combinations of multiple pesticides and ethanol [5, 13].

8. Management of poisoning incidents

Management of acute neonicotinoid insecticide poisoning is mainly symptomatic and supportive. Dermal and mucosal exposures should be decontaminated as soon as possible [13].

In case of coma and respiratory distress, intubation and assisted ventilation associated with hemodynamic support are required. The presence of solvents in liquid neonicotinoid formulas makes the activated charcoal and gastric lavage or vomiting ineffective, due to the risk of inhalation pneumonia [13]. Gastric lavage and activated charcoal should be avoided if corrosive injuries of the oral and gastrointestinal mucosa are found. Activated charcoal may hinder endoscopic evaluation of patients with corrosive lesions [13]. Prudent aspiration of the gastric contents can be considered, with respiratory protection, and if the ingested volume is high (over 100 ml), the ingestion period is short (less than 1 h) [13, 15]. The respiratory effects of neonicotinoids should be carefully monitored, particularly hypoventilation and respiratory failure. Patients with upper airway injuries such as hoarseness and stridor caused by irritant and corrosive effects of the solvent should probably undergo endoscopic assessment of vocal cordons [13].

Sometimes, organophosphorus intoxication may also be associated. In this case, acute poisoning may be manifested by miosis, bradycardia, hypersalivation and bronchorrhea. Because of these symptoms, atropine and oximes may be improperly used as an antidote. It is unknown whether these drugs are effective or may worsen the outcome of neonicotoid insecticide poisonings. In cases with life-threatening muscarinic manifestations (e.g., bronchorrhea with airway compromise), the use of atropine may be justified in neonicotinoid-poisoned patients [13, 44]. Oximes (e.g., pralidoxime) are usually either ineffective or contraindicated. In the absence of organophosphorus pesticides, oximes have a weak inhibitory effect on acetylcholinesterase activity and therefore may increase nicotinic effects (tachycardia, hypertension and muscle weakness) [5]. Because the severity of poisoning is not proportional to the plasma concentration of neonicotinoids, hemofiltration is ineffective in increasing their elimination [13, 43].

9. Prognosis and comparative mortality rates

The numbers of neonicotinoid poisonings have increased in the last decade, given that neonicotinoid insecticide is highly used. Respiratory, cardiovascular and certain neurological presentations (dyspnea/apnea, coma, tachycardia, hypotension, mydriasis and bradycardia) are symptoms of severe neonicotinoid intoxication [43]. Biochemical abnormalities and rhabdomyolysis have been reported as potentially serious complications that might lead to mortality [5].

Mortality through imidacloprid poisoning ranges from 0% to 4.2% in various studies. In a study in Taiwan, neonicotinoid poisoning mortality was 2.9%, inferior to that with organophosphates (12.3%) or carbamates (7.3%), but close to that with synthetic pyrethroids (3.1%) [47]. In the study in France conducted on 428 patients with acute neonicotinoid poisoning, six deaths were recorded [26]. Another study in Korea on 24 cases shows a mortality rate of 4.2% [48]. In addition to these studies on larger cohorts of patients, sporadic cases of acute neonicotinoid poisoning deaths are also reported in the literature (**Table 7**).

Authors, year of the study	Place of study	The type of neonicotinoid	Death numbers
Proença P et al., 2005 [36]	Portugal	Imidacloprid	2
Huang NC et al.,2006 [45]	Taiwan	Imidacloprid	1
Shadnia S et al., 2008 [40]	Iran	Imidacloprid	1
Yeh IJ et al., 2010 [44]	China	Imidacloprid	1
Iyyodurai R et al., 2010 [30]	India	Imidacloprid	1
Harish J et al., 2011 [49]	India	Imidacloprid	1
Fuke C et al., 2014 [49]	Japan	Imidacloprid	1
Vinod KV et al., 2015 [29]	India	Thiacloprid	1

Table 7. Deaths by acute poisoning with neonicotinoids reported in the literature.

10. Concluding remarks

Neonicotinoids act quite selectively on insects, but they are not free of human toxicity. Several cases of acute intoxication with such insecticides, sometimes severe, resulting in death, have been reported in the literature. The above review has highlighted the consequences of poisoning with these newer pesticides, not very well known at the moment. Therefore such information is valuable for clinicians, regulatory authorities and the public at large. Given the fact that these insecticides are increasingly being used in agriculture, horticulture and fish farming, but also for combating domestic pests, more studies on the human health effects of neonicotinoids exposure are needed and maybe some awareness programs about its toxicity should be implemented.

Author details

Nicolai Nistor[1,2], Otilia Elena Frăsinariu[1,2]* and Violeta Ştreangă[1,2]

*Address all correspondence to: otiliafrasinariu@gmail.com

1 "Grigore T. Popa" University of Medicine and Pharmacy Iasi, Iași, Romania

2 Regional Center of Toxicology, "St. Mary" Children's Emergency Clinic Hospital Iasi, Iași, Romania

References

[1] Konradsen F. Acute pesticide poisoning-a global public health problem. Danish Medical Bulletin. 2017;**54**(1):58-59

[2] Cimino AM, Boyles AL, Thayer KA, Perry MJ. Effects of neonicotinoid pesticide exposure on human health: A systematic review. Environmental Health Perspectives. 2017; **125**(2):155-161. DOI: 10.1289/EHP515

[3] Thany SH. Neonicotinoid insecticide: Historical evolution and resistance mechanism. In: Thany SH, editor. Insect Nicotinic Acetylcholine Receptors. New York: Springer Science; 2010:75-80

[4] Simon-Delso N, Amaral-Rogers V, Belzunces LP, Bonmatin JM, Chagnon M, Downs C, Furlan L, et al. Systemic insecticides (neonicotinoids and fipronil): Trends, uses, mode of action and metabolites. Environmental Science and Pollution Research. 2015;**22**:5-34. DOI: 10.1007/S11356-014-3470-Y

[5] Mohamed F, Gawarammana I, Robertson TA, Roberts MS, Palangasinghe C, Zawahir S, Jayamanne S. Acute human self-poisoning with Imidacloprid compound: A neonicotinoid insecticide. PLoS One. 2009;**4**(4):e5127. DOI: 10.1371/journal.pone.0005127

[6] Roberts JR, Karr JC. Pesticide exposure in children. Pediatrics. 2012;**130**(6):e1765-e1788. DOI: 10.1542/peds.2012-2758

[7] Fishel FM. Pesticide Toxicity Profile Neonicotinoid Pesticides. University of Florida, Florida; 2016. Available from: http://edis.ifas.ufl.edu/pi117

[8] Henry M, Béguin M, Requier F, et al. A common pesticide decreases foraging success and survival in honey bees. Science. 2012;**336**:348-350. DOI: 10.1126/science.1215039

[9] Fischer J, Müller T, Spatz A-K, et al. Neonicotinoids interfere with specific components of navigation in honeybees. PLoS One. 2014;**9**:e91364. DOI: 10.1371/journal.pone.0091364

[10] Proposition de resolution relative à la préservation des insectes pollinisateurs, de l'environnement et de la santé et à un moratoire sur les pesticides de la famille des néonicotinoïdes. 2014. Available from: https://www.senat.fr/leg/ppr13-643.pdf

[11] Woodcock BA, Bullock JM, Shore RF, Heard MS, Pereira MG, Redhead J, Ridding L, et al. Country-specific effects of neonicotinoid pesticides on honey bees and wild bees. Science. 2017;**356**(6345):1393-1395. DOI: 10.1126/science.aaa1190

[12] Tsvetkov N, Samson-Robert O, Sood K, Patel HS, Malena DA, Gajiwala PH, Maciukiewicz P, et al. Chronic exposure to neonicotinoids reduces honey bee health near corn crops. Science. 2017;**356**(6345):1395-1397. DOI: 10.1126/science.aam7470

[13] Phua DH, Lin CC, ML W, et al. Neonicotinoid insecticides: An emerging cause of acute pesticide poisoning. Clinical Toxicology. 2009;**47**:336-341. DOI: 10.1080/15563650802644533

[14] Kasiotis KM, Machera K. Neonicotinoids and their metabolites in human biomonitoring: A review. Hellenic Plant Protection Journal. 2015;**8**:33-45. DOI: https://doi.org/10.1515/hppj-2015-0006

[15] Testud F. Insecticides néonicotinoïdes. EMC—Pathologie professionelle et l'environnement. 2014;**9**(10):1-6

[16] Swenson TL. Neonicotinoid Insecticide Metabolism and Mechanisms of Toxicity in Mammals. Berkeley: University of California; 2013

[17] Casida JE. Neonicotinoid metabolism: Compounds, substituents, pathways, enzymes, organisms, and relevance. Journal of Agricultural and Food Chemistry. 2011;**59**(7):2923-2931. DOI: 10.1021/jf102438c

[18] Shi X, Dick RA, Ford AK, Casida JE. Enzymes and inhibitors in Neonicotinoid insecticide metabolism. Journal of Agricultural and Food Chemistry. 2009;**97**(11):4861-4866. DOI: 10.1021/jf900250f

[19] Sheets LP. Imidacloprid: A neonicotinid insecticide. In: Krieger RI, editor. Handbook of Pesticide Toxicology. 2nd ed. San Diego: Academic Press; 2001. pp. 1123-1130

[20] Gibbsons D, Morrissey C, Mineau P. A review of the direct and indirect effects of neonicotinoids and fipronil on vertebrate wildlife. Environmental Science and Pollution Research. 2015;**22**:103-118. DOI: 10.1007/s11356-014-3180-5

[21] Tomlin CDS. The Pesticide Manual, A World Compendium. 14th ed. Surry, England: British Crop Protection Council; 2006. pp. 598-599

[22] Chen M, Tao L, McLean J, Lu C. Quantitative analysis of neonicotinoid insecticide residues in foods: Implication for dietary exposures. Journal of Agricultural and Food Chemistry. 2014;**62**(26):6082-6090. DOI: 10.1021/jf501397m

[23] Kumar A, Verma A, Kumar A. Accidental human poisoning with a neonicotinoid insecticide, imidacloprid: A rare case report from rural India with brief review of literature. Egyptian Journal of Forensic Sciences. 2013;**3**(4):123-126. DOI: 10.1016/j.ejfs.2013.05.002

[24] IW W, Lin JL, Cheng CT. Acute poisoning with the neonicotinoid insecticide imidacloprid in N-methyl pyrrolidone. Journal of Toxicology: Clinical Toxicology. 2001;**39**(6):617-621

[25] Forrester MB. Neonicotinoid insecticide exposures reported to six poison centers in Texas. Human & Experimental Toxicology. 2014;**33**(6):568-573. DOI: 10.1177/0960327114522500

[26] Boels D, Chataignesr D. Expositions aux spécialités à base d'imidaclopride: synthèse des cas signalés aux centres antipoison français de 1999 à 2012;**2013**:1-44. Available from: http://www.centresantipoison.ne/CCTV/Imidaclopride_GT_Phytoveille_VF.pdf

[27] Viradiya K, Mishra A. Imidacloprid poisoning. Journal of the Association of Physicians of India. 2011;**59**:594-595

[28] Sibia RS, Kumar AS, Dhoot SR. Imidacloprid poisoning: A modern foe. International Journal of Research in Medical Sciences. 2014;**2**(2):752-754. DOI: 10.5455/2320-6012.ijrms20140573

[29] Vinod KV, Srikant S, Thiruvikramaprakash G, Dutta TK. A fatal case of thiacloprid poisoning. American Journal of Emergency Medicine. 2015;**33**:310.e5-310310.e6. DOI: http://dx.doi.org/10.1016/j.ajem.2014.08.013

[30] Iyyadurai R, George IA, Peter JV. Imidacloprid poisoning—Newer insecticide and fatal toxicity. Journal of Medical Toxicology. 2010;**6**(1):77-78. DOI: 10.1007/s13181-010-0041-6

[31] Agarwal R, Srinivas R. Severe neuropsychiatric manifestations and rhabdomyolysis in a patient with imidacloprid poisoning. The American Journal of Emergency Medicine. 2007;**25**(7):844-845. DOI: 10.1016/j.ajem.2006.11.044

[32] Sunny A, Chandirascharan VK, Mishra A, Jose N. Imidacloprid poisoning: Case report. Indian Journal of Forensic Medicine and Toxicology. 2015;**9**(2):1-4

[33] Radkika RH. Self poisoning by Imicon—a case report. International Journal of Advances in Case Report. 2017;**4**(2):64-67. DOI: http://dx.doi.org/10.21276/ijacr.2017.4.2.3

[34] Karatas AD. Severe central nervous system depression in a patient with acute imidacloprid poisoning. American Journal of Emergency Medicine. 2009;**27**(99):1171e5-1171e7. DOI: 10.1016/j.ajem.2009.01.006

[35] Pinar HU, Dogan R, Konul M, Karaca O. Acetamiprid poisoning followed by prolonged muscle weakness. Journal of the Turkish Society of Intensive Care. 2017;**15**:85-87

[36] Proença P, Teixeira H, Castanheira F, Pinheiro J, Monsanto EP, Vieira DN. Two fatal intoxication cases with imidacloprid: LC/MS analysis. Forensic Science International. 2005;**153**:75-80. DOI: 10.1016/j.forsciint.2005.04.015

[37] Estrada AF, Berrouet MC, Giraldo JA. Toxicidad por neonicotinoides: revisión de tema y reporte de dos casos. Medicina U.P.B. 2016;**35**(1):41-46. DOI: 10.18566/medupb.v35n1.a06

[38] Imamura T, Yanagawa K, Matsumoto N, Sakamoto T. Two cases of acute poisoning with acetamiprid in humans. Clinical Toxicology (Philadelphia, PA). 2010;**48**:851-853. DOI: 10.3109/15563650.2010.517207

[39] Agha A, Bella A, Aldosary B, Kazzi ZN, AlHumaidi MA. Imidacloprid poisoning presenting as leukoclastic vasculitis with renal and hepatic dysfunction. Saudi Journal of Kidney Diseases and Transplantation. 2012;**23**(6):1300-1303. DOI: 10.4103/1319-2442.103584

[40] Shadnia S, Moghaddam HH.Fatal intoxication with imidacloprid insecticide. American Journal of Emergency Medicine. 2008;**26**(5):634.e1-634634.e4. DOI: 10.1016/j.ajem.2007.09.024

[41] Chwaluk P. Acute inhalation imidacloprid poisoning—A case report. Przegląd Lekarski. 2010;**67**(8):619-620

[42] Lin PC, Lin HJ, Liao YY, Guo HR, Chen KT. Acute poisoning with neonicotinoid insecticides: A case report and literature review. Basic & Clinical Pharmacology & Toxicology. 2013;**112**:282-286. DOI: 10.1111/bcpt.12027

[43] Xing P, Xu J, Li L, Ma K. Acute severe multiorgan dysfunction syndrome with oral acetamiprid poisoning. Journal of the Formosan Medical Association. 2017;**116**(2):131-132. DOI: 10.1016/j.jfma.2016.06.008

[44] Yeh IJ, Lin TJ, Hwang DY. Acute multiple organ failure with imidacloprid and alcohol ingestion. The American Journal of Emergency Medicine. 2010;**28**(2):255.e1-255.e3. DOI: 10.1016/j.ajem.2009.05.006

[45] Huang NC, Lin SL, Chou CH, Hung YM, Chung HM, Huang ST. Fatal ventricular fibrillation in a patient with acute imidacloprid poisoning. The American Journal of Emergency Medicine. 2006;**24**(7):883-885. DOI: http://dx.doi.org/10.1016/j.ajem.2006.03.008

[46] Todani M, Kaneko H, Hayashida H, Tsuruta R, Kasaoka S, Maekawa T. Acute poisoning with neonicotinoid insecticide acetamiprid. Chūdoku Kenkyū. 2008;**21**(4):387-390

[47] Kim JC, So BH, Kim HJ, Kim HM, Park JH, Choi SM, Park KN, Chpoi KH. Clinical characteristics of patients with neonicotinoid insecticide poisoning. Journal of the Korean Society of Clinical Toxicology. 2010;**8**(9):24-29

[48] Harish J, Girish N, Nisarga R. Imidacloprid poisoning resulting in death. Pediatric Oncall. 2011;**8**(12). Available from: http://www.pediatriconcall.com/pediatric-journal/View/fulltext-articles/445/J/0/0/203/0

[49] Fuke C, Nagai T, Ninomiya K, Fukasawa M, Ihama Y, Miyazaki T. Detection of imidacloprid in biological fluids in a case of fatal insecticide intoxication. Legal Medicine (Tokyo). 2014;**16**(1):40-43

Chapter 7

Occupational Risk Factors for Acute Pesticide Poisoning among Farmers in Asia

Emine Selcen Darçın, Murat Darçın,
Murat Alkan and Gürdoğan Doğrul

Additional information is available at the end of the chapter

http://dx.doi.org/10.5772/intechopen.72006

Abstract

Types of pesticides are used in farming to increase the productivity and protection of crops or to control pests. However, exposure to acute pesticide poisoning is one of the most important occupational risk factors among farmers all over the world. They are directly exposed to high levels of pesticide poisoning when involved in the handling, spraying, mixing, or preparing of it. The low educational level, lack of information, training, judgment or experience, and the inability to read on pesticide safety are playing an important role for farmers' acute poisoning. On the other side, poor technology, inadequate personal protection, inappropriate type of clothing and equipment also leads to farmers' acute poisoning. Hence, this paper focuses on occupational risk factors for acute pesticide poisoning among farmers and their occupational safety. Discovering risk factors is also crucial for investigating health problems of farmers and its inevitable effects on their body. As it is seen from previous studies instead of field research such as deep interview on farmers' acute poisoning, data were mostly collected from hospitals. This study tries to emphasize the importance of field study to discover the risk factors for acute pesticide poisoning among farmers and their occupational safety in Asia.

Keywords: occupational risk factors, farmers, acute pesticide poisoning, occupational safety

1. Introduction

According to the World Health Organization, pesticides are chemical compounds that are used to kill pests, insects, rodents, fungi, and unwanted weeds. By their nature, pesticides are potentially toxic to humans which can also cause harm to human health [1]. The incorrect and unsafe use of pesticides can be a threat to human health [2]. They are mostly used for crop protection and to increase productivity in agriculture. Due to its widespread use in agriculture, occupational pesticide poisoning is likely to become a major health problem among agricultural workers all over the world. Since they directly contact with pesticides through spraying, mixing, handling, and preparing, farmers are at risk of exposure to pesticides. Hence, exposure to pesticides poisoning is an important occupational risk among farmers [3–5].

Farmers' low education level, lack of information and training on pesticide safety, poor spraying technology, and inadequate personal protection during pesticide use are the main reasons of poisoning [6]. These unsafe and misuses of pesticides can result in serious short-term or long-term health problems [7, 8]. Some of the symptoms of poisoning could affect the skin, nervous system, eyes, respiratory system, cardiovascular system, and gastrointestinal tract [9–11].

Discovering risk factors for acute pesticide poisoning of farmers is a very important issue for occupational safety. It will lead to decrease the number of poisoning cases. However, there have been very few researches that studied the risk factors for acute pesticide poisoning of farmers in agriculture. This chapter describes what the general risk factors of acute pesticide poisoning for farmers in Asia and the importance of their occupational safety are. Below, we present a description of pesticides and their mechanisms of actions.

2. What are pesticides?

Food and Agriculture Organization of the United Nations (FAO) defines that pesticide means any substance or mixture of substances intended for preventing, destroying, or controlling any pest. It also destroys vectors of human or animal disease; unwanted plants or animals causing harm during or otherwise interfering with the production, processing, storage, transport or marketing of food; agricultural commodities; wood and wood products or animal feedstuffs, or substances which may be administered to animals for the control of insects, arachnids, or other pests in or on their bodies. The term also comprises substances anticipated for use as a plant growth regulator, defoliant, desiccant or agent for thinning fruit or inhibiting the premature fall of fruit, and substances applied to crops either before or after harvest to protect the commodity from deterioration during storage and transport [12].

First of all, pesticides are designed to kill, prevent, destroy, repel, or mitigate living organisms such as pests (insects, mites, nematodes, weeds, and rats) [13], including insecticide, herbicide, fungicide, and various other substances used to control pests [14]. Pesticides are also used for crop protection, preservation of food and materials, and prevention of vector-borne diseases [15] like malaria, dengue, yellow fever dengue, leishmaniasis, and Japanese encephalitis [15, 16]. Briefly, it should be noted that:

- Insecticides (for killing insects) such as organochlorines, organophosphates, and carbamates. This category also includes insect repellents such as diethyltoluamide (DEET) and citronella.
- Herbicides or weed killers include substances such as paraquat, glyphosate, and propanil

WHO class	LD50 for the rat (mg/kg body weight)	
	Oral	Dermal
Ia. Extremely hazardous	<5	<50
Ib. Highly hazardous	5–50	50–200
II. Moderately hazardous	50–2000	200–2000
III. Slightly hazardous	Over 2000	Over 2000
U. Unlikely to present acute hazard	5000 or higher	

Table 1. Classification of pesticides [18].

- Fungicides (to kill mold or fungi): when applied to wood, they are called wood preservatives.
- Rodenticides to kill mice, rats, moles, and other rodents.
- Fumigants, which kill most organisms.
- Other products such as algaecides (to kill algae), miticides (to kill moths), and acaricides (to kill ticks) [17].

Secondly, pesticides are also responsible for thousands of acute pesticide poisoning and human injuries. Many people in developed and developing countries are affected by the negative effects of pesticides. This is mostly due to several reasons such as the lack of proper regulations, low education levels, little experience, and easy availability in markets [16].

The WHO issued classification of pesticides by hazard as seen in **Table 1**. The classification distinguishes between the more and the less hazardous forms of each pesticide in that it is based on the toxicity of the technical compound and on its formulations. Its classification ranges from extremely hazardous (class Ia) to slightly hazardous (class III) to unlikely to present acute hazard (class U) [18].

3. Acute pesticide poisoning

Acute pesticide poisoning has become a main health problem especially in developing countries with more than 300,000 deaths in a year. This is due to the poorer regulation, lack of surveillance systems, lack of experience or judgment, less enforcement, the inability to read, lack of training, and inadequate access to information systems [19]. Besides, the easy availability of highly toxic pesticides in farmers' homes has made pesticides the preferred means of suicide [20, 21].

It is not hard to diagnose symptoms of acute pesticide poisoning in humans due to their diversity and resemblance to other conditions. These symptoms could be classified as [9–11]:

- Skin: skin discomfort, rashes, blistering, burns, sweating, contact dermatitis, jaundice

- Nervous system: poor concentration, feelings of weakness, headache, dizziness, mood disturbances, depression, stupor, muscle twitching, seizures, paralysis, loss of consciousness, coma, excessive sweating, impaired vision, tremors, panic attacks, cramps
- Eyes: tearing, irritation, conjunctivitis
- Respiratory system: sore throat, runny nose, cough, pulmonary edema, difficulty breathing, respiratory failure
- Cardiovascular system: cardiac arrhythmias
- Gastrointestinal tract: nausea, vomiting, diarrhea, abdominal pain

Sometimes, symptoms of acute pesticide poisoning in humans do not become apparent for a long time. Age, body weight, sex, and metabolism all impact the health hazards at different levels. Due to its late effects, they can cause chronic illnesses. Besides general population, both male and female farm workers and children are at high risk to acute pesticide poisoning due to consumer goods or pesticide drift from farm fields. Mostly, women are the major workforce on plantations. They are exposed to pesticides due to mixing, handling, and spraying pesticides in the farm. It is well known that the harmful effects of toxins affect women workforce more than men due to their physiological makeup. According to a study carried on women sprayers, effects of pesticide exposure among them were fatigue, back pain, giddiness, difficulty in breathing, skin problems, nausea, eye irritation, headache, tight feeling in the chest, and swelling. They also stated that some side effects such as bleeding nose occurred initially upon spraying pesticides [22].

According to another study in Pakistan, it was reported upon the use of pesticides in cotton fields; all female workers suffered from headache, nausea, and vomiting [23]. While a study in Bangladesh reported the chronic illnesses on farm workers, about 85% of farm workers reported suffering gastrointestinal disorders during and after spraying, whereas 61, 63, and 47 of them reported, respectively, skin discomfort, eye problems, and feeling of weakness [24].

Moreover, children tend to be involved in more intense contact with their environment than adults. Therefore, they unintentionally ingest pesticides and are poisoned more often than grown-ups [25]. This incident generally occurs because of the unsafe storage and the different behaviors of young children who tend to put everything in their mouths and no ability to read labels and respond appropriately [26].

There have been several researches conducted in developing countries on acute pesticide poisoning. One of them is a study by Hoek and Konradsen in a rural area of Sri Lanka [27]. This study was conducted in two rural hospitals in Sri Lanka where 239 acute pesticide poisoning cases were examined. It reported that the large majority (84%) of incidents were intentional self-poisoning, with a case fatality rate of 18% due to endosulfan and paraquat. Ten of the non-intentional poisoning cases were due to exposure to the poison while spraying pesticides in the fields. Whereas 13% of the patients (31 out of the 239) reported a previous admission for pesticide poisoning, 20% reported a previous suicide attempt.

http://dx.doi.org/10.5772/intechopen.72006

4. Risk factors for acute pesticide poisoning among farmers in Asia

Pesticides play an important role in farming to increase the productivity of agriculture. However, globally acute pesticide poisoning is a major problem for those who are directly involved in the handling of pesticides, particularly farm workers in many developing countries. They routinely are exposed to high levels of pesticides. Farmers' exposure to acute pesticide poisoning occurs during the preparation of the pesticide spray. There are other ways that farmers are exposed to pesticide poisoning. One of them is during cleaning up of pesticide spraying equipment. Farmers who mix, load, and spray pesticides can be exposed to these toxins due to spills and splashes. Farmers can also be exposed to neighboring fields or by direct contact with pesticide residues on the crop or soil [28]. However, the unsafe, unconscious, indiscriminate, and extensive use of pesticides represents health problems [21]. There are many reasons of agricultural workers' exposure to acute pesticide poisoning. One of them is unsafe use or misuse of pesticides by farmers. Others are poor knowledge of storage, handling, and disposal [29]. Mostly hand pump is used as a spraying equipment by farmers. They complain of poor maintenance and leaks in the sprays. However, despite the fact that protective equipment, gear, and appropriate clothing were provided, farm workers did not use protective gear, as it was uncomfortable in the hot and humid conditions. Farm sprayers did not practice common hygiene such as washing their hands or their clothes after spraying [6, 22, 30].

According to a study, approximately 75% of pesticide usage in the United States occurs in agriculture. As such, agricultural workers are at greater risk of pesticide exposure than nonagricultural workers. The findings proved that acute pesticide poisoning in the agricultural industry would continue to be a crucial issue. Of the 3271 cases included in the analysis, 2334 (71%) were employed as farmworkers. The remaining cases were employed as processing/packing plant workers (12%), farmers (3%), and other miscellaneous agricultural workers (19%) [31].

Risk factors for acute pesticide poisoning among agricultural workers are also an important issue. A study explored work-related risk factors of acute occupational pesticide poisoning among male farmers in South Korea in 2011. In this study, a total of 1958 male farmers were interviewed. It suggested that the risk of acute occupational pesticide poisoning increased with lifetime days of pesticide application (OR, 1.74; 95% CI, 1.32–2.29). Reasons were not wearing personal protective equipment such as gloves (OR, 1.29) or masks (OR, 1.39), not following pesticide label instructions (OR, 1.61), applying the pesticide in full sun (OR, 1.48), and applying the pesticide upwind (OR, 1.54) which greatly increased risk of pesticide poisoning [32].

According to a research conducted in China, pesticide poisoning is an important health problem among Chinese farm workers. One thousand farmers were chosen from two villages. Farmers who reported risky behaviors such as not having personal protective equipment, having had a leaky knapsack, not avoiding physical contact with liquid pesticides, or continuing to apply pesticides when feeling ill had greatly higher risk of acute pesticide poisoning than farmers who did not report these behaviors (all $p \leq 0.01$) [33]. Data collection from 482 rice farmers in Thailand about risk factors for acute pesticide poisoning gave almost same results.

Pesticide exposure mostly caused from the misuse of pesticides including erroneous beliefs of farmers about pesticide toxicity, the use of faulty spraying equipment or lack of proper maintenance of spraying equipment, and protective gear and appropriate clothing during handling of pesticides [34].

5. Interventions for reducing risk factors for farmers' exposure to acute pesticide poisoning

Farmers are the major users of pesticides in agriculture. For this reason, they are more vulnerable to acute pesticide poisoning. There are many ways to reduce the farmers' exposure to acute pesticide poisoning. First of all, farmers must be aware of pesticide risks and its effect on health. The duty of national and international organizations, governments and pesticide industry is to disseminate educational materials of all types to pesticide users, farmers, farmer organizations, agricultural workers, unions, and other interested parties. Thus, pesticide users should learn educational materials before applying pesticides and should follow procedures [12]. Special educational programs can be set up by governments for farm workers prior to pesticide application. This procedure will provide knowledge on risks of pesticide poisoning use and also will decrease the pesticide exposure of farmers [35]. On the other side, protective and appropriate type of clothing and equipment must be used by farmers to prevent exposure to pesticides in all stages of pesticide spraying, mixing, and handling [28]. The United Nations Systems encourage international treaties to restrict export and sale of the most toxic pesticides. Many countries have signed them, but practically they are not implementing these agreements [16]. For this, all governments should develop a legal framework for the control of pesticides [36]. Lack of education, insufficient management, and inappropriate legal framework are the proximal causes of acute pesticide poisoning. Studies which were mentioned below illustrate the situation.

A study that was designed to assess participants' knowledge on the safety use of pesticides involved 300 farm workers working in India. As shown in **Table 2**, good knowledge on the safety use of pesticides was greatly influenced by the education level of farm workers. It is also seen that farmers lacked seriousness to practice safety measures despite their sufficient knowledge on the safety use of pesticides [35].

In the same study, there was a significant correlation (r, 0.525; $p < 0.001$) between the knowledge score and the practice score on protective measures.

Table 3 shows that 71.3% of the participants were reported wearing protective clothes and special gloves; 86% were reported wearing of special face mask; 46.1% of farmers were reported wearing face mask while working in the farm; 81.3% of them were reported not eating, drinking, and smoking during spraying; 66.7% of them were reported reading label instructions, 84.7% of the them were mentioned that they used leftover pesticide solutions on the same day, and 55.0% of the participants were reported knowing not to keep the leftover pesticide in a drinking container for later use while only 35% are following. Almost all (100%) participants stated that they wash hands after pesticide application [35].

	Education	N	Mean	Std. deviation	F-value	p-value
Knowledge on the safety use of pesticides	Up to primary	98	78.316	12.3771	6.328**	0.002
	Up to secondary	126	79.934	8.6792		
	10th and above	76	83.929	13.6800		
	Total	300	81.083	12.3728		
Practice on the safety use of pesticides	Up to primary	98	52.870	17.1966	0.233	0.793
	Up to secondary	126	52.034	10.3631		
	10th and above	76	51.563	10.2635		
	Total	300	52.188	12.9429		

*Significant @ 5% level.
**Significant @ 1% level.

Table 2. Knowledge and practice on the safety use of pesticides based on their education [35].

Safety practice	Level of practicing safety measures			Total
	Never	Sometimes	Always	
Wearing of protective clothes and gloves	12	111	91	214
	5.6%	51.9%	42.5%	71.3%
Wearing of special face mask	41	98	119	258
	15.9%	38.0%	46.1%	86.0%
Not eating, drinking, and smoking during the application of pesticides	20	95	129	244
	8.2%	38.9%	52.9%	81.3%
Reading and following label instructions	20	84	96	200
	10.0%	42.0%	48.0%	66.7%
Using leftover pesticide solution in the same day	4	166	84	254
	1.6%	65.4%	33.1%	84.7%
Washing hands after pesticide application	110	54	136	300
	36.7%	18.0%	45.3%	100.0%
Not keeping the leftover pesticide in drinking container	21	86	58	165
	12.7%	52.1%	35.2%	55.0%
Washing contaminated clothes separately	71	79	150	300
	23.7%	26.3%	50.0%	100.0%

Table 3. Safety practices in relation to pesticide knowledge [35].

Another research is carried out in Kuwait with a total of 250 participated farmers. According to the study, the majority (58%) of the farmers did not use any personal protective equipment when mixing or spraying pesticides. Farmers mentioned the reasons for not using personal protective equipment such as lack of availability when needed (35%), personal protective equipment being uncomfortable in the local hot and humid climate (90%), too expensive (65%), and slowing you down (29%). Younger and educated farmers were more likely to use personal protective equipment compared to older farmers. Farmers were asked if they take safety measures to reduce their risk of exposure to pesticides. The majority of respondents reported not eating (72%), drinking (65%), or smoking (59%) when mixing or applying pesticides. Over 70% of respondents, however, did not wash work clothing used while mixing or spraying pesticides separately from other cloths. Similarly, 46% of respondents reported that they did not consider wind direction when spraying pesticides [37].

The above findings suggest that governments and pesticide-producing industries should develop and promote the use of pesticide application methods and equipment that decreases risks to human health and expose to pesticide poisoning. Therefore, governments, pesticide industries, NGOs, and international organizations should work together to prevent the pesticide poisoning [12].

The initiative, Agricultural Worker Protection Standard (WPS), for example, is aimed at reducing the risk of pesticide poisoning among agricultural workers. It also offers occupational protections to over two million agricultural workers and pesticide handlers. It is intended to decrease the pesticide exposure incidents among farmworkers and their family members. The requirements in the WPS are intended to inform workers and handlers about pesticide safety and provide protections from potential exposure to pesticides. It keeps workers out of areas being treated with pesticides [38]. It is therefore a laudable intervention that should be continued and evaluated in order to learn from it and improve it.

6. Conclusion

Unsafe pesticide use and acute pesticide poisoning are major problems which affect the health of many farm workers all around the world. There are many reasons why acute pesticide poisonings are common among farmers. Some of main risk factors which results to occupational pesticide poisoning of farmers are an insufficient level of knowledge about pesticide use, wearing inappropriate personal protective equipment during spraying, and poor technology. Further studies should specially focus on occupational pesticide poisoning among farmers in order to determine possible short-term and long-term health effects and to develop preventive measures for it.

It is concluded from the existing studies that there are few studies that looked into the risk factors for occupational acute pesticide poisoning. More studies and researches are required in this field to create awareness among governments especially in developing countries. Governments and NGOs must be encouraged and asked for financial support by academicians for better and deep researches on occupational poisoning. It is also the duty of the governments to arrange special educational training programs for the farmers to increase their knowledge on the safety use of pesticide. This educational program will also help farmers to learn more about risk factors of poisoning and occupational safety. In addition, instead of obtaining from hospitals, data must be obtained from quantitative research methods to learn more about the real reasons of occupational poisoning.

http://dx.doi.org/10.5772/intechopen.72006

Author details

Emine Selcen Darçın[1]*, Murat Darçın[2], Murat Alkan[2] and Gürdoğan Doğrul[2]

*Address all correspondence to: darcin@gazi.edu.tr

1 Gazi University, Ankara, Turkey

2 Gendarmerie and Coast Guard Academy, Ankara, Turkey

References

[1] WHO. Improving Availability of Information about Human Exposures to Pesticides [Internet]. 2017. Available from: http://www.who.int/ipcs/poisons/pesticides/en/ [Accessed: 20-07-2017]

[2] Damalas CA. Understanding benefits and risks of pesticide use. Scientific Research and Essays. 2009;**4**:945-949

[3] Wesseling C, Aragón A, Castillo L, Corriols M, Chaverri F, de la Cruz E, Keifer M, Monge P, Partanen TJ, Ruepert C, van Wendel de Joode B. Hazardous pesticides in Central America. International Journal of Occupational and Environmental Health 2001;**7**: 287–294

[4] Konradsen F, van der Hoek W, Cole DC, Hutchinson G, Daisley H, Singh S, et al. Reducing acute poisoning in developing countries—Options for restricting the availability of pesticides. Toxicology 2003;**192**:249–261

[5] Coronado GD, Thompson B, Strong L, Griffith WC, Islas I. Agricultural task and exposure to organophosphate pesticides among farm workers. Environmental Health Perspectives. 2004;**112**:142-147

[6] Hurtig AK, Sebastian MS, Soto A, Shingre A, Zambrano D, Guerrero W. Pesticide use among farmers in the Amazon Basin of Ecuador. Archives of Environmental Health. 2003;**14**(58): 223-228

[7] Soares W, Almeida RMVR, Moro S. Rural work and risk factors associated with pesticide use in Minas Gerais, Brazil. Cadernos de Saúde Pública. 2003;**19**:1117-1127

[8] Remor AP, Totti CC, Moreira DA, Dutra GP, Heuser VD, Boeira JM. Occupational exposure of farm workers to pesticides: Biochemical parameters and evaluation of genotoxicity. Environment International. 2009;**35**:273-278

[9] Reigart JR, Roberts JR, editors. Recognition and Management of Pesticide Poisoning. 5th ed. Washington: Environmental Protection Agency [Internet]; 1999. Available from: http://npic.orst.edu/rmpp.htm Accessed: 12-08-2017

[10] Bödeker W. Zur Häufigkeit tödlicher und nichttödlicher Pestizidvergiftungen: eine Betractung nationaler und internationaler Morbiditäts- und Mortalitätsstatistiken. En: Bödeker W, Dümmler C., Hrsg. Pestizide und Gesundheit. Karlsruhe, Alemania: Verlag C. F. Müller; 1990. pp. 89–118

[11] Alavanja MCR, Hoppin JA, Kamel F. Health effects of chronic pesticide exposure: Cancer and neurotoxicity. Annual Review of Public Health. 2004;**25**(1):155-197

[12] FAO. International Code of Conduct on the Distribution and Use of Pesticides: Guidelines on Compliance and Enforcement of a Pesticide Regulatory Programme [Internet]. 2006. Available from: www.fao.org/WAICENT/FAOINFO/AGRICULT/AGP/ AGPP/Pesticid/Code/ Download/Compliance06.pdf [Accessed: 20-07-2017]

[13] Watts M. Highly Hazardous Pesticides in the Pacific, National Toxics Network, New Zealand [Internet]. 2016. Available from: http://www.ntn.org.au [Accessed: 20-07-2017]

[14] EPA. What is a Pesticide [Internet]. 2017. Available from: https://www.epa.gov/ minimum-risk-pesticides/what-pesticide [Accessed: 20-07-2017]

[15] National Resource Council. Pesticides in the Diets of Infants and Children. Washington, DC: National Academy Press; 1993

[16] Jers E. Pesticides: Pesticides Are Responsible for Millions of Human Poisonings and Hundreds of Thousands Deaths each Year [Internet]. 2014. Available from: http://www.globalhealthminders.dk/ghm-emerging-issue-brief-pesticides/ [Accessed: 20-07-2017]

[17] WHO. Children's Health and the Environment. WHO Training Package for the Health Sector [Internet]. 2008. Available from: http://www.who.int/ceh/capacity/Pesticides.pdf [Accessed: 01-10-2017]

[18] WHO. The WHO Recommended Classification of Pesticides by Hazard and Guidelines to Classification. Geneva: World Health Organization [Internet]; 2009. Available from: http://www.who.int/ipcs/publications/pesticides_hazard/en/ [Accessed: 28-07-2017]

[19] Thundiyil JG, Stober J, Besbelli N, Pronczuk J. Acute pesticide poisoning: A proposed classification tool. Bulletin of the World Health Organization. 2008;**86**(3):205-212

[20] Konradsen F. Acute pesticide poisoning—A global public health problem. Danish Medical Bulletin. 2007;**54**:58-59

[21] Jeyaratnam J. Acute pesticide poisoning: A major global health problem. World Health Statistics Quarterly. 1990;**43**:139-144

[22] Pesticide Action Network (PAN) Asia and the Pacific. Poisoned and Silenced: A Study of Pesticide Poisoning in the Plantations [Internet]. 2002. Available from: www.panap.net [Accessed: 20-07-2017]

[23] Tahir S, Anwar T. Assessment of pesticide exposure in female population living in cotton growing areas of Punjab, Pakistan. Bulletin of Environmental Contamination and Toxicology. 2012;**89**:1138-1141

[24] Miah SJ, Hoque A, Paul A, Rahman A. Unsafe use of pesticide and its impact on health of farmers: A case study in Burichong Upazila, Bangladesh. IOSR Journal of Environmental Science, Toxicology and Food Technology. 2014;**8**(1):57-67

[25] UNEP. Childhood Pesticide Poisoning: Information for Advocacy and Action. Châtelaine, Switzerland: United Nations Environment Programme [Internet]; 2004. Available from: http://www.who.int/ceh/publications/en/pestpoisoning.pdf [Accessed 20-07-2017]

[26] David Suzuki Foundation. Northern Exposure: Acute Pesticide Poisonings in Canada [Internet]. 2007. Available from: http://www.davidsuzuki.org/publications/downloads/2007/DSF-pesticide-poisoning.pdf [Accessed 12-07-2017]

[27] van der Hoek W, Konradsen F. Risk factors for acute pesticide poisoning in Sri Lanka. Tropical Medicine & International Health 2005;**10**(6):589–596

[28] Damalas CA, Koutroubas SD. Farmers' exposure to pesticides: Toxicity types and ways of prevention. Toxics. 2016;**4**(1):1-10

[29] Karunamoorthi K, Mohammed M, Wassie F. Knowledge and practices of farmers with reference to pesticide management: Implications on human health. Archives of Environmental & Occupational Health. 2012;**67**:109-116

[30] Damalas CA, Georgiou EB, Theodorou MG. Pesticide use and safety practices among Greek tobacco farmers: A survey. International Journal of Environmental Health Research. 2006;**16**(5):339-348

[31] Calvert GM, Karnik J, Mechler L, Beckman J, Morissey B, Sievert J, Barrett R, Lackovic M, Mabee L, Schwartz A, Mitchell Y, Moraga-McHaley S. Acute pesticide poisoning among agricultural workers in the United States, 1998–2005. American Journal of Industrial Medicine. 2008;**51**(12):883-898

[32] Kim JH, Kim J, Cha ES, Ko Y, Kim DH, Kim DH, Lee WJ. Work-related risk factors by severity for acute pesticide poisoning among male farmers in South Korea. International Journal of Environmental Research and Public Health. 2013;**10**:1100-1112

[33] Zhang X, Zhao W, Jing R, Wheeler K, Smith GA, Stallones L, Xiang H. Work-related pesticide poisoning among farmers in two villages of southern China: A cross-sectional survey. BMC Public Health. 2011;**11**:429-436

[34] Raksanam B, Taneepanichskul S, Siriwong W, Robson M. Factors associated with pesticide risk behaviors among rice farmers in rural community, Thailand. Journal of Environment and Earth Science. 2012;**2**(2):32-39

[35] Kumari PL, Reddy KG. Knowledge and practices of safety use of pesticides among farm workers. Journal of Agriculture and Veterinary Science. 2013;**6**(2):1-8

[36] Food and Agriculture Organization of the United Nations (FAO). Guidelines for Legislation on the Control of Pesticides [Internet]. 1989. Available from: http://www.fao.org/fileadmin/templates/agphome/documents/Pests_Pesticides/Code/Old_guidelines/LEGIS.pdf [Accessed: 01-10-2017]

[37] Jallow MF, Awadh DG, Albaho MS, Devi VY, Thomas BM. Pesticide knowledge and safety practices among farm workers in Kuwait: Results of a survey. International Journal of Environmental Research and Public Health. 2017;**14**(4):3-15

[38] United States Environmental Protection Agency (EPA). Agricultural Worker Protection Standard (WPS) [Internet]. 2017. Available from: https://www.epa.gov/pesticide-worker-safety/agricultural-worker-protection-standard-wps [Accessed: 20-07-2017]

Chapter 8

Activating Carbon Fibers and Date Pits for Use in Liver Toxin Adsorption

Ameereh Seyedzadeh, Asel Mwafy,
Waleed Khalil Ahmed, Kamala Pandurangan and
Ali Hilal-Alnaqbi

Additional information is available at the end of the chapter

http://dx.doi.org/10.5772/intechopen.71891

Abstract

Acute liver failure (ALF) is a rare, potentially fatal complication of severe hepatic illness. It is a syndrome that triggers a cascade of events, leading to multiple organ failures and often death. The work aimed at demonstrating the usefulness of activated raw date pits and carbon fiber reinforced polymers (CFRP) in the management of ALF. The activated carbons produced are used for adsorption of albumin bound toxins from the liver of patients with ALF. The liver is not cured, however, patients are given the time they need to find a suitable donor. Initially, date pits are milled and epoxy is removed from the CFRP. Both materials then undergo pyrolysis and activation treatments. The activated carbon fiber (ACF) and powdered activated carbon (PAC) resulting are tested using FTIR and TGA analysis. FTIR spectrums provide information about functional groups present in the samples and TGA graphs illustrate weight loss as treatment temperature increases. From the data analysis carried out, it appears that the process of recycling both; date pits and CFRP was successful. This confirms the ability of PAC and ACFs to adsorb toxins and as potential candidates for consideration in the search for effective treatment options for liver failure.

Keywords: carbon fiber, pyrolysis, chitosan, adsorption, activation

1. Introduction

Acute liver failure (ALF) is a rare, potentially fatal complication of severe hepatic illness resulting from various causes; it is a devastating syndrome that triggers a cascade of events, leading to multiple organ failure and often death. The work presented below aimed at demonstrating the usefulness of activated raw date pits and carbon fiber reinforced polymers (CFRP) in the management of acute liver failure. Date pits are the seeds of *Phoenix dactylifera* L. *(Arecaceae)* that have been used in Arabic traditional medicine for centuries to treat diabetes. In the following pages, an overview is presented with a focus on artificial liver support systems including the roles of bilirubin toxin, activated charcoal and purified water.

1.1. Liver failure

Acute liver failure occurs when patients' livers cease to remove all the toxins in the blood stream therefore an increase in the level of toxins becomes an issue. Some of these toxins bind to certain proteins in order to travel through the blood stream without poisoning other cells and tissues [1]. Due to this strong bond between proteins, such as albumin serum and toxins, it is hard to eliminate them using conventional dialysis [2]. This is because dialysis is only capable of removing water-soluble toxins. However, date seeds are listed in folk remedies for treatment of various infectious diseases, diabetes, hypertension and cancer due to their hepatoprotective effects attributed to the antioxidant and free radical scavenging activities. In the absence of effective means to remove toxins from the liver, liver support devices are utilized to provide patients with the stability they need to either recover or the time they need for transplantation [3]. Liver support devices are categorized into Artificial liver support devices (ALSD) and Bio-Artificial liver support devices (BLSD). The difference being that ALSD are purely mechanical, or in other words; not cell based, while BLSD include a cell element allowing the device to act as a replacement for some of the most important functions in the liver. Payable to this, ALSD act as a bridge to transplantation and do not have the ability to allow the existing liver to recover. On the other hand, BLSD, while acting as a detoxifier also provides the ability to salvage the liver [4].

An example of an ALSD is MARS (Molecular Adsorbent Recirculating System), which is a device used to remove albumin-bound toxins by selectively adsorbing them through membranes in the machine. The toxins are adsorbed onto the surfaces of materials like activated carbon through the membranes [5]. Removing toxins in this manner is crucial for patients with end-stage liver failure due to the single option being liver transplant but lack of donors and the need for a suitable donor with the right blood type in time makes the situation life threatening [6]. The ability to remove these toxins is a temporary fix which gives patients the time they need to find a suitable donor [7]. Carbon is treated to form activated carbon (AC), which is characterized by low-volume pores and a large surface area. AC is one of the best adsorbents due to its large surface area that can be greater than 1000 m^2/g, leading to its broad uses in many purification and medical applications.

1.2. Bilirubin toxin

Bilirubin toxin binds to a certain protein called albumin to travel through the blood stream. Such a bond is hard to break [8]. Thus, many researchers studied the effect of increasing the albumin concentrations on bilirubin adsorption [9]. This was accomplished by many different group studies. Annesi and his team [10] tested for bilirubin as well as tryptophan toxin adsorption using several AC samples with a particle size of 0.3 - 0.5mm. Results showed that the presence of higher albumin concentrations played a role in decreasing the bilirubin adsorption. This indicates that in devices similar to MARS, the problem of adsorbing albumin over bilirubin might occur. However, in such a study the influence of changing AC concentrations on the efficiency of bilirubin adsorption was not considered. This means that the negative effect of increasing the albumin concentrations on bilirubin adsorption can be solved. Using higher concentration of AC is one of the possible solutions in which the effect of albumin concentrations will no longer affect the efficiency of bilirubin adsorption. Another very effective method could be coating the AC samples with high binding affinity solutions such as chitosan gel.

In addition, previous studies showed that granular AC does not have a high adsorption capacity for bilirubin toxin. Thus, preparing AC in powder form by grinding it will play a vital role in increasing the adsorption capacity of bilirubin toxin [11]. Using granular AC has its own drawbacks in which it does not utilize its full capabilities. This is due to the very small surface area and pore structure of the granular AC as opposed to the powdered AC which has such a high adsorption capacity. By comparing the granular and powdered AC, it can be clearly seen that the adsorption properties depend on two very essential and important elements which are the particle size and internal surface area.

Nikolaev et al. [12] studied the efficiency of adsorbing bilirubin toxin of different types of AC. The different types of AC which were used in this research are Nitrogen based granular carbons, AC based on pyrolysis and fibrous AC. The tests were carried out for different particle sizes ranging between 7 and 9 μm of fibrous AC and 0.5–1.0 mm for activated carbon which was prepared using the pyrolysis technique.

Furthermore, a previous study used surface modified chitosan beads to examine their binding affinities for bilirubin in buffer solutions as compared to AC. Throughout conducting this study, it was observed that chitosan beads adsorbed a bilirubin average of 1.18 mg/g of chitosan beads whereas AC adsorbed 0.74 mg/g [13]. Based on the information provided, it can be clearly concluded that combining powdered AC which has a porous structure and large surface area as well as high adsorption capacity with chitosan's high binding affinities for bilirubin could provide a large adsorption capacity for bilirubin. In other words, combining both could play an important role in increasing and enlarging the adsorption capacity for bilirubin than each functional alone. This method is still under testing in order to use it for the adsorption of protein bound toxins from the liver.

To test for bilirubin adsorption using AC, an albumin-bound bilirubin solution is prepared and mixed with PBS solution to form a stock which is left to stabilize for six hours. PBS is a solution similar to blood plasma which will provide an in lab alternative to using blood for testing. Bilirubin binds to high and low affinity sites on albumin. The AC is expected to adsorb the bilirubin bound to the low affinity sites. The stock will then be serially diluted into different concentrations at a PH of 7.4. a control is taken from each concentration as well as samples containing different amounts of AC. The samples are retained in amber bottles to avoid photo degradation of the bilirubin and are placed in a shaking water bath set at 140 rpm and 37°C. A spectrophotometer is then used to test for the albumin and bilirubin present in each sample every hour for the first four hours then after 16 hrs. Between readings, bottles are kept in a shaking water bath. The readings are taken for two wavelengths; 416 nm for bilirubin testing and 350 nm for albumin testing. The albumin readings are expected to remain stable since AC adsorbs bilirubin and not albumin. Bilirubin on the other hand is expected to decrease with time in the bottles containing the AC.

1.3. Activated carbon

1.3.1. Date pit activated carbon

AC can be prepared from many different raw materials depending on availability, surface area, pore size distribution and porous texture [14]. Some examples are wood, coal, coconut, rice husk, shells of plants, stones of fruits, asphalt, metal carbides, carbon blacks, and polymer scraps [15]. Due to the abundance of date palm biomass in the UAE, it can be used to prepare AC. Date pits have a mass varying between 10 and 15% of the total date fruit mass. Payable to their high nutritional value, date pits' utilization is highly requested by the date processing industries in raising their value-added products [16].

1.3.2. Activated carbon fiber

Carbon fiber reinforced polymers (CFRP) are widely used in many industries, most important of which are the aerospace and automobile industries [17]. This is due to their lightweight, very high strength and ability to endure impact [18]. Around 20% of yearly prepreg carbon fiber production goes to use in the aerospace field as well as 30% being facilitated to the automobile industry [19]. An increasing number of aircraft structures have become highly dependent on the use of these materials. Some of which are the Boeing 787 Dreamliner and Airbus A380 and A350 [20].

With an increase in demand for CFRP comes a larger amount of scrap generated. Scrap sources include end of roll, trim, out-timed and out-of-spec waste. Many manufacturers deal with this waste by disposing of it into landfills [21]. This is not only harmful for the environment but is also costly for manufacturers [22]. Therefore, methods of recycling these CFRP are being researched and some are being implemented on an industrial scale. Recycling CFRP can either be done thermally or chemically [23].

1.4. Applications of activated carbon fiber

In today's world, activated carbon fiber (ACF) is a highly versatile material which has been a pioneer within a broad range of applications [24]. What was stated as an exotic material many years ago is nowadays playing an intrinsic role in our daily lives [25]. As outlined below, several applications of ACF will be discussed.

1.4.1. Medical applications

In the medical field, activated carbon fiber has many remarkable uses. It is normally linked with the adsorption of organic toxins in which it is widely used as an antitoxin in the treatment of kidney and liver disease. In other words, for blood dialysis in the treatment of liver and kidney disease, ACF is used as a filtering medium that adsorbs toxins from the blood stream of patients' bodies. Other uses in the medical field include the treatment of cholestasis during

http://dx.doi.org/10.5772/intechopen.71891

pregnancy as well as lowering cholesterol levels. Several studies have been carried out on the possibility of utilizing ACF in the medical field. It was found that ACF can be used as an anti-flatulent in the abdominal radiography process. Other than that, activated carbon in general is a significant ingredient for stomach remedies. It helps in controlling diarrhea and flatulence, as well as lowering the toxin levels throughout the body.

1.4.2. Purification of water

Water makes up more than two thirds of human body weight and the earth's surface. This is evidence that water is one of the most essential substances on earth. In fact, if there was no water there would be no life on earth. However, that same water might be harmful to the human body if it was not purified. Thus, water purification is an important industry requirement in which water undergoes a number of treatments to be usable and drinkable. Water purifiers are designed to remove impurities and contaminants from water. Several materials are used in water purifiers to help removing these contaminants. ACF can be used as a media for water purification. It is a porous material with a high adsorption capacity by which it could adsorb the pollutants perfectly. Recently some studies have shown that ACF is popular in water purification industry and that is due to removing heavy metals like lead, as well as dissolving chemicals and some types of parasites.

2. Methods of recycling CFRP and removing epoxy

2.1. Recycling CFRP

There are three possible methods of recycling CFRP which include mechanical, thermal and chemical recycling. Mechanical recycling mainly involves size reduction methods, such as cutting, trimming or shredding. Thermal recycling comprises of material treatment at very high temperatures. The type of thermal recycling of interest in this work is pyrolysis, where the material is heated in a furnace in the presence of Nitrogen gas. Furthermore, the chemical recycling process revolves around the removal of the matrix using chemical dissolution reagents [26].

2.2. Removing epoxy from carbon fiber

Carbon fiber reinforced polymers (CFRPs) are composite materials that are often coated by epoxy layers. These epoxy layers add to the carbon fiber properties in which it has been proved through different studies that epoxy contributes in the enhancement of the chemical resistance, strength and durability of the composite materials [27]. Although, the use of epoxy resin is beneficial in many aspects, it originates difficulties related to the removal of this very strong resin. Therefore, many methods are followed in order to remove epoxy from carbon fiber [28]. Using acetone as a solvent to dissolve the epoxy is one of the approaches that is followed during the curing process. A certain amount of acetone is added to the carbon fiber to dissolve an epoxy resin. In other words, acetone/epoxy solutions of different concentrations are prepared. The solution is then sonicated and stirred for an hour. After that, the mixture is exposed to heating at a certain temperature. Lastly, hardener is added to the mixture. Other studies showed how adding acetone might impact the characteristics of epoxy. According to these authors, the occurrence of residual solvent might lead to some significant changes in the mechanical and physical properties as well as the thermal degradation.

In contrast, FTIR results showed that the presence of acetone does not affect the chemical properties of the material. According to the literature, it can be seen that a more efficient method of removing epoxy has been applied. This technique is based on using thermal processes in order to remove the epoxy from the carbon fiber. Thermal processes could include more than one method and technique such as pyrolysis. Pyrolysis is one of the most studied thermal processes due to its popularity in the commercial scale [29]. The process operates at different temperature ranges depending on what type of resin is used. For example, epoxy resin tends to be stronger than other types of resin which means it might require higher temperatures to be fully removed. One of the main drawbacks of using this technique is the remaining resin residue such as char. This char contaminates the fibers and thus a post treatment is needed to burn it. However, exposing this composite material to high temperatures during the treatment might lead to a significant reduction in the properties of the material. Different group works have studied the effect of raising the temperature on the properties of the carbon fiber. The results showed that for some types of fiber such as glass fibers a temperature of 1300°C is needed in order to remove the char completely and to produce a perfectly clean one but a reduction by up to 85% of the tensile strength was observed [30]. Thus, in order to produce an acceptable strength for the carbon fibers a maximum pyrolysis temperature in the range of 500–550°C is advisable.

Chitosan can be used in many different applications. In biomedical applications, Chitosan can act as an interaction site in order to increase the adsorption capacity [31]. Therefore, in this work chitosan was used in the coating process in which both activated carbon fiber (ACF) and date pit activated carbon (DPAC) samples were coated with Chitosan [32]. The chitosan used in coating both materials contains amino (−NH2) and hydroxyl (−OH) groups on its chains [33]. These groups accomplished the main benefit of using chitosan. In other words, these groups helped in forming AC with a large adsorption capacity [34].

Chitosan is a natural source that is available abundantly in nature. It can be produced and found naturally in the cell walls of fungi, the shells of crustaceans and the shells of insects [35]. It is produced commercially in many different forms. Chitosan powder is one of the forms which can be used and found in the market [36]. Thus, in this work the chitosan powder is used in making chitosan gel which will be used to coat the samples of ACF and DPAC.

This work focuses on removing the epoxy from CFRP and activating, both date pit powder and CFRP at different temperatures. This will allow a comparison of the results under different conditions to find the optimum activating temperature for the materials. Chitosan gel is then prepared by mixing chitosan powder and dilute acetic acid. The resulting solution is used to coat both types of charcoal. It is expected that coating will increase the adsorption efficiency of the materials by providing a high binding affinity for carbon fiber. The resulting samples are all compared to conclude which material has a higher bilirubin adsorption capacity and the optimum activation temperature for the DPAC and ACF.

Further studies will later be conducted regarding the use of the different types of charcoal produced for the adsorption of albumin-bound bilirubin. Batch tests will be carried out on different samples to test for the effect of coated AC dosage on the adsorption capacity of the materials. Moreover, the contact time between the coated AC and bilirubin toxin will be tested to determine whether increasing the contact time will increase the amount of bilirubin adsorbed.

3. Experimental processing

3.1. Materials

The aim of this work is to use thermal treatment by pyrolysis to remove the epoxy from the CFRP and prepare the material for activation. According to literature, some drawbacks to pyrolysis may be faced, including the loss of mechanical properties such as tensile strength and elasticity. Furthermore, the fibers released are likely to be covered in char, a black residue formed during the thermal degradation of the resin.

Several materials were utilized in the preparation, pyrolysis and activation processes of the CFRP.

To prepare the CFRP sheets, obtained from the aerospace industry, for pyrolysis, the sheets of material are shredded into strips. This is to enable their placement in the furnace to carry out the thermal treatments. The steps toward activated carbon fiber are pyrolysis and activation, both carried out in a furnace (GSL – 1500X). the samples of CFRP are separately placed in the steel roll inside the furnace. For the pyrolysis process, nitrogen gas (N_2) is passed through the sample and for activation, carbon dioxide (CO_2) is passed into the steel roll. In order to control the operation temperatures inside the furnace, it is connected to a laptop with the PT software installed. The temperature program to be run is added to this software and the temperature rises and falls are monitored on the screen.

Following pyrolysis, samples of the treated carbon fiber are immersed in acetone to indicate the presence or absence of epoxy. In accordance to later tests, if the acetone turned into a yellow color, this is an indication of the presence of epoxy in the sample.

3.2. Procedural setups

3.2.1. Pyrolysis

The carbon fiber reinforced polymer is waste product obtained from the aerospace industry. It is attained in sheets, which are shredded before carrying out treatment and tests. The method followed for activating the material is physical activation to avoid contamination or poisoning in case the activated carbon fiber is to be used for purification or medical purposes. Physical activation involves a two-step process; pyrolysis and activation.

The aim of pyrolysis is to remove the epoxy in the material as well as provide an inert atmosphere for activation to take place. The process involves passing nitrogen gas through the sample. The shredded CFRP is added to the steel roll, which is then inserted into the furnace. The steel roll is positioned correctly using a marked rod and the furnace is closed from both ends with tubes through which the nitrogen gas will flow. The gas enters and leaves the furnace passing through the CFRP sample. To ensure that approximately the right amount of gas is passing through the sample, the outlet tube is connected to a tilted water bottle and the bubbles created are observed. To change the gas flow rate, the valve on the nitrogen gas cylinder is controlled.

Passing an inert gas through the sample aims at removing impurities, such as hydrogen and oxygen to create a more stable and heat resistant compound composed mainly of carbon. The pyrolysis treatment is carried out by increasing the temperature inside the furnace while passing the gas through the steel roll. The temperature is kept at its peak for a specific period of time before it is dropped back to room temperature. To control the temperature rises and falls, the furnace is connected to a laptop with the PT software installed where a simple program is entered for the various temperatures and durations.

To find the optimum temperature for the pyrolysis and activation processes, they are executed at various temperatures; 600, 800 and 1000°C. Tests are later used to decide which treatment temperature is most effective.

3.2.2. *Acetone test*

One of the biggest challenges faced in this work is the removal of the epoxy in the material. This is because the exact nature of the epoxy is unknown due to restrictions from the aircraft manufacturers. Therefore, acetone testing is used after the pyrolysis process as a step to ensure that the epoxy has been eliminated from the material. Approximately 20 ml of acetone are added to a beaker and a sample of the material which has undergone pyrolysis treatment is added to the beaker and left to soak overnight. It is expected that the acetone of the sample containing epoxy turns yellow, as opposed to clear for the sample which contains no epoxy. This test is done on samples treated at all temperatures prior to activation.

3.2.3. *Activation*

During the next stage, carbon dioxide gas is passed through the sample to allow some carbon to react with it producing carbon monoxide gas, as shown in Eq. (1), which is then removed from the system through the water bottle with the excess gas. This process is known as gasification and develops porosity in the material by removing some carbon atoms. The furnace is operated in a similar way to the pyrolysis process with the only difference being the gas utilized. Since pyrolysis treatments will be carried out at three different temperatures of 600, 800 and 1000°C, the same will be done with the activation treatment.

$$C + CO_2 \rightarrow 2CO \tag{1}$$

It is expected, according to previous literature, that the carbon fiber will have a larger adsorption capacity of toxins than powdered activated carbon. In order to prove this, the adsorption capacity of the activated carbon fiber will be tested and compared with the adsorption capacity of activated date pit powder.

3.2.4. *Chitosan gel preparation and coating*

Chitosan gel is used to coat a sample of the DPAC to allow for comparisons with the ACF and uncoated DPAC. To prepare the chitosan gel, 198 ml of water are mixed with 2 ml of acetic acid in a reagent bottle to form dilute acetic acid. The outcome is a 1% concentrated acetic acid by volume. 100 ml of the solution is then measured using a measuring cylinder and poured into a beaker with a magnet placed inside and put on a magnetic stirrer to stir and heat the solution first. 0.5 g of chitosan powder is gradually added to the stirring diluted acid, to avoid splashes, clumping and achieve a more even distribution. The magnetic stirrer is set at a temperature around 45°C. Approximately an hour later, when the chitosan gel has reached the desired consistency, 5 g of the activated carbon are weighed and added gradually to the gel after turning off the heater so the mixture is only stirring. The carbon is then left to coat overnight as it stirs (for about 24 hours). The coating procedure is carried out three times while oven drying between each coating. This is done to ensure that the DPAC is fully coated [8].

3.3. Experimental techniques used

For determining the characterization of activated carbon fiber, FTIR and TGA analysis are conducted.

3.3.1. *FTIR (Fourier transform infrared spectroscopy)*

The main benefits of using a Fourier Transform Infrared (FTIR) spectroscopy is that it is quick and takes measurements in a matter of seconds. It also has a very high sensitivity due to the extremely delicate detectors employed in the device. Infrared spectroscopy gives information about the chemical structure and functional groups of raw materials and the prepared activated carbon. The data obtained presented information about the interaction and polymeric association between chitosan and carbon. The Infra-red transmission spectra were recorded with a Perkin Elmer spectrophotometer ranging from 400 to 4000 cm^{-1} using the KBr technique.

3.3.2. *TGA test*

TGA (Thermogravimetric analysis) is an essential method used in materials characterization. It is a technique in which the mass of a substance is measured as a function of temperature or time as the sample is monitored under a controlled atmosphere. This technique provides useful information about chemical phenomena such as solid–gas reactions and thermal decomposition, as well as physical phenomena including phase transitions, absorption and desorption. A typical TGA analyzer consists of a sample pan that is backed by a precision balance inside a furnace. The temperature inside the furnace is programmed under a controlled temperature. The mass of the sample is monitored during the experiment. This experiment may occur under different conditions in which it could be conducted under a variety of atmospheres including: inert gas, carburizing gases, ambient air, vapors and vacuum. Also, the experiment might take place under a variety of pressures such as high vacuum, high pressure, and constant pressure. The data collected from the thermal reactions which occur inside the TGA are represented into a plot. That plot is indicating the thermal curve which is displayed as time or temperature in the x-axis and as weight (mg) or weight percent (%) in the y-axis. The TGA thermal curve provides different useful information about the characteristics of the materials. The purity of the sample is one of the characteristics that can be determined using the TGA thermal curve. This can be accomplished by calculating the formula weight through substituting the atomic mass in the formula and then comparing the measured values with the calculated ones. To further characterize the sample, an extrapolated onset temperature that represents the temperature at which the weight loss starts can be calculated. Another useful calculation that illustrates one of the characterization of the sample is the peak calculation of the first derivative of the weight loss curve. The peak of the 1st derivative shows the inflection point which is basically represents the point of greatest rate of change on the weight loss curve. The temperature range at which thermolysis would be performed is determined by analyzing the samples thermogravimetrically.

4. Results and discussion

4.1. FTIR analysis

4.1.1. Date pits activated carbon

FTIR Analysis, was conducted for further identification of the functional groups present in activated carbon. **Figure 1** depicts the corresponding FTIR range of the date pit activated carbon that primarily concludes that phenols, carboxylic acids, and carbonyl functional groups are the ones present, all of which are categorized as typical acidic functional groups.

Furthermore, the spectrum consisted of an IR band of around 3427 cm^{-1} which is assigned to a vibration stretch of hydroxyl group denoted as OH. Additionally, C=O group frequency is observed at a wavelength of 1720 cm^{-1} while aliphatic groups at around 2923 and 2855 cm^{-1}, along with 1033 cm^{-1} which corresponds to C—O stretching, as tabulated in **Table 1**. In elucidating chitosan coated carbon's FTIR spectra that merely represent the adsorption of both chitosan and carbon, it has been noted, as **Figure 1** demonstrates, that the stretching vibration of O—H and N—H functional groups are observed at a frequency of 3433 cm^{-1}. The bands at around 2923 and 2855 cm^{-1} correspond to the asymmetric and symmetric stretching. Moreover, the peaks in the range of 1630, 1157, 1381, 1017 and 890 cm^{-1} assigned to N—H bending, C—N stretching, O—H in plane bending, C—C—C Skeletal in the backbone and CH_3—C—OH stretching respectively as recorded in **Table 1**. Bands around 647 and 496 cm^{-1} indicate the presence of OH and C—C bending vibrations respectively [19].

4.1.2. Activated carbon fiber

Fourier Transform Infrared Spectroscopy (FTIR) analysis is done in order to identify the functional groups associated with the activated carbon fiber. The **Figure 2** illustrates the FTIR specterum obtained from the carbon fiber before and after activation at different temperatures of 500, 600, 800 and 1000°C. The spectrum shows an IR band of 3600 and 3200 cm^{-1} is assigned

http://dx.doi.org/10.5772/intechopen.71891

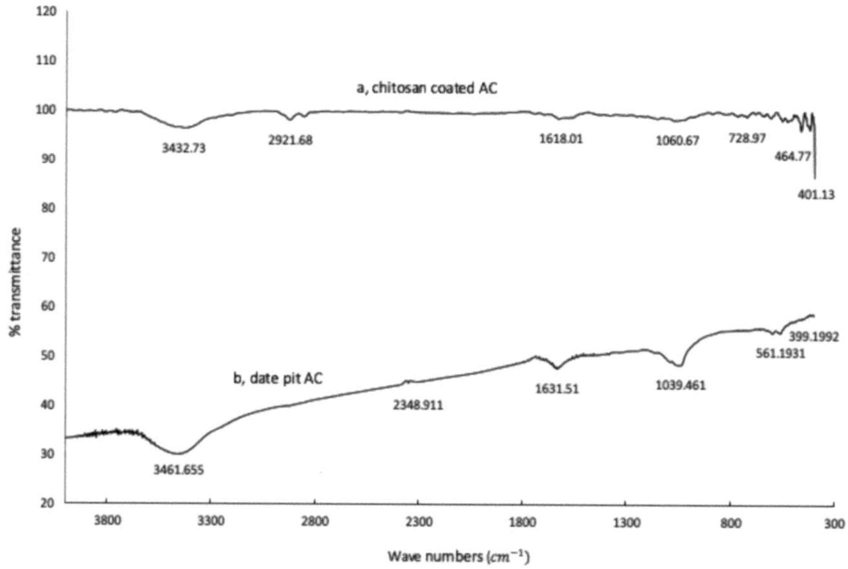

Figure 1. FTIR spectrum of the date pit activated carbon.

to the hydroxyl (OH) group and the peak at 2329 cm^{-1} is related to the C ≡ C stretching as the data in **Table 1** presents. Furthermore, the frequency observed at a wavelength of 1843 cm^{-1} is due to the CHO stretching. 1450–1479 cm^{-1} are related to the vibrations of the CH bonds. Peaks at 1068–1148 cm^{-1} and 1565cm^{-1} are attributed to the vibrations at C—O—C and N-H stretching respectively. Moreover, the non-symmetric vibration absorption of C=O is illustrated in the peak at 1840 cm^{-1}, as well as the stretching vibration of the C=O or C=N present at 1750–1640 cm^{-1}. The peaks at around 1403 and 650 cm^{-1} are due to the CH_2 bending and OH bending vibration frequency respectively. According to the data illustrated for the ACF, it is observed that the spectrum at different temperatures portrays similar patterns but the intensity of the absorption bands is increased as the treatment temperature is increased.

4.2. TGA (Thermogravimetric analysis)

4.2.1. Date pits activated carbon

Thermogravimetric analysis (TGA) and differential thermogravimetric analysis (DTG) profiles of the DP-AC are shown in **Figure 3**. The TGA curve gives an approximation about the weight loss of the sample with respect to temperature, while the DTG curve indicates the decomposition temperature as well as the oxidation temperature of the sample. The first decomposition stage occurred between 21.5 °C ≈ 99°C where a weight loss of 10.4% was observed. This loss was due to the release of surface bounded water and volatile matters. The highest rate of degradation in this stage was indicated by the peak on the DTG curve at a maximum rate of decomposition temperature of 54°C. The next stage showed a slower rate of weight loss with only 10.6% change over a wide range of temperature between 100°C up to 900°C. Most of the weight loss in this stage was due to the decomposition of hemicellulose and cellulose constituents. While for temperatures above ≈ 450°C, the weight loss was due to decomposition of

Functional Group	Wavelength
Activated Carbon Fiber	
OH	3600 cm^{-1} – 3200 cm^{-1}
C≡C stretching	2329 cm^{-1}
CHO stretching	1843 cm^{-1}
CH bonds	1450 cm^{-1} – 1479 cm^{-1}
C-O-C vibrations	1068 cm^{-1} – 1148 cm^{-1}
N-H stretching	1565 cm^{-1}
C=O	1840 cm^{-1}
C=N	1750 cm^{-1} – 1640 cm^{-1}
CH_2 bending	1403 cm^{-1}
OH bending vibration	650 cm^{-1}
Chitosan Coated AC	
N-H bending	1630 cm^{-1}
C-N stretching	1157 cm^{-1}
O-H bending	1381 cm^{-1}
C-C-C	1017 cm^{-1}
CH_3-C-OH	890 cm^{-1}
OH	647 cm^{-1}
C-C	496 cm^{-1}
Date Pit AC	
OH	3427 cm^{-1}
C=O	1720 cm^{-1}
C-O	1033 cm^{-1}
Aliphatic Groups	2923 cm^{-1} – 2855 cm^{-1}

Table 1. Functional groups associated with wavelength bands.

lignin. At temperature 900°C, the amount of ash residual was 79% which is considered as indication for the thermal stability of the material (date pits activated carbon) under investigation over a broad range of temperatures.

4.2.2. Activated carbon fiber

Thermogravimetric analyses (TGA) were conducted in a TA (schimadzu Q40) equipment. The samples of the activated carbon fiber were heated up to 600°C at a heating rate of 10°C/min under nitrogen atmosphere (flow rate 100 mL/min). Using the data obtained, TGA curves were prepared as shown in **Figure 4**. The TGA curve produced shows the weight loss versus time curves for several temperatures. The temperatures at which the activated carbon fibers were prepared during the pyrolysis are indicated in **Figure 4**. Based on **Figure 4**, it can be clearly

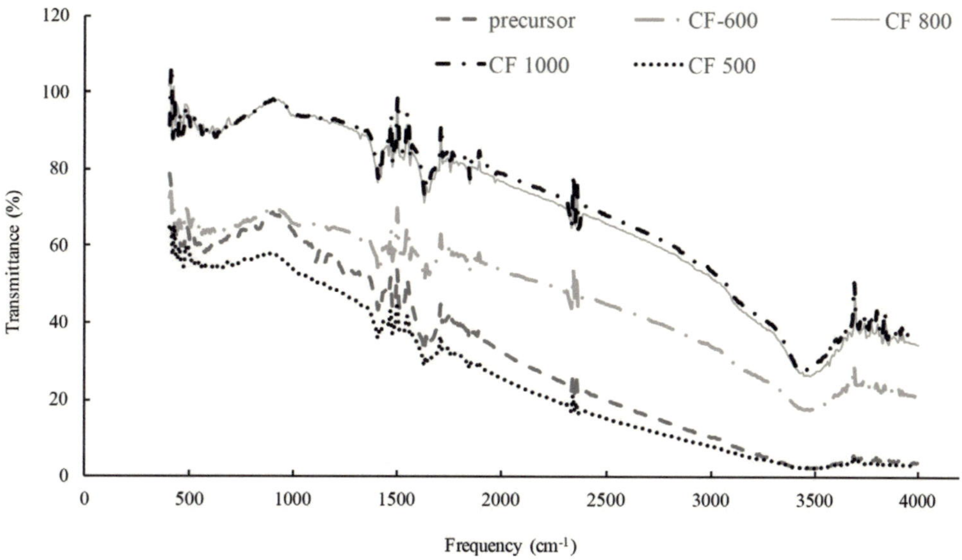

Figure 2. FTIR spectrum of the activated carbon fiber.

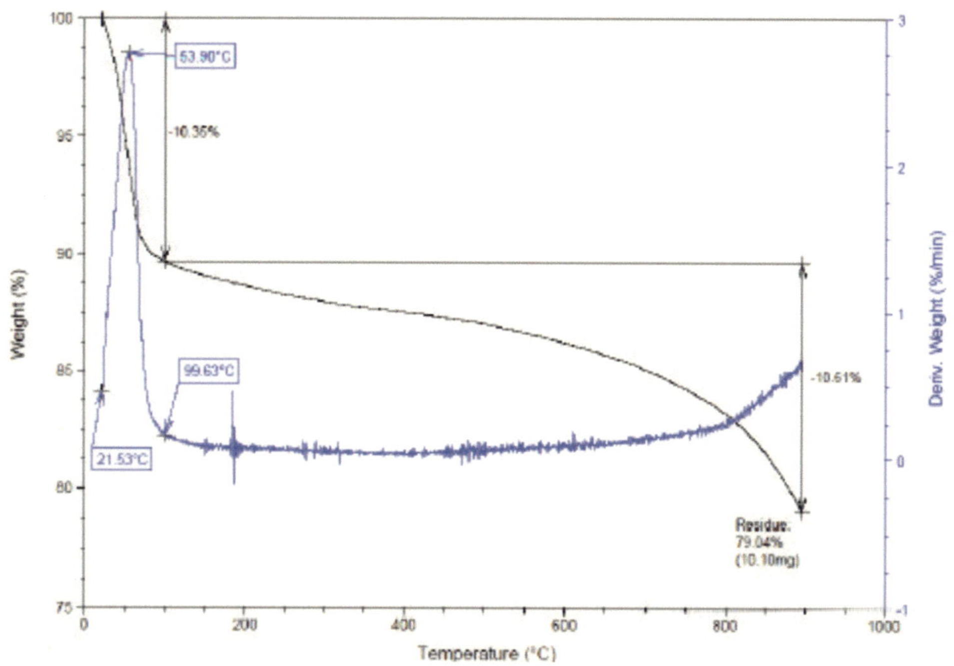

Figure 3. TGA profile of date pit activated carbon.

seen that the TGA test was done for several samples of activated carbon fiber at different temperatures. These temperatures are 500, 600, 800 and 1000°C. TGA curve shows a weight loss due to the release of moisture at 200°C. Only one prominent weight loss peak around 300

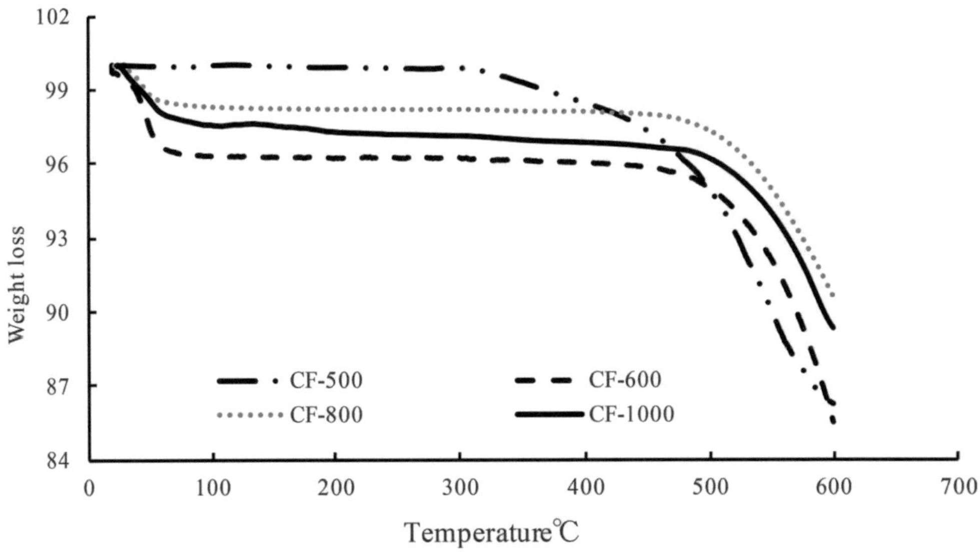

Figure 4. TGA profile of activated carbon fiber.

to 550°C was observed in the derivative mass loss curve. The corresponding weight loss between 300 to 550°C is related to the pyrolysis of the material. Similar patterns were observed for all the samples at various temperatures.

FTIR results give information about the functional groups present on the two materials; DPAC and ACF. This test allows for comparisons between the composition and makeup of the activated carbon. The TGA tests allow observations related to the material behavior under temperature conditions and drawing conclusions based on the variation of the activated material. Consequently, these assessments acknowledge important aspects of the ACs and provide a means for their comparisons. However, the adsorption capacity for bilirubin was not tested and therefore, direct conclusions regarding which material is a better adsorbent for bilirubin could not be drawn. Therefore, this test will be studied and conducted in further research.

5. Conclusion

The results presented above show that activation of date pits and CFRP was successful. The preparation of ACs from date pits and CFRPs and their characterization pave the way for their applications in the field of clinical practice, notably, for the adsorption of bilirubin, which is considered a toxin secreted by patients suffering from liver failure.

Data generated from the processes of activation and characterization showed that the rates of absorption for activated carbon fiber materials, as expected, were higher as compared to the date pits AC. This was noticed by the visibly larger peak frequencies on the FTIR graphs indicating higher absorption of the CFs. Furthermore, TGA graphs illustrated higher thermal properties meaning that the CF is a better absorbent.

These findings also confirm the ability of date pits AC and CFRPs as adsorbent of toxins and potential candidates for consideration in the search for effective treatment options for liver failure.

Acknowledgements

The authors would like to thank UAEU for their support of the project. This work has been financially funded by the SURE program at UAE University, Al Ain.

Author details

Ameereh Seyedzadeh, Asel Mwafy, Waleed Khalil Ahmed, Kamala Pandurangan and Ali Hilal-Alnaqbi*

*Address all correspondence to: alihilal@uaeu.ac.ae

Department of Mechanical Engineering, College of Engineering, United Arab Emirates University, Al Ain, UAE

References

[1] Annesini M, Piemonte V, Turchetti L. Removal of albumin-bound toxins from albumin-containing solutions: Tryptophan fixed-bed adsorption on activated carbon. Chemical Engineering Research and Design. 2010;**88**(8):1018-1023

[2] Magosso E, Ursino M, Colì L, Baraldi O, Bolondi L, Stefoni S. A modeling study of bilirubin kinetics during molecular adsorbent recirculating system sessions. Artificial Organs. 2006;**30**(4):285-300

[3] Ding W, Zou L, Sun S, Li W, Gao D. A new method to increase the adsorption of protein-bound toxins in artificial liver support systems. Artificial Organs. 2014;**38**(11):954-962

[4] McKenzie TJ, Lillegard JB, Nyberg SL, editors. Artificial and Bioartificial Liver Support. Seminars in Liver Disease. Thieme Medical Publishers. 2008;**28**(02):210-217

[5] Puri P, Anand AC. Liver support devices. MEDICINE. 2012;**22**

[6] Shinke K, Ando K, Koyama T, Takai T, Nakaji S, Ogino T. Properties of various carbon nanomaterial surfaces in bilirubin adsorption. Colloids and Surfaces B: Biointerfaces. 2010;**77**(1):18-21

[7] Nieuwoudt MJ. Bio-Artificial Liver Support System: An Evaluation of Models Used in Demonstrating or Improving Metabolic and Clinical Efficacy. University of Pretoria; 2010

[8] Asano T, Tsuru K, Hayakawa S, Osaka A. Bilirubin adsorption property of sol-gel-derived titania particles for blood purification therapy. Acta Biomaterialia. 2008;**4**(4):1067-1072

[9] Puppalwar P, Goswami K, Dhok A. Review on "evolution of methods of bilirubin estimation". IOSR Journal of Dental and Medical Sciences. 2012;**1**(3):17-28

[10] Annesini M, Carlo C, Piemonte V, Turchetti L. Bilirubin and tryptophan adsorption in albumin-containing solutions I: Equilibrium isotherms on activated carbon. Biochemical Engineering Journal. 2008;**40**(2):205-210

[11] Ash S, Sullivan T, Carr D. Sorbent suspension vs. sorbent columns for extracorporeal detoxification in hepatic failure. Therapeutic Apheresis and Dialysis. 2006;**10**(2):145-153

[12] Nikolaev V, Sarnatskaya V, Sigal V, Klevtsov V, Makhorin K, Yushko L. High-porosity activated carbon for bilirubin removal. The International Journal of Artificial Organs. 1991;**14**(3):179-185

[13] Chandy T, Sharma C. Polylysine-immobilized chitosan beads as adsorbents for bilirubin. The International Journal of Artificial Organs. 1992;**16**(6):568-576

[14] Phalakornkule C, Foungchuen J, Pitakchon T. Impregnation of chitosan onto activated carbon for high adsorption selectivity towards CO2: CO2 capture from biohydrogen, biogas and flue gas. Journal of Sustainable Energy & Environment. 2012;**3**(4):153-157

[15] Cobb A, Warms M, Maurer EP, Chiesa S. Low-tech coconut shell activated charcoal production. International Journal for Service Learning in Engineering. 2012;**7**(1):93-104

[16] Hossain MZ, Waly MI, Singh V, Sequeira V, Rahman MS. Chemical composition of date-pits and its potential for developing value-added product-a review. Polish Journal of Food and Nutrition Sciences. 2014;**64**(4):215-226

[17] Jiang G, Pickering SJ, Lester E, Blood P, Warrior N, editors. Recycling Carbon Fibre/Epoxy Resin Composites Using Supercritical Propanol. 16th International Conference on Composite Materials, Kyoto, Japan;. Japan: Japan Society for Composite Materials Kyoto; 2007

[18] Witik RA, Teuscher R, Michaud V, Ludwig C, Månson J-AE. Carbon fibre reinforced composite waste: An environmental assessment of recycling, energy recovery and landfilling. Composites Part A: Applied Science and Manufacturing. 2013;**49**:89-99

[19] López FA, Rodríguez O, Alguacil FJ, García-Díaz I, Centeno TA, García-Fierro JL, et al. Recovery of carbon fibres by the thermolysis and gasification of waste prepreg. Journal of Analytical and Applied Pyrolysis. 2013;**104**:675-683

[20] Feraboli P, Kawakami H, Wade B, Gasco F, DeOto L, Masini A. Recyclability and reutilization of carbon fiber fabric/epoxy composites. Journal of Composite Materials. 2012;**46**(12):1459-1473

[21] Nilakantan G, Olliges R, Su R, Nutt S, Center MGC, editors. Reuse Strategies for Carbon Fibre-Epoxy Prepreg Scrap. Orlando, FL: CAMX Conference Proceedings; 2014

[22] McConnell VP. Launching the carbon fibre recycling industry. Reinforced Plastics. 2010;**54**(2):33-37

[23] Costa ML, Botelho EC, JMFd P, Rezende MC. Characterization of cure of carbon/epoxy prepreg used in aerospace field. Materials Research. 2005;**8**(3):317-322

[24] Lee T, Ooi C-H, Othman R, Yeoh F-Y. Activated carbon fiber-the hybrid of carbon fiber and activated carbon. Reviews on Advanced Materials Science. 2014;**36**(2):118-136

[25] Pimenta S, Pinho ST. Recycling carbon fibre reinforced polymers for structural applications: Technology review and market outlook. Waste Management. 2011;**31**(2):378-392

[26] Yang Y, Boom R, Irion B, van Heerden D-J, Kuiper P, de Wit H. Recycling of composite materials. Chemical Engineering and Processing Process Intensification. 2012;**51**:53-68

[27] Loos MR, Coelho LAF, Pezzin SH, Amico SC. The effect of acetone addition on the properties of epoxy. Polímeros. 2008;**18**(1):76-80

[28] Oliveux G, Dandy LO, Leeke GA. Current status of recycling of fibre reinforced polymers: Review of technologies, reuse and resulting properties. Progress in Materials Science. 2015;**72**:61-99

[29] Jiang G, Pickering SJ, Lester EH, Turner T, Wong K, Warrior N. Characterisation of carbon fibres recycled from carbon fibre/epoxy resin composites using supercritical n-propanol. Composites Science and Technology. 2009;**69**(2):192-198

[30] Pickering SJ. Recycling technologies for thermoset composite materials—Current status. Composites Part A: Applied Science and Manufacturing. 2006;**37**(8):1206-1215

[31] Luk CJ, Joanne Y, Chunwah MY, Chiwai K, Kimhung LA. Comprehensive study on adsorption behaviour of direct, reactive and acid dyes on crosslinked and non-crosslinked chitosan beads. Journal of Fiber Bioengineering and Informatics. 2014:35-52

[32] Kyzas GZ, Bikiaris DN. Recent modifications of chitosan for adsorption applications: A critical and systematic review. Marine Drugs. 2015;**13**(1):312-337

[33] Okoya AA, Akinyele AB, Amuda OS, Ofoezie IE. Chitosan-grafted carbon for the sequestration of heavy metals in aqueous solution. American Chemical Science Journal. 2016;**11**(3):1-14

[34] Luk CJ, Yip J, Yuen CM, Kan C, Lam KA. Comprehensive study on adsorption behaviour of direct, reactive and acid dyes on crosslinked and non-crosslinked chitosan beads. Journal of Fiber Bioengineering and Informatics. 2014;**7**(1):35-52

[35] Kyzas GZ, Dimitrios NB. Recent modifications of chitosan for adsorption applications: A critical and systematic review. Marine Drugs. 2015;**13**:312-337

[36] Moussaoui Y, Mnasri N, Elaloui E, Salem RB, Lagerge S, de Menorval L, editors. Preparation of Chitosan Gel. EDP Sciences: EPJ Web of Conferences; 2012

Section 3

Forensic Toxicology Topics

Chapter 9

Simplified Analysis of Toxic Gaseous Substance in Forensic Practice: Experiences from Japan

Hiroshi Kinoshita, Naoko Tanaka, Ayaka Takakura,
Mostofa Jamal, Asuka Ito, Mitsuru Kumihashi,
Shoji Kimura, Kunihiko Tsutsui, Shuji Matsubara and
Kiyoshi Ameno

Additional information is available at the end of the chapter

http://dx.doi.org/10.5772/intechopen.70029

Abstract

Toxicological examination in forensic practice is important for the proper diagnosis of acute poisoning. We have discussed the properties and features of poisoning incidents due to gaseous substances and elaborated on the simplified analytical techniques and apparatus used for their identification and quantitation for forensic purposes. Briefly, we have explained the simplified analysis of toxic gaseous substances such as carbon monoxide, hydrogen cyanide, hydrogen sulfide, and helium in blood. The techniques used include color testing, gas chromatography, detector tube, oximeter, and spectrophotometric method. In doing so, we have shared our experiences and highlighted the fact that the analysis of gaseous substances can be performed using readily available laboratory tools and equipment. We have emphasized the need and usefulness of the reference data tables for guiding forensic diagnosis. We hope that the above overview will assist other colleagues to implement such simplified techniques for the advancement of forensic medicine practice.

Keywords: toxicological examination, toxic gaseous substances, simplified analysis

1. Introduction

Toxicological examination in forensic practice is important for the proper diagnosis of acute poisoning [1]. The forensic pathologist requests toxicological analysis to forensic toxicologist in case of poisoning or poisoning suspected cases. It will usually consist of two-stage testing at autopsy [2]. The first step is usually performed as a screening test. The second step is required for the identification and quantification of its causative agent following the confirmatory test. Toxic gaseous substances are one of the targets for toxicological examination in a daily forensic practice. Simplified analysis of gaseous substances involves both first and second step of toxicological examination in forensic practice.

In the present chapter, we share our experiences about the analysis of gaseous substances such as carbon monoxide, hydrogen sulfide, cyanide, and helium.

2. Autopsy and subsequent toxicological examination in gas-related poisoning incidents

Gaseous substances can cause acute poisoning. They get absorbed into the body by inhalation. Most of them do not produce specific symptoms but they can induce dizziness, lethargy, headaches, and suffocation. There is no specific finding at autopsy in most poisoning cases [1, 2]. Most of gaseous substances cause little or no tissue damages. However, there will be observed unique findings in some poisoning cases, such as cherry red appearance of postmortem lividity in carbon monoxide poisoning, bright pink lividity with bitter almond odor in cyanide poisoning, and dark green coloration and rotten egg smell in hydrogen sulfide poisoning [2]. Nonspecific findings such as generalized organ congestion and pulmonary edema may be observed in most cases [1]. The presence of gaseous poisons is usually indicated by the circumstances of the incident, and involvement of gaseous substances is sometimes indicated by circumstantial evidence [3].

Although detailed management is out of scope of this chapter, it is sufficient to mention that the management of poisoning by gaseous substances involves the use of antidotes when available; decontamination; artificial respiration with demand-valve resuscitators, bag-valve-mask devices; administration of hyperbaric oxygen; performance of cardiopulmonary resuscitation (CPR); and close observation and monitoring of vital signs.

In our laboratories, toxicological examination is routinely performed on a daily basis—from the screening test using immunoassay kits to subsequent identification and quantification using gas chromatography mass spectrometry or liquid chromatography mass spectrometry techniques. Since the physiological effects of most gaseous substances correlate with the concentration in blood, it becomes the best indicator of toxicity [4]. As numerous reference tables for fatal levels of chemicals have been reported [5–9], forensic diagnosis is made in reference to the values reported in the data tables. In addition, several other factors have to be considered for toxicological evaluation; these include the properties of the sample, diffusion and redistribution, degradation, and metabolism [1, 2, 10, 11]. In the light of the above, we have instituted simplified analysis techniques for gaseous substances; these techniques provide a lot of information promptly that aid forensic diagnosis. In the following paragraphs, we describe these techniques for each of the main gaseous substances.

http://dx.doi.org/10.5772/intechopen.70029

3. Specific substances and its simplified analysis methods

3.1. Carbon monoxide (CO)

CO is an odorless, nonirritable, and colorless gas and is slightly lighter than air (specific gravity for the air; 0.97). It is mainly produced by incomplete combustion of fuels or carbon compounds [8, 12]. Its common sources are vehicle exhaust, smoke from fire, and improperly maintained heating systems. CO is the leading cause of poisoning death in Japan [13–15], and also a common cause of poisoning in the United States [16, 17]. The annual number of victims by CO poisoning is about 2000–4000 in Japan, including accidental or suicidal cases [13–15]. CO is absorbed from the lung into the bloodstream. As the affinity of CO for hemoglobin is 230–270 times greater than that of oxygen, it binds to hemoglobin in erythrocyte, and forms carboxyhemoglobin (CO-Hb) [12, 18, 19]. The formation of CO-Hb (represented as a percentage of the total hemoglobin) in blood depends on various factors such as the concentration of inspired CO, duration of CO exposure, pulmonary ventilation, exercise, and health status [12, 18]. The toxicity of CO is thought to be tissue hypoxia due to the formation of CO-Hb. Its binding is a reversible process; however, as the binding between CO and hemoglobin is strong, the CO elimination half-life is long, about 4–5 hours under room air ventilation for a resting adult at sea level. The formation of CO-Hb decreases the capacity of oxygen transport, and it causes insufficient oxygen supply in tissues [12, 18, 19].

The hypoxia due to CO-Hb formation causes signs and symptoms. Clinical symptoms roughly correlate with CO-Hb levels (**Table 1**). The CO-Hb concentration of nonsmoking healthy subjects is 1–3%, and around 5–8% in smokers. No symptom is observed below 10% of CO-Hb levels. Neurological symptoms such as headache, dizziness, nausea, and weakness are observed in CO-Hb level from 10 to 30%. Increase of respiration and heart rate, syncope, and confusion are observed in 30–50% of CO-Hb level. When the level of CO-Hb exceeds 50%, it becomes life-threatening. It is noteworthy that the value of CO-Hb is important for the diagnosis of CO-poisoning or fire-related death [12, 18, 19]. In addition to hemoglobin, CO

CO-Hb (%)	Clinical symptom
0–10	No symptom
10–20	Headache, ear ringing, fatigue
20–30	Headache, weakness, nausea, vomiting
30–40	Severe headache, dizziness, nausea, vomiting
40–50	Syncope, confusion, increased respiration and heart rate, muscle weakness
50–60	Coma, convulsions, depressed respiration
60–70	Coma, convulsions, cardiorespiratory depression, often fatal
70+	Respiratory failure, death

Table 1. Correlation of carboxyhemoglobin (CO-Hb) levels to clinical symptoms.

combines with heme-proteins such as myoglobin and cytochrome oxidase, and it may cause the impairment of cardiac and neurological functions [12, 18].

The most characteristic appearance of the body in poisoning case is a cherry red color of the skin. It is usually observed in cases where CO-Hb exceeds 30% [1]. At autopsy, the common findings include discoloration of blood, organs, and muscle that become cherry red color, as a result of CO-Hb and carboxymyoglobin. Other autopsy findings such as pulmonary edema and generalized organ congestion are also observed [1].

With regard to the identification and quantification of CO, several methods and techniques have been reported [20]. Spectrophotometric methods and gas chromatography techniques are widely used. The CO-Hb is relatively stable under storage in cool and dark conditions [18, 21–23]. It is important to note that postmortem production of CO has been reported in some conditions, and therefore, it is recommended not to use body cavity fluids such as pleural effusion for the measurement of CO in severe putrefied case [24–28].

For identification purposes, the qualitative test for CO includes color test and microdiffusion tests. Color test is a simple procedure where a blood sample mixed with 0.01 M ammonia solution (1:20) [29] or a few drops of blood are added to some 10% sodium hydroxide solution [1]. This test is based on the fact that CO-Hb is relatively tolerant to alkaline condition. However, as other simple methods have been established, color testing for CO poisoning is now rarely required and not recommended [1, 29]. The microdiffusion test using Conway cell [30] or on the filter paper [31] have been reported. It is based on reaction with palladium chloride. This is still the most widely used method since it was invented by Conway in 1944.

With regard to quantification, spectrophotometric method, gas chromatography, detection tube, and oximeter are used. The spectrophotometric method is the most popular, and various assay procedures have been reported. CO-Hb could be determined by the changes of absorption spectrum in either Soret (410–425 nm) [32–34] or visible region (500–600 nm) [30, 35–38]. In our laboratories, we perform the measurement of the spectrum of blood sample by adding sodium hydrosulfite. The addition of sodium dithionite reduces oxyhemoglobin without affecting the CO-Hb. This procedure is simple, and it does not need an extraction from the sample. **Figure 1** shows the spectra of blood samples from a normal nonsmoker (CO-Hb: 0%) and CO poisoning victim (CO-Hb: 68 and 95%, respectively). Twin-peaked spectrum was observed in CO poisoning sample.

The CO is extracted and introduced in gas chromatography. Various methods and apparatus have been reported for its extraction [39–44]. And the released CO is detected by the thermal conductivity detector (TCD) [39–42, 44], or the flame ionization detector with the catalytic reduction of the CO to methane [43]. As this method is a direct measurement of CO contents in the sample as well as a measurement of the hemoglobin, two measures represent the percentage of CO-Hb. Application of gas chromatography equipped with semiconductor detector has been reported for forensic practice [45]. This gas chromatography system (sensor gas chromatography, sGC) is highly sensitive for CO and has some advantages such as portability and easy handling. This apparatus does not need a gas cylinder as it uses the room air as the career gas. Although it is not commonly in use, further application in the field of forensic medicine would be expected.

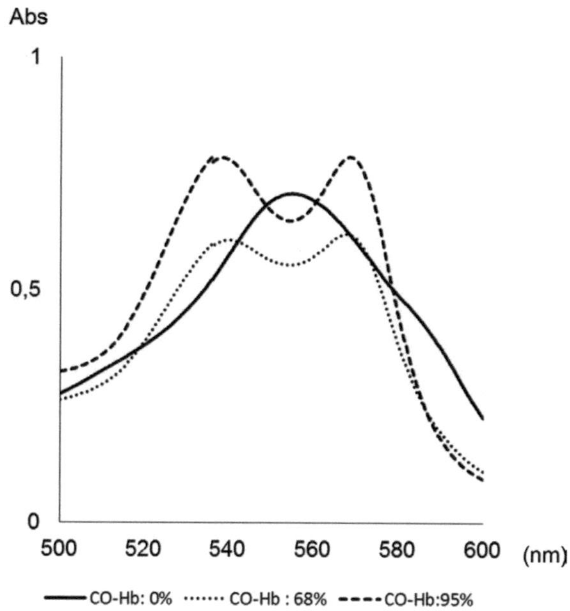

Figure 1. Spectra of blood sample from CO-Hb: 0, 68, and 95%, respectively.

The detector tube method is widely used for the determination of various gaseous substances [46, 47]. It is also applied for the quantitation of CO in blood [48]. This apparatus consists of a CO-separator tube, CO-detector tube, and aspirating pump. The CO-separator tube is packed with silica gel particles coated with ferricyanide [48]. The CO-detector tube is packed with silica gel particles coated with sulfite palladium potassium [46, 49]. These tubes and pump are connected in series. The CO in blood is released following the injection of blood sample (200 μL) in CO-separator tube, and the released CO gas is detected by the CO-detector tube, followed by the aspirating of the pump. As the detector tube is easy to carry at the scene where an incident has taken place or to a point-of-care testing, it is applied to not only screening test, but also for quantitation.

Oximeter is routinely used for laboratory test [50, 51], and it is also applied in forensic medicines [52–64]. This instrument uses seven wavelengths in the visible region for the determination of various hemoglobin species, such as oxyhemoglobin, CO-Hb, reduced hemoglobin, and methemoglobin. It automatically analyzes the proportion of each species of hemoglobin and oxygen contents. This oximeter system (**Figure 2**) requires 50 μL of blood for a single measurement, and it may be a valid option in case of difficult blood sampling due to severe blood loss. As there are many advantages such as no necessity of sample preparation, easy handling, and portability, it is suitable for forensic practice. In a recent study, it has been reported that squeezed splenic blood can be used as an alternative specimen for CO-Hb measurement using oximeter [65].

3.2. Cyanide

Hydrogen cyanide (molecular weight, 27; boiling point, 25.7°C) is a colorless gas or liquid, with a bitter almond like odor [8, 12]. Cyanide is used for various purposes, such as fumigate,

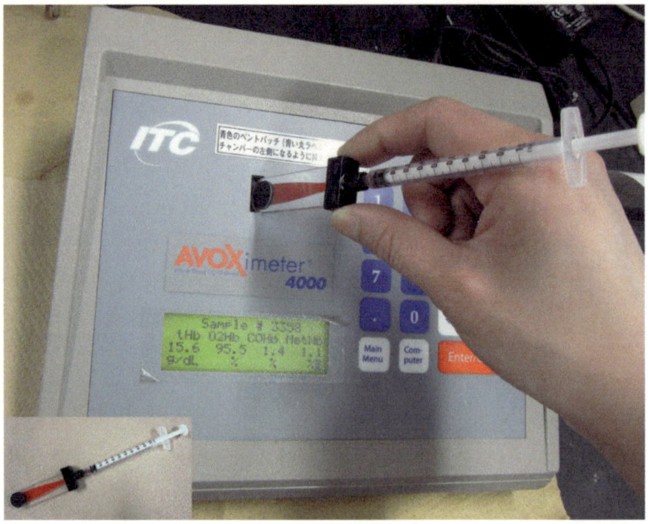

Figure 2. Portable oximeter (AVOX 4000) and its operation. Sample cartridge is shown in lower left-hand corner.

fungicide, insecticide, metal polishes, and electroplating. Hydrogen cyanide is present in fire smoke from burning nitrogen-containing plastics. Poisoning occurs by hydrogen cyanide gas inhalation or ingestion of cyanide salts. It is a highly toxic substance with a rapid onset of toxic effects as it is absorbed quickly from lung or the stomach [12]. Cyanide binds to heme iron in cytochrome complex, and it inhibits cellular respiration. The symptoms of acute poisoning include headaches, tachypnea, dizziness, coma, seizure, and death within 10–20 minutes in severe cases [12].

At autopsy, the appearance of the body is slightly bright pink. This is thought to be due to the presence of excess oxyhemoglobin [1]. Moreover, because cyanide inhibits cellular respiration, tissue oxygen consumption would be decreased. The stomach wall is damaged by the alkaline nature of stomach contents in case of cyanide salt ingestion [1]. It is well known that almond-like odor is one of the characteristics of cyanide poisoning [1, 8, 12, 19]. However, it can be detectable only approximately in one-third to half of the victims [19, 66], as this characteristic depends on the genetic trait [1]. Other autopsy findings are nonspecific in cyanide poisoning [1].

Cyanide level in blood is useful to confirm its toxicity [12]. The blood sample should be taken from the peripheral sites in case of cyanide salt ingestion, to exclude the effect of postmortem diffusion [66]. The normal blood cyanide level is 0.016 μg/mL for nonsmoker and 0.041 μg/mL for smoker. Cyanide concentration of less than 0.2 μg/mL in blood does not usually elicit any symptom [12]. Fatal concentration of cyanide in blood has been reported to be not lower than 3–5 μg/mL [67]. Lethal dose of potassium cyanide ingestion for adults is 200–300 mg.

For identification purposes, various methods have been devised. Color and microdiffusion tests are the most common [67, 68]. The Schöenbein-Pagenstecher method, using guaiac-cupper paper, is employed as a preliminary test [68]. This coated paper turns blue in the presence of

http://dx.doi.org/10.5772/intechopen.70029

cyanide. This method is user-friendly and highly sensitive for cyanide. However, since it is difficult to store the guaiac-cupper paper for a long period, we prepare it immediately before examination. Other color test or commercially available test tube methods and test papers have also been used to test cyanide in blood samples [29, 66]. The microdiffusion test using Conway cell (pyridine-pyrazolone method) have been reported [67]. Although this method is also highly sensitive for cyanide, and also used as a quantitative examination, its main drawback is that it is relatively time-consuming.

For quantitative testing, gas chromatography and detection tube are employed in our laboratories. To do so, cyanide is extracted from the sample by adding the concentrated phosphoric acid or sulfuric acid, and detected by nitrogen phosphorus detector (NPD) or flame thermoionic detector (FTD), equipped with a gas chromatography device [69, 70]. Application of sGC has also been reported for cyanide measurement [71]. The sGC system is also highly sensitive for cyanide and has some advantages such as it is easy to operate and portable. Further application would be expected in the field of forensic medicine (**Figure 3**).

The detector tube is also used for the quantitation of cyanide in blood [46, 47, 72]. This apparatus consists of a cyanide-separator tube, cyanide-detector tube, and aspirating pump. These tubes and the pump are connected in series. The cyanide-separator tube is packed with silica gel particles coated with sulfuric acid, and the released cyanide gas is detected by the cyanide-detector tube, followed by the aspirating of the pump (**Figure 4**). The cyanide-detector tube is packed with silica gel particles coated with mercuric chloride and pH indicator [46], and the hydrochloric acid formation by the reaction between cyanide and mercuric chloride was observed. Because the detector tube is easy to handle and portable, it can be carried to the scene of accident or poisoning and at the point of care, and it is well applied in forensic medicine practice.

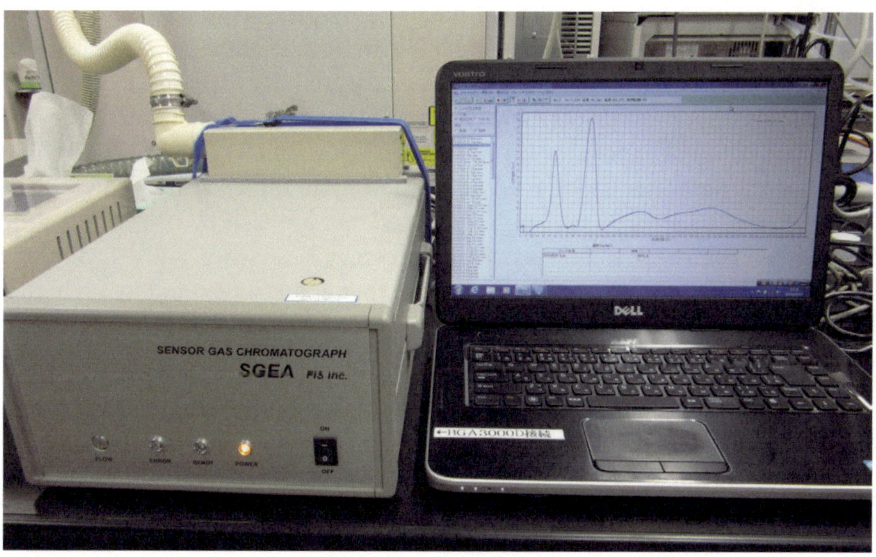

Figure 3. Equipment of the sensor gas chromatography for hydrogen cyanide quantification.

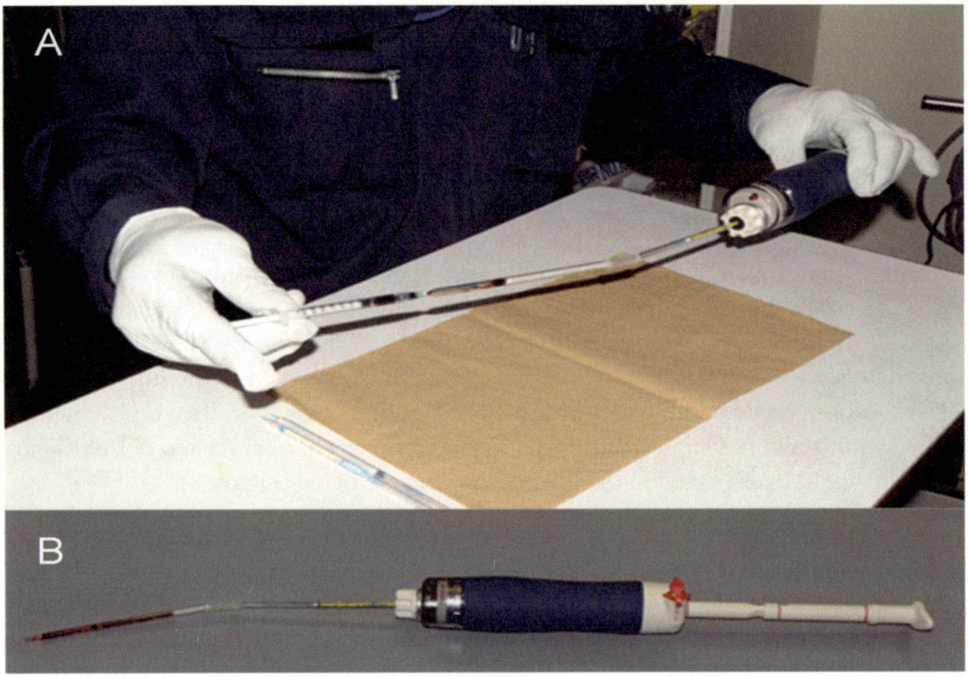

Figure 4. Procedure of the measurement of hydrogen cyanide in blood using detector tube (A). The detector tube is connected to the aspirating pump and separator tube (B).

3.3. Hydrogen sulfide (H_2S)

The H_2S is a gas with a rotten egg smell. It is colorless, flammable, and heavier than air (specific gravity for the air, 1.19) [8, 12]. It is formed as a by-product of the chemical industry. It occurs in volcanic gases and hot springs, and it is also formed at the process during putrefaction of organic substances. It is highly toxic and causes cellular asphyxia by the inhibition of cytochrome oxidase, like cyanide. Its toxicity depends on various factors such as its concentration in air and duration of exposure [12]. An odor is detectable at a concentration of 0.2 ppm in air, but olfactory paralysis is observed at 100–150 ppm. Inflammatory conditions such as rhinitis, pharyngitis, bronchitis, and pulmonary edema are also observed as a result of its irritant properties [12]. The systemic toxicity is shown by headaches, nausea, vomiting, dizziness, loss of consciousness, and respiratory failure that are observed following high levels of H_2S exposure (above 500 ppm); unfortunately, most fatalities occur at the scene [12].

Nonspecific findings such as generalized organ congestion and pulmonary edema can be observed. The dark-greenish discoloration of cerebral gray matter, organ, and skin with rotten egg smell has been reported [1, 12].

The blood sulfide concentration is less than 0.05 μg/mL in normal healthy subjects [8]. Fatal concentration of sulfide in blood has been reported to be not lower than 0.13–0.45 μg/mL [73]. Since the formation of sulfide by postmortem degradation of protein has been reported, the interpretation of the results requires caution and expertise [12].

http://dx.doi.org/10.5772/intechopen.70029

As a qualitative test for H_2S, color testing is commonly used. The lead acetate paper is used as a preliminary test [66, 68]. The sample is mixed with sulfuric acid and heated, then the lead acetate paper is suspended; if the paper turns black, it indicates the presence of H_2S. This procedure is easy to perform [66].

As a quantitative test for H_2S, gas chromatography and detection tube are used. The gas chromatography method measures extracted H_2S using flame photometric detector (FPD) [74, 75]. The detector tube is also used for the quantitation of H_2S in blood [46, 47, 76]. This apparatus consist of a H_2S-separator tube, H_2S-detector tube, and aspirating pump. As explained previously, these tubes and pump are connected in series. The H_2S-separator tube is packed with silica gel particles coated with phosphoric acid, and the released H_2S gas is detected by the H_2S-detector tube, followed by the aspirating of the pump. The H_2S-detector tube is packed with silica gel particles coated with lead acetate [46, 49], and the indicator range is then observed. As this method is easy to operate and portable, it can be carried to the scene or point of care, and it is well suited for forensic practice.

3.4. Helium

Helium (He), a colorless and odorless inert gas, acts as a simple asphyxiant agent. It causes oxygen depletion by the replacement of the inspired air [77]. It has highly diffusive properties and low solubility in water. It is used as a career gas for party balloons or cryogenic liquids. Medically, mixture gas of He and oxygen improve the oxygen flow in patient with upper airway obstruction [78].

The identification and quantification of helium in forensic samples is usually performed using a headspace gas chromatography with TCD detector or gas chromatography mass spectrometry [79–84]. It has been reported that lung tissue, intratracheal, and stomach gas are suitable matrices for the analysis of the inert gases [79–84]. The gas sampling at the time of autopsy is relatively easy, it is a good practice to consider gas sampling in case helium exposure is suspected.

3.5. Other toxic gases

There are a lot of toxic gases that cause tissue damages, such as ammonia gas or chlorine gas [19]. These gases are widely used as industrial chemicals and cause irritation and inflammation at the points of contact. They may cause tissue necrosis in severe cases. Although the incidence of poisoning cases by these gases is relatively low, the detector tube method is often used as one of the simplified analytical methods.

4. Conclusion

We have discussed the properties and features of poisoning incidents due to gaseous substances and elaborated on the simplified analytical techniques and apparatus used for their identification and quantitation for forensic purposes.

In doing so, we have shared our experiences and highlighted the fact that the analysis of gaseous substances can be performed using readily available laboratory tools and equipment. We have emphasized the need and usefulness of the reference data tables for guiding forensic diagnosis.

We hope that the above overview will assist other colleagues to implement such simplified techniques for the advancement of forensic practice.

Acknowledgements

This work was supported by JSPS KAKENHI Grant-in-Aid for Scientific Research (C) Number 15K08873.

Author details

Hiroshi Kinoshita[1]*, Naoko Tanaka[1], Ayaka Takakura[1], Mostofa Jamal[1], Asuka Ito[1], Mitsuru Kumihashi[1], Shoji Kimura[1], Kunihiko Tsutsui[2], Shuji Matsubara[3] and Kiyoshi Ameno[1]

*Address all correspondence to: kinochin@med.kagawa-u.ac.jp

1 Department of Forensic Medicine, Faculty of Medicine, Kagawa University, Kagawa, Japan

2 Health Sciences, Faculty of Medicine, Kagawa University, Kagawa, Japan

3 Community Health Care Education Support Center, Postgraduate Clinical Education Center, Kagawa University Hospital, Kagawa, Japan

References

[1] Knight B. Forensic Pathology. 2nd ed. London: Arnold; 1996

[2] Skopp G. Postmortem toxicology. Forensic Science Medicine and Pathology. 2010;**6**:314-325

[3] Moffat AC, Osselton MD, Widdop B. Forensic toxicology. In: Moffat AC, Osselton MD, Widdop B, editors. Clarke's Analysis of Drugs and Poisons in Pharmaceuticals, Body Fluids and Postmortem Materials. London: Pharmaceutical Press; 2004. pp. 80-93

[4] Poklis A. Forensic toxicology. In: Eckert WG, editor. Introduction to Forensic Sciences. 2nd ed. Boca Raton: CRC Press; 1997. pp. 107-132

[5] Stead AH, Moffat AC. A collection of therapeutic, toxic and fatal blood drug concentration in man. Human Toxicology. 1983;**3**:437-464

[6] Winek CL, Wahba WW, Winek CL Jr, Balzer TW. Drug and chemical blood-level data 2001. Forensic Science International. 2001;**122**:107-123

[7] Moffat AC, Osselton MD, Widdop B. Monographs analytical and toxicological data. In: Moffat AC, Osselton MD, Widdop B, editors. Clarke's Analysis of Drugs and Poisons in Pharmaceuticals, Body Fluids and Postmortem Materials. London: Pharmaceutical Press; 2004. pp. 567-1721

[8] Baselt RC. Disposition of Toxic Drugs and Chemicals in Man. 8th ed. Foster City: Biochemical Publications; 2008

[9] Schulz M, Iwersen-Bergmann S, Andresen H, Schmoldt A. Therapeutic and toxic blood concentrations of nearly 1,000 drugs and other xenobiotics. Critical Care. 2012;**16**:R136. DOI: 10.1186/cc11441

[10] Jones GR. Postmortem toxicology. In: Moffat AC, Osselton MD, Widdop B, editors. Clarke's Analysis of Drugs and Poisons in Pharmaceuticals, Body Fluids and Postmortem Materials. London: Pharmaceutical Press; 2004. pp. 94-108

[11] Kennedy MC. Post-mortem drug concentrations. Internal Medicine Journal. 2010;**40**:183-187

[12] Elenhorn MJ, Barceloux DG. Medical Toxicology Diagnosis and Treatment of Human Poisoning. New York: Elsevier; 1988

[13] Ministry of Health, Labour and Walfare. Vital Statistics of Japan. Tokyo: Health, Labour and Walfare Statistics Association; 1998-2015

[14] Tsunoda N. Drug and toxic poisoning in recent Japan. Journal of Health Science. 1999;**45**:356-366

[15] Ito T, Nakamura Y. Death from carbon monoxide poisoning in Japan between 1968-2007 through data from vital statistics. Journal of Japanese Society for Emergency Medicine. 2010;**13**:275-282

[16] Centers for Disease Control and Prevention (CDC). Carbon monoxide exposures—United States, 2000-2009. Morbidity and Mortality Weekly Report. 2009;**60**:1014-1017

[17] Anderson AR, Centers for Disease Control and Prevention (CDC). Top five chemicals resulting in injuries from acute chemical incidents—Hazardous substances emergency events surveillance, nine states, 1999-2008. MMWR Supplements. 2015:**64**;39-46

[18] World Health Organization. Environmental Health Criteria 213, Carbon Monoxide. 2nd ed. Geneva: World Health Organization; 1999

[19] Powers RH, Dean DE. Forensic Toxicology Mechanism and Pathology. Boca Raton: CRC Press; 2016

[20] Akane A, Fukui Y. A review on the development of carboxyhemoglobin analysis. The Research and Practice in Forensic Medicine. 1985;**28**:185-190

[21] Kunsman GW, Presses CL, Prodriguez P. Carbon monoxide stability in stored postmortem blood samples. Journal of Analytical Toxicology. 2000;**24**:572-578

[22] Hampson NB. Stability of carboxyhemoglobin in stored and mailed blood samples. American Journal of Emergency Medicine. 2008;**26**:191-195

[23] Tanaka N, Ameno K, Jamal M, Kumihashi M, Miyatake N, Kinoshita H. Effects of sampling methods and storage on the value of oxyhemoglobin ratio and carboxyhemoglobin ratio. The Research and Practice in Forensic Medicine. 2012;**55**:51-55

[24] Kojima T, Yashiki M, Une I, Nishiyama Y. Post-mortem formation of carbon monoxide in a drowned body. Nihon Hoigaku Zasshi. 1980;**34**:163-168

[25] Kojima T, Nishiyama Y, Yashiki M, Une I. Postmortem formation of carbon monoxide. Forensic Science International. 1982;**19**:243-248

[26] Kojima T, Yashiki M, Une I. Experimental study on postmortem formation of carbon monoxide. Forensic Science International. 1983;**22**:131-135

[27] Kojima T, Yashiki M, Okamoto I, Noda J, Une I, Miyazaki T, Chikasue F. Postmortem formation of carbon monoxide in blood and body cavity fluids of rats drowned and kept immersed in fresh water. Hiroshima Journal of Medical Sciences. 1984;**33**:591-594

[28] Kojima T, Okamoto I, Yashiki M, Miyazaki T, Chikasue F, Degawa K, Oshida S, Sagisaka K. Production of carbon monoxide in cadavers. Forensic Science International. 1986;**32**:67-77

[29] Uges DRA. Hospital toxicology. In: Moffat AC, Osselton MD, Widdop B, editors. Clarke's Analysis of Drugs and Poisons in Pharmaceuticals, Body Fluids and Postmortem Materials. London: Pharmaceutical Press; 2004. pp. 3-36

[30] Pharmaceutical Society of Japan. Toxic gas testing method. In: Standard Method of Chemical Analysis in Poisoning—With Commentary. 4th ed. Tokyo: Nanzando; 1992. pp. 57-73

[31] Miyaishi S, Moriya F, Yamamoto Y, Ishizu H. A simple method of semi-quantitative determination of carboxyhemoglobin for the use at the scene of postmortem inspection. The Research and Practice in Forensic Medicine. 1992;**35**:141-145

[32] Akiya S, Tanimura A. Microdetermination of carbon monoxide-hemoglobin. Yakugaku Zasshi. 1952;**72:**453-454

[33] Kozuka H, Niwase T, Taniguchi T. Spectrophotometric determination of carboxyhemoglobin. Journal of Hygiene Chemistry. 1969;**15**:342-345

[34] Ishizawa F. A study on the spectrophotometric determination of carboxyhemoglobin in blood—"isosbetic point" method. Nihon Hoigaku Zasshi. 1981;**35**:191-200

[35] Yamamoto K. Spectrophotometric two-wavelength method for COHb determination—with special reference to van Kampen's method. Nihon Hoigaku Zasshi. 1976;**30**:299-305

[36] Hayashi T, Yamaguchi H, Nanikawa R. A spectrophotometric determination of CO-Hb in blood on the basis of difference in absorbancy of deoxy- and carboxy-hemoglobin. Nihon Hoigaku Zasshi. 1977;**31:**234-240

[37] Katsumata Y, Aoki M, Sato K, Suzuki O, Oya M, Yada S. A simple spectrophotometry for determination of carboxyhemoglobin in blood. Journal of Forensic Sciences. 1982;**27**:928-934

[38] Ishizu H, Ameno S, Yamamoto Y, Okamura Y, Shogano N. A simple spectrophotometric method for CO-Hb determination in blood and its application in legal medicine. Acta Criminologicae et Medicinae Legalis Japonica. 1982;**48**:187-196

[39] Miyauchi C, Sakaki K. An improved method for gas chromatographic quantification of carboxyhemoglobin in blood. Nihon Hoigaku Zasshi. 1974;**28**:59-64

[40] Hishida S, Mizoi Y. Studies on the quantitative determination of carbon monoxide in human blood by gas chromatography. Nihon Hoigaku Zasshi. 1976;**30**:319-326

[41] Sakata M, Haga M. Determination of carbon monoxide in blood by head space analysis. The Journal of Toxicological Sciences. 1980;**5**:35-43

[42] Takahashi S, Kumabe Y, Itoh N, Kuwahara C, Matsubara K, Hata M, Fukui Y. Gas chromatographic analysis of carbon monoxide in the blood with the use of ultrasonic irradiation. Nihon Hoigaku Zasshi. 1980;**34**:556-562

[43] Guillot JG, Weber JP, Savoie JY. Quantitative determination of carbon monoxide in blood by head-space gas chromatography. Journal of Analytical Toxicology. 1981;**5**:264-266

[44] Lewis RJ, Johnson RD, Canfield DV. An accurate method for the determination of carboxyhemoglobin in postmortem blood using GC-TCD. Journal of Analytical Toxicology. 2004;**28**:59-62

[45] Tanaka N, Kinoshita H, Takakura A, Jamal M, Kumihashi M, Uchiyama Y, Tsutsui K, Ameno K. Application of sensor gas chromatography for the determination of carbon monoxide in forensic medicine. Current Study of Environmental and Medical Sciences. 2014;**7**:9-11

[46] Komyo Rikagaku Kogyo. Gas Detector Tube System Handbook. 4th ed. Tokyo: Komyo Rikagaku Kogyo; 2003

[47] Ishizawa F, Fujita T, Iseki K, Hori T, Saito T, Usui K, Hatano Y, Nozawa M, Tominaga A. Screening of poisonous substances by detector tube. Chudoku Kenkyu. 2015;**28**:266-272

[48] Ishizawa F, Misawa S. A handy and simple apparatus for the quantitative determination of COHb in blood. Acta Criminologicae et Medicinae Legalis Japonica. 1986;**52**:26-32

[49] Pharmaceutical Society of Japan. Standard Methods of Analysis for Hygienic Chemists—With Commentary (1990). Tokyo: Kanehara Shuppan; 1990

[50] Mahoney JJ, Vreman HJ, Stevenson DK, Van Kessel AL. Measurement of carboxyhemoglobin and total hemoglobin by five specialized spectrophotometers (CO-oximeters) in comparison with reference methods. Clinical Chemistry. 1993;**39**:1693-1700

[51] Touger M, Gallagher EJ, Tyrell J. Relationship between venous and arterial carboxyhemoglobin levels in patients with suspected carbon monoxide poisoning. Annals of Emergency Medicine. 1995;**25**:481-483

[52] Okada M, Okada T, Ide K. Utilization of a CO-oximeter in the medico-legal field. Nihon Houigaku Zasshi. 1985;**39**:318-325

[53] Ohshima T, Takayasu T, Nishigami J, Lin Z, Kondo T, Nagano T. Application of hemoglobin analysis by CO-oximeter to medico-legal practice with special reference to diagnosis of asphyxia. Nihon Houigaku Zasshi. 1992;**46**:382-388

[54] Higuchi T, Noguchi K, Maeda H. An evaluation of analyzed data of hemoglobin derivatives by CO-oximeter in medico-legal autopsy. Nihon Houigaku Zasshi. 1992;**46**:416-418

[55] Maeda H, Fukita K, Oritani S, Nagai K, Zhu BL. An evaluation of post-mortem oxymetry in fire victims. Forensic Science International. 1996;**81**:201-209

[56] Oritani S, Nagai K, Zhu BL, Maeda H. Estimation of carboxyhemoglobin concentrations in thermo-coagulated blood on a CO-oximeter system: An experimental study. Forensic Science International. 1996;**83**:211-218

[57] Maeda H, Fukita K, Oritani S, Ishida K, Zhu BL. Evaluation of post-mortem oxymetry with reference to the causes of death. Forensic Science International. 1997;**87**:201-210

[58] Shimizu K, Mizukami H, Fukushima T, Sasaki M, Shiono H. Use of a CO-oximeter for forensic diagnosis of hypothermia. Nihon Houigaku Zasshi. 1998;**52**:196-201

[59] Brehmer C, Iten PX. Rapid determination of carboxyhemoglobin in blood by oximeter. Forensic Science International. 2003;**133**:179-181

[60] Watanabe N. Medico-legal application of hemoglobin analysis using CO-oximeter. Hokkaido Igaku Zasshi. 2003;**78**:557-566

[61] Olson KN, Hillyer MA, Kloss JS, Geiselhart RJ, Apple FS. Accident or arson: Is CO-oximetry reliable for carboxyhemoglobin measurement postmortem? Clinical Chemistry. 2010;**56**: 515-520

[62] Tanaka N, Ameno K, Jamal M, Ohkubo E, Kumihashi M, Kinoshita H. Application of oximeter AVOX 4000 for the determination of CO-Hb in the forensic practice. The Research and Practice in Forensic Medicine. 2010;**53**:39-43

[63] Fujihara J, Kinoshita H, Tanaka N, Yasuda T, Takeshita H. Accuracy and usefulness of the AVOXimeter 4000 as routine analysis of carboxyhemoglobin. Journal of Forensic Sciences. 2013;**58**:1047-1049

[64] Tanaka N, Ameno K, Jamal M, Kumihashi M, Miyatake N, kinoshita H. Effects of sample dilution on the value of carboxyhemoglobin ratio. Japanese Journal of Forensic Pathology. 2014;**20**:39-40

[65] Tanaka N, Kinoshita H, Jamal M, Takakura A, Kumihashi M, Miyatake N, Ameno K. Squeezed splenic blood sampling as an alternative method for carboxyhemoglobin measurement. Romanian Journal of Legal Medicine. 2015;**23**:106-108

[66] Braithwaite RA. Metals and anions. In: Moffat AC, Osselton MD, Widdop B, editors. Clarke's Analysis of Drugs and Poisons in Pharmaceuticals, Body Fluids and Postmortem Materials. London: Pharmaceutical Press; 2004. pp. 259-278

[67] Seto Y. Cyanide. In: Suzuki O, Watanabe K, editors. Drugs and Poisons in Humans, A Handbook of Practical Analysis. Berlin: Springer-Verlag; 2002. pp. 113-122

[68] Department of Legal Medicine, Hiroshima University. Simple Laboratory Procedure of the Drug and Poisons. Tokyo: Jiho; 2001

[69] Yoshida M, Watabiki T, Ishida N. The quantitative determination of cyanide by FTD-GC. Nihon Houigaku Zasshi. 1989;**43**:179-185

[70] Seto Y, Tsunoda N, Ohta H, Shinohara T. Determination of blood cyanide by headspace gas chromatography with nitrogen-phosphorus detection and using a megabore capillary column. Analytica Chimica Acta. 1993;**276**:247-259

[71] Tanaka N, Hanada M, Hirano S, Takakura A, Jamal M, Ito A, Kumihashi M, Tsutsui K, Kimura S, Ameno K, Ishimaru I, Kinoshita H. Determination of cyanide by sensor gas chromatography. Japanese Journal of Forensic Pathology. 2016;**22**:79-82

[72] Ishizawa F, Misawa S. The handy and simple apparatus for the quantitative determination of hydrogen cyanide in blood. Nihon Houigaku Zasshi. 1987;**41**:88-92

[73] Kage S. Hydrogen sulfide and its metabolite. In: Suzuki O, Watanabe K, editors. Drugs and Poisons in Humans, A Handbook of Practical Analysis. Berlin: Springer-Verlag; 2002. pp. 101-111

[74] Fukui Y, Kagawa M, Takahashi S, Hata M, Matsubara K. Analysis of sulfur compounds in biological materials by gas chromatography with flame photometric detector. Nihon Houigaku Zasshi. 1980;**34**:575-581

[75] Tanaka E, Nakamura T, Terada M, Misawa S, Suzuki Y, Kuroiwa Y. The determination of hydrogen sulfide in fluid and tissue samples by gas chromatography with flame photometric detector. Eisei Kagaku. 1987;**33**:149-152

[76] Norimine E, Ishizawa F, Miyata K, Ishiwata T, Yoshida T, Honda K. Development of detection kit for hydrogen sulfide in blood. Chudoku Kenkyu. 2009;**22**:234-235

[77] Kinoshita H, Tanaka N, Jamal M, Takakura A, Kimura S, Tsutsui K, Ameno K. Atomspheric asphyxia: Pathophysiology and forensic diagnosis. In: Santos AR, editor. Asphyxia Risk Factors, Prevalence and Neurological Impacts. New York: Nova Science Publishers Inc; 2015. pp. 73-83

[78] Berganza CJ, Zhang JH. The role of helium gas in medicine. Medical Gas Research. 2013;**3**:18

[79] Yoshitome K, Ishikawa T, Inagaki S, Yamamoto Y, Miyaishi S, Ishizu H. A case of suffocation by an advertising balloon filled with pure helium gas. Acta Medica Okayama. 2002;**56**:53-55

[80] Auwaerter V, Grosse Perdekamp M, Kempf J, Schmidt U, Weinmann W, Pollak S. Toxicological analysis after asphyxia suicide with helium and a plastic bag. Forensic Science International. 2007;**170**:139-141

[81] Tanaka N, Kinoshita H, Jamal M, Kumihashi M, Tobiume T, Tsutsui K, Ameno K. Usefulness of intratracheal gas analysis in an autopsy case of helium inhalation. Romanian Journal of Legal Medicine. 2013;**21**:237-238

[82] Tanaka N, Takakura A, Jamal M, Kumihashi M, Ito A, Ishimoto S, Tsutsui K, Kimura S, Ameno K, Kinoshita H. Stomach gas as a useful matrix for detecting ante-mortem gas exposure. A case of asphyxia by helium inhalation. Romanian Journal of Legal Medicine. 2016;**24**:21-22

[83] Oosting R, van der Hulst R. Peschier L, Verschraagen M. Toxicological findings in three cases of suicidal asphyxiation with helium. Forensic Science International. 2015;**256**:38-41

[84] Malbranque S, Mauillon D, Turcant A, Rouge-maillart C, Mangin P. Quantification of fatal helium exposure following self-administration. International Journal of Legal Medicine. 2016;**130**:1535-1539

Chapter 10

Optical Express Methods of Monitoring of Pathogens in Drinking Water and Water-Based Solutions

Tatiana Moguilnaya and Aleksey Sheryshev

Additional information is available at the end of the chapter

http://dx.doi.org/10.5772/intechopen.70236

Abstract

Hygienic standards to the quality of potable water require continuous monitoring of the absence of pathogenic microorganisms directly in water flow. Despite a great number of laboratory devices for checking the quality of potable water, there are no express analyzers for monitoring of pathogenic organisms, which could be embedded directly into the automatic checkout systems. The reasons of it are low concentration of pollutions and the presence of additional effects, which impede automatic data processing. The new method, the express analysis of pathogens in water, was developed. It shall be mentioned that the proposed method of express diagnostics allows detection of infectious agents in the water in minutes based on nonlinear effects. This research has, hopefully, laid the foundation for development of a prototype for determination of the content of the genetically modified soy in meat products. The inventive methods can be recommended for DNA diagnostics in medicine ,veterinary sciences and insanitation. The main advantage of this method is that there is no need for DNA isolation. It is sufficient to create a suspension of the product by centrifugation.

Keywords: express diagnostics, viruses, pathogens, laser monitoring, colloidal solution

1. Introduction

Hygienic standards to the quality of potable water require continuous monitoring of the absence of pathogenic microorganisms directly in water flow. Despite a great number of laboratory devices for checking the quality of potable water, there are no express analyzers for monitoring of pathogenic organisms, which could be embedded directly into the automatic checkout systems. The reasons of it are low concentration of pollutions and the presence of additional effects, which impede automatic data processing. At present, monitoring of microbiological parameters of the composition of drinking water is of great importance. Water supply systems are the key to ensuring the livelihoods of cities, in connection with which the issue of realizing the control of drinking water parameters directly in the pipeline flow in real time is becoming increasingly acute. To solve this problem, it is necessary to implement continuous monitoring, including super-toxicants in drinking water. At the same time, much attention is paid to the development of fundamentally new and highly effective detection and control systems for the spread of pathogenic microorganisms. The problem is complicated by the fact that the maximum permissible concentration of pathogenic microorganisms can be within even a few molecules.

To date, the control is performed by the laboratory methods. That process takes from several hours to several days, depending on the method. In addition, these tests must be conducted in laboratory conditions by highly qualified personnel. That necessitates the development of a device that can be integrated into an automated line for monitoring drinking water. For example, the PCR method is an excellent diagnostic method, but it requires preliminary DNA isolation. The method of luminescent analysis using fluorescent markers requires very specialized sample preparation.

Thus, the problem of real-time assessing quality of drinking water to guarantee the absence of hazardous biological and chemical substances, even in small and ultrasmall concentrations, is becoming increasingly important. The content of pathogenic microorganisms in water can vary from 10^{-8} up to 105 mg/m^3. Although there are a great number of laboratory devices for checking the quality of potable water, there are no express analyzers for monitoring of pathogenic microorganisms that could be embedded directly into the automatic checkout systems. The optical phenomena of stimulated scattering in water solutions, which contain DNA, are investigated insufficiently.

Yet such research would be of great interest for the development of automatic control systems of potable water. Laser methods are widely applied to the analysis of structures of multicomponent liquids and are thus useful as a tool for the determination of low concentrations. In this chapter we describe new methods of express monitoring of viruses and pathogenic organisms in water and aqueous solutions based on nonlinear effects. We also describe a modified PCR method of diagnosis of genetically modified foods. The proposed methods can be recommended for the diagnosis of DNA, in the field, in medicine and veterinary sciences, in sanitary epidemiological studies to detect agents of dangerous infections in the event of potential bioterrorist attacks

1.1. Aim and objectives of our studies

The purpose and objectives of our research are to determine in spectra what kind the optical parameters allows us to diagnostic patogens with a probability of not less than 95%. To do this, no less than 1500 spectra were obtained for each of the pathogens studied. A large amount of experimental material allowed to create software that automatically determines the type of pathogen and signals its presence.

http://dx.doi.org/10.5772/intechopen.70236

2. Methods and findings

As a preliminary to a detailed description, a comparative analysis of the methods is given in **Table 1**. This comparative analysis is shown to highlight the benefits of our method, which will allow automated monitoring of pathogens. It should be noted that the certification of the method was carried out on the laboratory basis of the State Research Center for Applied Microbiology and Biotechnology (Obolensk, Moscow Region) and at the All-Russian Research Institute of Veterinary Sanitation, Hygiene and Ecology of the Russian Academy of Agricultural Sciences. Approbation of the device was carried of the double-blind method. The double-blind method is an experimental procedure in which neither the representatives of the testing organization nor the researchers know what is in the tested samples. The double-blind method is used to avoid the appearance of the effects of the experimenter's prejudice relative to the studied characteristic (the Rosenthal effect) and to eliminate the possibility of distorting the results of the experiment of the knowledge effect of what is required of the subject.

In **Table 2**, results of comparison of tests by a double-blind method against a standard test method are shown. It should be noted also that we studied transmission IR spectra of a number of pathogen (salmonella, viruses of herpes genitaler, hepatitis A and C, grippe A and B) solutions and luminescence of nanomarkers. In our experiments, the laser radiation passed through a quartz cell with water solutions of the pathogens, nanosilver,

Method	Need for sample preparation	Special laboratory conditions	Use of reagents	Duration of the measurement	Duration of result processing
1. Agglutination method	Yes	Yes	Yes	1 h	1 day
2. Immune deposition	Yes	Yes	Yes	20–60 min	1 day
3. Immunobloom	Yes	Yes	Yes	2–4 h	1 day
4. Method of a fixation of the complement	Yes	Yes	Yes	1 h	1 day
5. Phagocytic activity test	Yes	Yes	Yes	24 h	2 days
6. Immune-enzyme analysis	Yes	Yes	Yes	2–4 h	1 day
7. Neutralization method	Yes	Yes	Yes	4–7 days	5–8 days
8. Method of the luminescence	No	Yes	No	15 min	30 min
9. The method of stimulated luminescence and SBS	No	No	No	2 min	1 min

Table 1. Comparison of methods by duration and sophistication.

Pathogen/the method and result of research	Test/ positive	Device/ positive	Test/ negative	Device /negative duration of the measurement	Test/false negative	Device/false negative	Test/false positive	Device/false positives
E. coli 12571 agglutination method	20 yes	20 yes	20 yes	1 h	0	0	0	0
Enterococcus faecalis	20 yes	20 yes	20 yes	20–60 min	0	0	0	01
Shigella flex 3 immunobloom	10 yes	10 yes	10 yes	2–4 h	0	0	0	01
Method of a fixation of the complement	10 yes	10 yes	10 yes	1 h	0	0	0	01
Kolifag MS-2 phagocytic activity test	5yes	5yes	10yes	24 h	0	0	0	01
Staphylococcus aureus by immune-enzyme analysis	5 yes	5 yes	5 yes	2–4 h	0	0	0	02

Table 2. Comparison of results by methods used by duration and false positive.

or nanomarkers. We found that exciting radiations with wavelengths 1017 and 810 nm induce the stimulated Brillouin scattering (SBS) in spectra of the water containing DNA. We believe that the power threshold for the onset of this effect is achieved by adding a forced radiation luminescence and laser radiation. A comparative analysis of the methods is given in **Table 1**. Comparative analysis shows that our method (9) is promising for automated monitoring of pathogens.

2.1. Basic concepts of methods for monitoring pathogens in water

2.1.1. Overview of bioluminescence

Bioluminescence is a form of chemiluminescence where light energy is released by a chemical reaction. The reaction can occur either inside or outside the cell. Chemiluminescence occurs like many chemical reactions, for example, by recombination of free radicals or the oxidation reaction. In this case, as in the bioluminescence reaction, released energy is not dissipated as heat, as is the case during most of the exothermic chemical reactions, and consumed in the formation of one of the reaction products in an excited electronic state. Emitting light during the chemiluminescent reaction is necessary to satisfy at least two conditions: Firstly, the energy released during the reaction must exceed about 41–71.5 kcal/mol, and, secondly, the energy difference between the ground and excited states that the reaction product should be less than the enthalpy of the chemical reaction. Under these conditions, it can be formed with a sufficiently high transition of oxidized luciferin in the excited state and the subsequent transition of it to the ground state with the emission of photons

http://dx.doi.org/10.5772/intechopen.70236

The ratio of the number of emitted photons to the total number of elementary events is called the quantum yield of the reaction. The quantum yields of bioluminescence, unlike most chemiluminescent reactions, are very high, reaching values of 0.1–1. Chemiluminescence is rarely carried out for the reaction processes in aqueous solutions at neutral pH at such a quantum yield Bioluminescent process power radiation depends on the difference in energy between the oxidized forms of the ground and excited states of luciferin. This power is related to the radiation frequency by the relation ΔE = hv; On half the width of the radiation band, which has a width usually about 50 nm (**Figure 1a**) [1].

2.1.2. Overview on stimulated Brillouin scattering

The stimulated Brillouin scattering (SBS) is a nonlinear process that can occur in liquid media at large intensity. The mechanism of the appearance of Brillouin radiation arises from the photon-phonon interaction. The basic mechanism of SBS phenomenon is illustrated in **Figure 1b**. In scattering effects, energy gets transferred from one light wave to another wave at a longer wavelength or lower energy. The lost energy is absorbed by the molecular vibrations, or phonons, in the medium. Stimulated scattering is affected by the threshold level. The SRS is a nonlinear parametric interaction between light and molecular vibrations. Optical phonon participates in SRS, but acoustic photon participates in SBS. Due to SRS power transferred from shorter wavelength channels to the longer wavelength channels. SRS occurs in both directions, either forward or backward direction. The input signal from the laser source is the pump signal and generates a new wave due to scattering in the medium. This wawe is called the Stokes wave. SBS occurs only in the backward direction; for example, when input power exceeds threshold power, Stokes power shifted to the backward direction. Pump wave losses power, while Stokes wave gains power. The pump wave creates acoustic wave in transmission medium through a process called electrostriction. The interaction between pump wave and acoustic wave creates the generation of back propagating optical wave which is called Stokes wave. When acoustic waves travel through the transparent liquid media, they induce spatially periodic local compressions and expansions which in turn cause local increases and decreases in the refractive index. This phenomenon is known as photoelastic effect altered to a degree such that a significant portion of the optical signal is back-scattered. So, we can say that the acoustic wave alters the optical properties of the fiber, including the refractive index. This fluctuation of refractive index scatters the incident wave and creates Stoke wave which

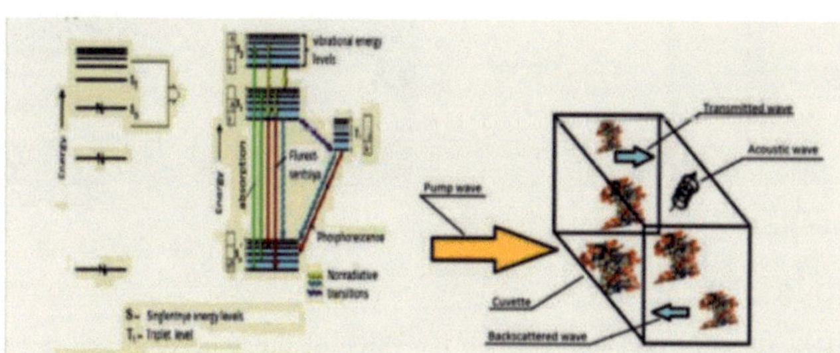

Figure 1. Comparison of the phenomenon of luminescence (a) and stimulated Brillouin scattering (b).

propagates in the opposite direction. The magnitude of the photoelastic effect increases with increasing input optical power. If the input power reaches the threshold level of SBS and the refractive index is variable, then an acoustic wave appears. Modern research shows that water has a quasi-crystalline structure. Similar effects were observed in the liquid and solid [2].

Our investigations showed the occurrence of luminescence mainly in solutions containing DNA or fluorescent markers. Brillouin scattering was observed in solutions containing low concentrations of particles, including nanoscale. Based on these investigations, we developed the method of monitoring nanoparticle sizes, composition, chemical reactions, and transition processes occurring in solutions. At present we are creating series of devices for monitoring MPC (maximum permissible concentration) in tap water by using the proposed method.

2.2. Description of the monitoring of pathogens in water by resonance laser spectroscopy techniques

We used a specially designed testing bench and the scheme of experimental setup shown in **Figure 1**. We analyzed about 700 spectra for each of the pathogens. Pathogens that we studied are shown in **Table 1**. We excited viruses and bacteria suspensions with a laser beam having wavelengths of 810 and 1017 nm and then evaluated the forward-scattering spectra. The testing bench consists of the following components: (1) the block of the three of semiconductor laser sources with wavelengths λ1 = 1017 nm, λ2 = 810 nm, and λ3 = 670 nm; (2) the quartz cuvette; (3) spectrum analyzer "Agilent" with the spectral resolution 0.05 nm, equipped with the microcomputer for processing spectra; (4) and (5) waveguides for the radiation input-output ; and (6) the computer equipped with original software for processing spectra (**Figure 1a**, **b**). The laser radiation passed through a waveguide into the cuvette with the sample. Sometimes, we used an additional laser with a wavelength λ4 = 532 nm. That source enhanced the intensity of luminescence. The radiation, which passed through the cuvette and the output waveguide, was analyzed by a spectrum analyzer (**Figure 2**).

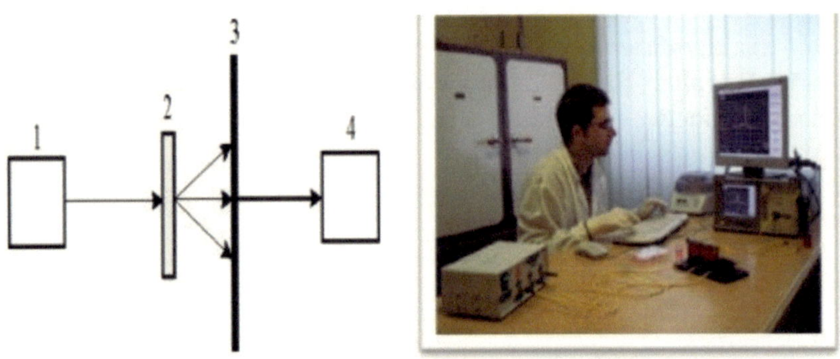

a b

Figure 2. (a) The experimental setup: (1) the block of the three of the semiconductor laser sources with exciting wavelengths λ_1 = 1017 nm, λ_2 = 810 nm, and λ_3 = 670 nm; (2) the quartz cuvette; (3) spectrum analyzer "Agilent"; and (4) computer equipped with original software for processing spectra.; (b) photo.

http://dx.doi.org/10.5772/intechopen.70236

This radiation was registered in short-range IR. Experiments were repeated, at least, 40 times for statistical significance. Spectral characteristics were measured for a range of concentrations of pathogens, from 10 to 10^9 (cells/ml). The data were placed into a spectra database. We developed the coherent spectroscopic method for the monitoring of the pathogenic organisms directly in water pipeline, genetically modified products, and nanostructured materials in colloidal solution. The method is based on an analysis of spectral characteristics of stimulated radiation, passed through the solution. Spectra were analyzed by the spectrum analyzer "Agilent" (USA) with spectral resolution 0.5 nm or by the spectrum analyzer "AQ6370C," which provides spectral resolution, ±0.01 nm and 0.02 nm; maximum input power, +20 dBm; and a sensitivity level of input power, −90 dBm. The input-output waveguides bring the exciting and passing radiations from laser to the cell and from cell to the analyzer, respectively.

We found that exciting radiations with wavelengths 1017 and 810 nm induce the stimulated Brillouin scattering in spectra of the water containing pathogen DNAs. We revealed that peak positions and widths of "fingerprints" for pathogens under study and optical densities of these bands were proportional pathogen content, if their content was less 15%. Thus, Stokes and anti-Stokes bands of the stimulated Brillouin scattering can be used to recognize the pathogens. Nonlinear effects like SBS arise due to the density of radiation in this solution [3]. The similar density of radiation is reached due to a combination of the luminescence fields and laser radiation [2] giving the characteristic peak. The modal frequency of this peak depends on the type of DNA accordingly. The strains of viruses were obtained from the Museum of the State Scientific Center. We investigated the inelastic scattering spectra from water solutions of many pathogens (**Table 3**). Traditional methods for detection of microorganisms are based on the enumeration of bacterial cells after their cultivation on a nutrient media. This method is sensitive, inexpensive, and simple, but it takes at least several days for completion. Two known methods for reducing the detection time—immunoassay and polymerase chain reaction—are complicated. At the present time, the problem of automatic monitoring of characteristics of drinking water directly within a water steam is particularly acute. Two resonance control techniques could be particularly instrumental in finding solution of that problem—spectroscopy of Raman scattering and stimulated Brillouin scattering. The utilization of Raman scattering spectroscopy technique requires transferring an enormous amount of energy for extracting an informative signal, which is considerably lower than the noise [4]. At present laser-based technology requires no consumables, or reagents are currently being developed [2]. A new method for detection of live or dead pathogens in water is described below. It is based on the diagnostics of nonlinear effects, which comprises two phenomena: an induced luminescence of DNA under the influence of laser radiation and a stimulated Brillouin scattering (SBS) [5]. The following model parameters were selected for the identification: of the peaks positions of the spectral line, corresponding to a pathogen and the difference between two wavelengths corresponding, respectively, to the laser mode maximum and of the peak of a spectral line of Stokes . Previously, we studied the spectra of virus [6]. The present work is focused on studying spectra of bacteria. The induced luminescence of DNA under the influence of laser radiation differs from ordinary luminescence in their characteristics [1]. Luminescence phenomenon was observed if the laser power is below the threshold of the Brillouin scattering effect.

Viruses		Bacteria	
1	Herpes simplex virus	17	*Mycobacterium tuberculosis avium*
2	Herpes zoster virus	18	*Mycobacterium tuberculosis bovis*
3	Herpes genitaler virus	19	*Mycoplasma hominis*
4	Epstein-Barr virus	20	*Neisseria gonorrhoeae*
5	Cytomegalovirus	21	*Neisseria meningitidis*
6	Hepatitis A virus	22	*Peptostreptococcus anaerobius*
7	Hepatitis B virus	23	*Proteus mirabilis*
8	Hepatitis C virus (genotype 1B)	24	*Staphylococcus aureus*
9	Hepatitis D virus	25	Streptococcus ß-hemolytischer
10	AIDS virus	26	*Streptococcus pneumoniae*
Bacteria		27	*Streptococcus viridans*
11	*Compylobacter jejuni*	**Fungus and parasites**	
12	*Chlamydia psittaci*	28	*Candida albicans*
13	*Chlamydia trachomatis*	29	*Gardia lamblia* intestinalis
14	*Enterococcus*	30	*Plasmodium malariae*
15	*Helicobacter pylori*	31	*Trichomonas vaginalis*
16	*Mycobacterium tuberculosis* hominis		

Table 3. Pathogens included in the experiment.

2.3. Investigation of luminescence in the water solution

2.3.1. Description of the experiment

We studied the luminescence of the hepatitis C virus. For this we used a source with a power below the threshold. The virus was diluted in the different media (physiology liquor, water, alcohol) in proportions of the greatest possible (10^{10} cells/ml) concentration, intermediate (10^5 cells/ml) concentration, and minimum concentration (10^1 cells/ml) of a virus in liquor. We used a strain of HCV genotype 1b isolated from a patient with hepatitis C. Then we cleaned and Concentration of the hepatitis virus in solution . At the initial stage of the purification of the culture medium containing the virus was removed from the cell pellet using low-speed centrifugation. To reduce the loss of infectivity and minimize proteolysis of proteins, centrifugation was performed at 4 C. The supernatant was completely removed, and the precipitate was resuspended by adding the virus into each centrifuge cup 1 ml NTE buffer pH 7.4. Then, the contents were combined, and the resulting cup material was further resuspended in a Dounce homogenizer (Dounce Tissue Homogenizers). Then, for destruction of virus aggregates, resulting suspension was sonicated for 1 min at setting Soniprep 150 (Sanyo).

To obtain a viral suspension of high purity, zonal ultracentrifugation method was used in a sucrose density gradient. Two solutions were prepared by sucrose (Sigma-Aldrich, USA) in NTE buffer at pH 7.4 at a concentration of 10 and 50%. For this we used three basic solutions Sucrose with a concentration of 20%, 30, 40%.

http://dx.doi.org/10.5772/intechopen.70236

The gradient was prepared by laminating successive to each other 50, 40, 30, 20, and 10% sucrose solution in amounts of 6 ml each tube to nitrocellulose followed by diffusion at 4 C for 12 h. The solution containing the virus was layered gently onto the surface gradient in the volume of 1 ml in each tube. We carried out the study of the dynamics of change in the intensity of luminescence. To do this, we utilized the laser, with the power being two times lower than the SBS phenomena threshold.

We continuously measured the spectral characteristics by the analyzer. The reference time started after the cuvette with a given concentration of the bacteria was placed in the optical path. The saved spectra retained their timing marks. We found that frequency of mode has a time drift (**Figure 3**).We observed two peaks in 1–2 s; then both peaks merged into one, and after 3–4 s, the luminescence disappeared.

2.3.2. Spectra of viruses

We investigated scattering, arising at the passage of laser radiation through colloidal solution (water, alcohol, physical solution) and fine-dispersed phase. We studied transmission spectra of a substance containing DNA: solutions of viruses and microorganisms.

Two shifted and one unshifted frequency components relative to laser frequency were detected in these spectra. The center of our attention was placed on the shifted component study, due to the fact that the analysis of processes in the fine-dispersed phase information is simple. We observed that the shifted components occur as in the Stokes and anti-Stokes ranges. On our opinion spectra of some samples under study are the spectra of Brillouin scattering as the distance between the central and the shift components does not depend on the excitation source wavelength. In other spectra we observed the spectral distributions of induced super fluorescence in liquids. In this case, the intensity of the shifted spectral distribution was higher than the intensity of the spectral distribution of laser radiation by several orders of magnitude, and the width of the spectral peak was decreased sharply. In both cases the width of the Lorentzian component, selected from such shifted spectral distribution, is proportional to the size of the particles, even if the solution contains impurities mainly proteinaceous.

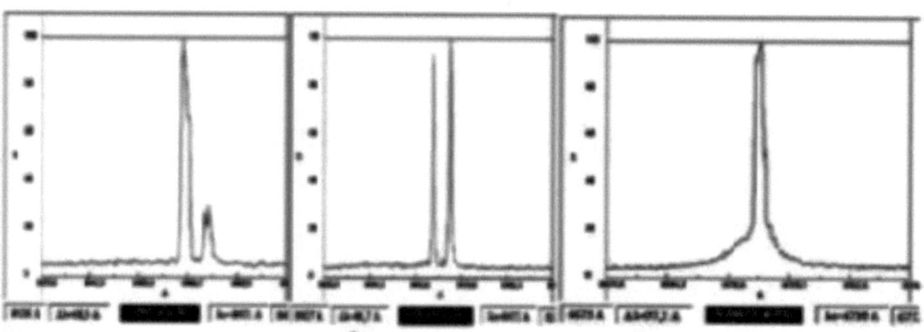

a b c

Figure 3. Intensity of stimulated luminescence of hepatitis C in the physiological solution from time (a) 30 s, (b) 1 min, and (c) 2 min.

We find out that the peak intensity of shifted distribution does not always have the logarithmic dependence on composition (**Figure 4**). We created autocorrelation functions of such dependencies. Our investigations showed the occurrence of super luminescence mainly in solutions containing DNA or fluorescent markers. Brillouin scattering was observed in solutions containing low concentrations of particles, including nanoscale.

2.3.3. Spectra of bacteria

We studied the inelastic scattering spectra from water solutions, containing *Escherichia coli* with concentration from 10 cells/ml to 10^9 cells/ml, as well as from a mix of *E. coli, B. subtilis var. niger, Shigella flexneri*, and the latex beads. The strains of *E. coli, B. subtilis var. niger*, and *Sh. flexneri* were obtained from the Museum of the State Scientific Center of Applied Microbiology and Biotechnology .The bacterial cultures were grown at 37°C for 48 h under aerobic conditions on a solid nutrient media (agar Hottinger, pH 7.2). Suspensions with bacterial cells (10^9 cells/ml) were prepared in 2 ml of 0.9% NaCl solution by using industry standard samples with 10-unit turbidity. Then, suspensions were diluted with distilled water to final concentrations ranging from 1×10^8 to 1×10^2 cells/ml. Every sample was tested by placing 0.1 ml of bacterial suspension into the appropriate solid nutrient medium. And then, the number of colonies was calculated after 48 h incubation period at 37 ± 1°C. At least 30–50 colonies must be growing on the agar medium. The suspensions of bacterial cell (*B. subtilis var. niger* and *Shigella flexneri*) were prepared for the analysis as 2 ml of 0.9% NaCl samples with the concentrations of 10^5 and 10^3 cells/ml. For assessing the sensitivity, we used bacterial suspensions of live microorganisms with seven concentrations —1×10^2, 1×10^3, 1×10^4, 1×10^5, 1×10^6, 1×10^7, 1×10^8 cells/ml—and the suspensions of *E. coli* microorganisms with the same concentrations but inactivated for 30 min at 1000C. For assessing the specificity, we used the mixes of *E. coli* and *Sh. flexneri* microorganisms with the concentration of 1×10^4 cells/ml and with the ratios,

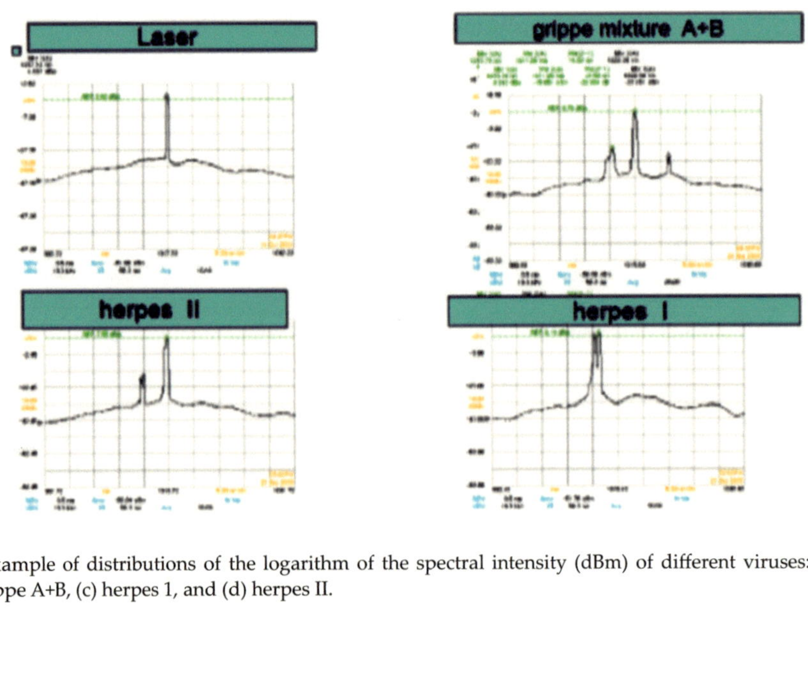

Figure 4. Example of distributions of the logarithm of the spectral intensity (dBm) of different viruses: (a) laser, (b) mixture grippe A+B, (c) herpes 1, and (d) herpes II.

respectively, of 1:3, 1:1, and 3:1. We also used mixes of *E. coli* and latex particles with the same concentrations and the same respective ratio concentration.

The spectra of bacteria, unlike viruses [4], often have several maxima (**Figure 4**). However, as a rule, only one peak has an intensity maximum at the same frequency in different solutions, such as water or physiological solution. And, the position of only one peak depends on the concentration.

The logarithm of the intensity at that frequency is a linear function of the concentration up to a level of 10^5 of cells/ml. However, the intensity is not an informative parameter, because it will depend on a power of IR source (**Figure 5**). At the same time, for the developed method, the difference between the frequencies (wavelengths) of the maximum of the Lorenz component of a laser mode and the maximum of the Lorenz component of a Stokes component was found to be an informative parameter [1]. However, the Stokes component exists no more than 20 min in the spectrum. Obviously, pathogen DNA will be destroyed during this time. For a practical application, we can use the difference between the frequency maximum of the laser mode and the frequency maximum of the fundamental mode of the bacteria (**Figure 6**) exceeded 10^2 cells/ml; its respective peak appeared in the anti-Stokes region. We examined the forward-scattering spectra for the mixes containing two or more pathogens (**Figure 6**). The average difference between wavelength of the peak maximum of the laser mode and the peak of Stokes components was equal to 1 ± 0.03 nm, which considerably exceeded the spectral resolvability of the device. The signal from pathogen organism was observed in the limited time interval.

To do this, we utilized the laser, with the power being two times lower than the SBS phenomena threshold. We continuously measured the spectral characteristics by the analyzer. The reference time started after the cuvette with a given concentration of the bacteria was placed in the optical path. The saved spectra retained their timing marks. We found that frequency of mode has a time drift. This process was continued until the intensity of the Stokes component had been reduced to the level of noise. Obviously, this effect was caused by DNA damage. It has been found that Stokes component appeared much earlier, within 25–30 seconds after the start of irradiation of the object, at moderate concentrations of 10^4 to 10^6 cells/ml. In the case of low solutions with concentrations, up to 10^6, the signal existed longer than in the case of higher concentrations. We believe that at low concentrations the scattering of a signal delay is caused by a

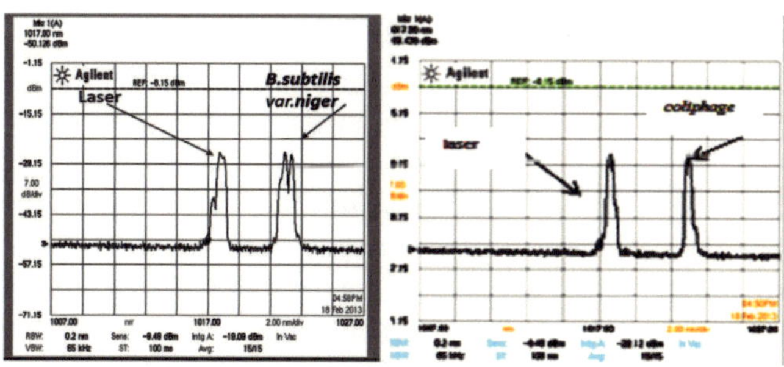

(a) (b)

Figure 5. Example of distributions of the logarithm of the spectral intensity (dBm) for *B. subtilis var. niger*: (a) concentration of 10^3 cells/ml and (b) bacteriophage (coliphage) concentration of 10^3 cells/ml.

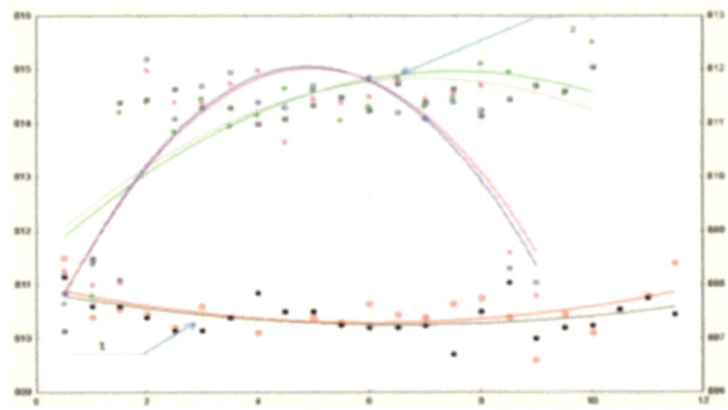

Figure 6. The logarithm of the intensity of the laser mode (1) and Stokes component (2) vs. laser exposure time for the living *E. coli*: laser with λ2 = 810 nm; log of intensity Stokes component (2); – – concentration 10^3 cells/ml; – – concentration live 10^5 cells/ml; – – concentration live 10^7 cells/ml; log of intensity laser mode (1) in the presence of *E. coli*; – – concentration live 10^3 cells/ml; – – concentration live 10^7 cells/ml.

nonuniform distribution of contaminated DNA in the volume of a tested specimen. The rapid decay indicates that fewer cells are rapidly destroyed by the action of coherent radiation. In the case of extremely high concentrations, we believe that the increase in the threshold in a signal generation was due to an increase in the required power of the exciting radiation of the pump. Most likely, that was because the destroyed cells were also absorbing the stimulating radiation, but they were not contributing to the formation of resonance scattering. For more details, please refer to [7].

Spectra from suspensions of the mix of pathogens with the latex beads have two Stokes components. One of them appears without delay in time, and its intensity was independent of the concentration of the latex beads. The intensity of bead component has several orders of magnitude lower than one of the pathogens. However, we did not detect the anti-Stokes component of the peaks corresponding to the dispersion of latex beads. In this case, we did not observe any change in the magnitude of this component in time.

To identify the main informative parameters of the method, the experimental samples were statistically processed. Initial comparative analysis was based on Student's t-test [6].

We developed a proprietary software for the diagnostics of the pathogens [8]. The informative parameters for diagnostics were (a) the reference spectra previously registered in the database and preprocessed based on statistical analysis of the spectral distribution of the pathogen; (b) the difference between the lengths of the laser mode high waves and Stokes (anti-Stokes component); and (c) the number of peaks in the distribution of the Stokes spectrum. Statistical analysis indicated that the above algorithm of recognition is capable of detecting the presence of bacteria spectrum with 0.95 probability [6, 9]. The pathogen monitoring method has developed. We obtained a large amount of experimental data and conducted statistical analysis aiming to determine the probability of detection of spectra by Student's t-test. We have studied the dynamics of the spectra for a number of direct dispersion of bacteria. In addition, we have studied the dynamics of changes in the spectra for solutions containing live bacteria and dead cells. The analysis of these dynamics demonstrated that dead cells do not produce luminescence. The peak of a Stokes component of dead cell is formed by the energy transfer from the laser mode. Central peak frequency of a Stokes component at a concentrations above 102 cells/ml is displaced into the anti-Stokes region (1010 nm), which utilized laser with λ1 = 1017 nm. On the basis of these results, the method and the corresponding device have been developed. That device was tested on a water supply pipeline.

2.4. Detection of live and dead bacteria

Accurate determination of live and dead bacteria is important in many microbiology applications. Traditionally, viability in bacteria is synonymous with the ability to form colonies on solid growth medium. Alternative methods, such as fluorescent in situ hybridization (FISH); nucleic acid amplification techniques such as real-time quantitative PCR (RT-qPCR or qPCR), reverse transcriptase PCR (RT-PCR), and propidium monoazide-PCR cannot be used for continuous monitoring, as they require complex sample preparation [9]. These traditional methods are time-consuming, and they do not provide real-time results or timely information required in the industrial applications. We have developed a method of detection of live and dead cells of pathogenic organisms. Separately, we have studied the luminescence of live and dead cells. To do this, we took the spectral distribution at a pump power slightly below the threshold. Linear relationship between intensity and the concentration for luminescence was not observed.

We conducted studies that determine the difference in spectra between live and dead pathogens, and detoxification of organism suspensions of microorganisms was disinfected by boiling for 30 min. We have found that the dead cells do not produce luminescence. We researched the difference in time dynamics of appearing spectral line for live and dead pathogens. In the first 2 or 3 min, we did not observe Stokes component for dead cells (**Figure 9**). Over time, the peak in the Stokes region appeared, and the intensity of the laser mode decreased (**Figures 8** and **10**). The peak of the Stokes component is a result of energy transfer from the laser mode. The fall of the laser intensity modes was observed in lasers with both employed wavelengths: λ2 = 840 nm and λ1 = 1017 nm. However, in the second case, the drop in intensity was stronger, and the frequency maximum of the second mode was observed in anti-Stokes region (1010 nm). Due to this study, it was possible to identify live and dead *E. coli* cells in the solutions with previously undetected pathogenic components.

2.5. Spectroscopic methods for monitoring genetically modified products

At the present time, the areas under the transgenic crops are being increased all over the world. Thus, 60% of all the areas allocated for cultivation of soy are occupied by the plants containing the transgenic lines of this product. Genetically modified organisms are the live organisms, which due to introduction of alien genes acquired new phenotypic properties. Usage of living modified organisms (viable crops) in the territory of the Russian Federation is forbidden by the law, and only import of the vegetative raw materials processed in appropriate way is permitted

Today, the most effective control method is the method of PCR (polymerase chain reaction), allowing not only to detect the presence of GMO in products but also to determine their quantity. Medical practice widely employs invasive methods of infectious disease detection based on the analysis of blood samples with the help of polymerase chain reaction and immune-enzyme analysis (IEA). The use of these methods for express diagnostics in mass screening implies a number of problems: the need of a special laboratory equipment according to sanitary and epidemiological standards, expensive test systems, and time that is necessary to get results (from several hours to several days). These factors hamper rapid epidemiological interventions in case of spreading infections as viral hepatitis and immunodeficiency virus and call for updating of the present and development of new diagnostic methods. Improvement of express diagnostics includes possibility to use the method in field conditions, its economical efficiency, high capacity, and quick results.

Unfortunately, the PCR method of analysis has its drawbacks. It requires difficult, long preparation of tests, expensive equipment, and specially equipped premises. All this does not allow us to use the PCR method for a mass express screening of products.

2.5.1. *Overview on PCR method*

Polymerase chain reaction (PCR) is an experimental method of the molecular biology, allowing us to achieve a substantial growth of the small concentrations of certain fragments of nucleic acids (DNA) in a biological material (test). The method relies on thermal cycling, consisting of cycles of repeated heating and cooling of the reaction for DNA melting and enzymatic replication of the DNA. Primers (short DNA fragments) containing sequences complementary to the target region along with a DNA polymerase, which the method is named after, are key components to enable selective and repeated amplification. As PCR progresses, the DNA generated is itself used as a template for replication, setting in motion a chain reaction in which the DNA template is exponentially amplified. PCR can be extensively modified to perform a wide array of genetic manipulations. PCR is not generally considered to be a recombinant DNA method, as it does not involve cutting and pasting DNA, only amplification of existing sequences.

In the first step, the two strands of the DNA double helix are physically separated at a high temperature in a process called DNA melting. In the second step, the temperature is lowered, and the two DNA strands become templates for DNA polymerase to selectively amplify the target DNA. The selectivity of PCR results from the use of primers that are complementary to the DNA region targeted for amplification under specific thermal cycling conditions. PCR amplifies a specific region of a DNA strand (the DNA target). The PCR was carried out in an amplifier, a device, which ensures a periodic cooling and heating of the test tubes, usually with the accuracy not less than 0.1°C. Modern amplifiers allow us to set complex programs, including with a possibility of "a hot start." For real-time PCR, special devices are produced equipped with a fluorescent detector.

When chains are disengaged, the temperature is lowered, so that the primers could contact a one-chained matrix. This stage is called hybridization. The temperature of the hybridization depends on the composition of the primers and is usually 4–5°C below the temperature of their fusion. Duration of the stage is 0.5–2 min. A wrong choice of a temperature results either in a bad linkage of the primers with a matrix (if the temperature is too high) or in a linkage in a wrong place and appearance of nonspecific products (if the temperature is too low).

By using a primer, the DNA polymerase makes a copy of a matrix chain. This is a stage of elongation. The polymerase begins a synthesis of the second chain from the primer's 3′-end, which has bonded a matrix, and moves along the matrix in the direction from 3′ to 5′. The temperature of the elongation depends on a polymerase. The frequently used polymerases Taq and Pfu are most active at 72°C. The period of elongation depends on both the kind of DNA polymerase and on the length of an amplificated fragment. Usually, the period of elongation is accepted as equal to 1 min per each thousand of base pairs. When all the cycles are finished, an additional stage of the final elongation is often done to complete the construction of all the one-chained fragments. This stage lasts 7–10 min. The quantity of the specific product of the reaction (limited by primers) theoretically increases proportionally to 2n, where n is the number of reaction cycles.

DNA markers are based on PCR primers. For real-time analysis, special DNA amplifiers with an optical unit are used to detect fluorescence within the reaction tube during the reaction. For real-time analysis, special DNA amplifiers with an optical unit are used to detect fluorescence within the reaction tube during the reaction [7]. These amplifiers are known as markers.

Now, carrying out of an express analysis is essentially impossible, because a preliminary extraction of a DNA of an investigated product is necessary. This can be done only in the conditions of a special laboratory. This is due to the fact that, if the lab ware or reactants are polluted by the products of the other reactions or other protein molecules, the results will be incorrect. Special premises are necessary for cleaning of the nucleic acids and for the analysis of the products of amplification. Considerable time is also necessary for a periodic heating of the tests. If the latter problem is solved, the division of DNA and cleaning of the nucleic acids essentially do not allow us to develop an express analyzer working directly with a product.

2.5.2. Description of the experiment

This experiment was conducted in order to develop a prototype of an express analyzer of a genetically modified soy. To do so, a certain number of problems are needed to be solved such as ensuring optical control of the parameters of soy in a multicomponent environment containing parasitic parameters of DNA, optimizing heat exchange system in a real-time mode, and developing an optical scheme for reading of the informative parameters and a signal processing system with account of the errors. With the above aims in mind, we undertook a research of the markers applied for carrying out of the reaction. In order to obtain a stimulated luminescence, the light-emitting diode pumping was replaced with a laser pumping, which resulted in an increase of the marker's own luminescence by more than an order. We replaced the lamp in the optical unit with a laser in order to reduce noise. The equipment for removing and analyzing the spectral characteristics and spectra of the inelastic scattering of marker are shown in **Figure 7**. We modified the experimental setup described in Part 2 a little.

We used an additional laser with a wavelength of 532 nm to enhance luminescence of the marker and achieve the SBS threshold.

As our previous research has shown, there is a protein luminescence (meat, milk) in the visible spectral range. The protein luminescence is absent in the near-IR range radiations. Also, the power of a luminescent marker is insignificant, and it is necessary to carry out rather many PCR reactions. The luminescence of an extraneous protein does not allow us to carry out diagnostics because of an inadmissible signal/noise ratio. Thus, if we analyze the spectrum of the investigated object in the near infrared region, we can confine ourselves to centrifuging the sample for uniform distribution in solution.

Also, spectral distributions during excitation of the markers by two types of lasers, with the wavelength corresponding to the wavelength exciting a marker and the wavelength lying within the range of the registration of the radiation, are obtained. An example of the of spectral intensity distribution (dBm) marker HEX-1030 with laser pumping with an operating wavelength $\lambda 3$ = 1016nm and laser pumping with an operating wavelengths $\lambda 3$ = 1016nm and $\lambda 4$ = 532 nm is shown in **Figure 8a** and **b** accordingly. The research also demonstrated that in the frequency range of about 1.01 microns, a peak of the inelastic scattering appears, proportional to keeping of a marker in a solution. Since luminescence in this area should fall, the reasons for occurrence of this peak are most likely connected with SBS effect. The maximum peak power increases by more than 1 dBm, if we used laser pumping of two lasers. We assumed that the difference in the position of the laser maximum and Stokes intensities in the spectra of the inelastic light scattering in the natural and modified soy is connected with the change of the molecular structure of the genetically modified samples, which in turn leads to a change of the electronic power levels of the biological objects (**Figure 9**).

Thus, the registration of the position of the maximum and the intensity of the inelastic diffused light in the field of inelastic scattering of light in the field of 850–1100 nm can be used as informative parameters for determination of the genetically modified soy. The spectral distributions of the inelastic scattering can serve as informative parameters for determination of the presence of a genetically modified product.

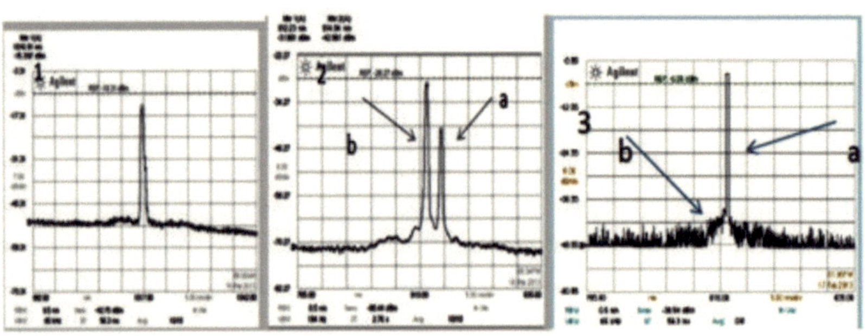

Figure 7. An example of the spectral intensity distributions (dBm); a(2) live *E. coli*; b(3) dead *E. coli*. Arrow "a" shows the peak corresponding to indicate *E. coli* laser mode; arrow "b."

http://dx.doi.org/10.5772/intechopen.70236

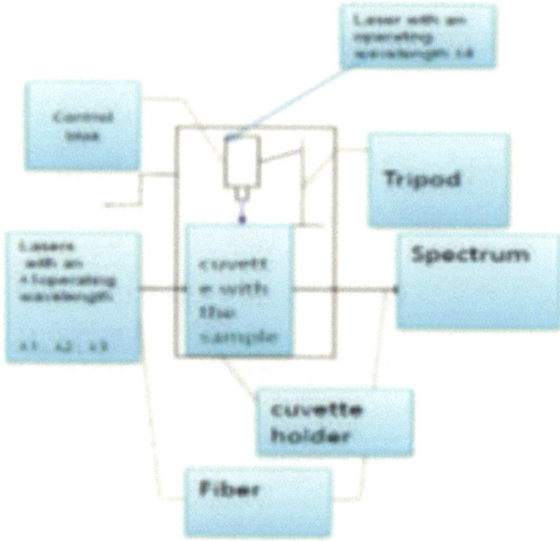

Figure 8. The equipment analyzing the spectral characteristics λ_4 = 532 nm or 488 nm, 633 nm λ_1 = 674 nm, λ_2 = 810 nm, and λ_3 = 1010 nm HEX-1030 laser with an operating wavelength λ_3= 1016nm.

The maximum peak power increases by more than 1 dBm, if we use laser pumping of two lasers. However, for practice, only one laser can be used. The spectrum analyzer can be replaced with a photodetector, if you control only one component. This allows you to develop cheap devices. We developed an experimental sample of a device using one laser in the near-field region (**Figure 10**).

The spectrometer was replaced by a receiver. We did not isolate soy DNA. We received a soybean mixture with water and centrifuged. Intensity of the inelastic scattering of the natural and genetically modified soy in absolute and relative figures is shown in **Figure 9a, b**. So, we

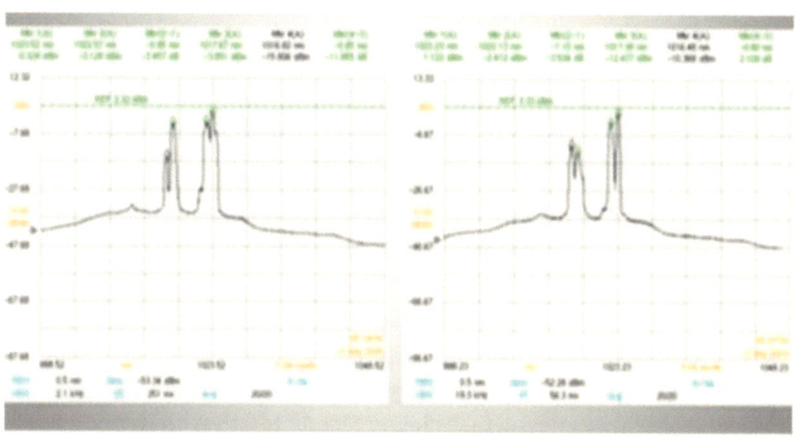

Figure 9. Marker HEX-1030 (a) laser pumping with an operating wavelength λ_3 = 1016 nm; and (b) laser pumping with an operating wavelengths λ_3 = 1016 nm and λ_4 =532 nm.

have also established the new method for rapid analysis of genetically modified soy in meat products detected by a modified PCR fluorescent method.

2.5.3. Comparison of standard PCR method and a modified PCR method

Table 4 compares the two methods. Analysis shows that our method can be the basis of devices working outside the laboratory, directly in shops and cafes.

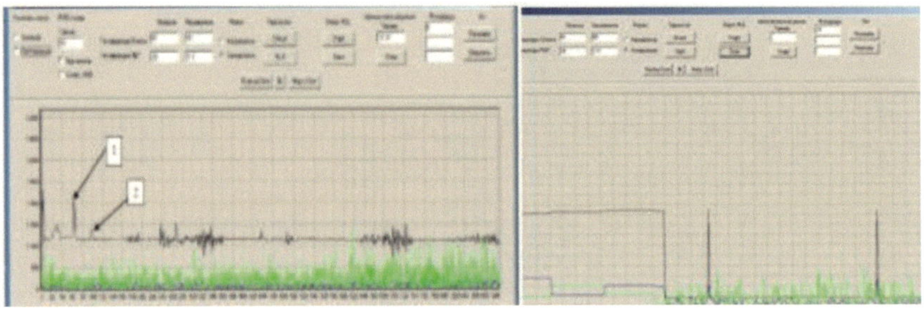

Figure 10. Distribution of signals in the presence of genetically modified soybean: (1) laser signal and (2) marker signal.

Standard PCR	Modified PCR method
The need for DNA extraction	Diagnosis is made immediately in the sample
The need to organize specialized laboratories	The need to organize specialized laboratories
Reaction time (1 h)	Reaction time (1 min)

Table 4. Comparison of standard and modified PCR methods.

3. Discussions

Traditional methods for detection of microorganisms are based on the enumeration of bacterial cells after their cultivation on a nutrient media. This method is sensitive, inexpensive, and simple, but it takes at least several days for completion.

Two known methods for reducing the detection time—immune assay and polymerase chain reaction—are complicated. In addition to the fact that this method requires the isolation of DNA, it also uses various sets of reagents to identify and differentiate the tested pathogen. For example, there are the set of reagents for the detection and differentiation of DNA from bacteria of the genus *Shigella* spp. and enteroinvasive *E. coli* (EIEC), *Salmonella* (*Salmonella* spp.), and thermophilic *Campylobacter* spp., modified with specific primers to *B. subtilis var. nigger*). In environmental objects and clinical material by polymerase chain reaction (PCR) with hybridization-fluorescent detection, "AmpliSens® *Shigella* spp. and EIEC/*Salmonella* spp./*Campylobacter* spp.-FL" and "AmpliSens® *Bacillus* anthracis-FRT" are often used in practice.

The PCR Stafipol-RV kit is designed to quantitatively detect the in vitro DNA of the causative agent of *Staphylococcus aureus* in a biological material by polymerase chain reaction with a fluorescent detection of the result in real time.

Another set of reagents is used to quantify the hepatitis C virus (HCV) RNA by polymerase chain reaction (PCR) with hybridization-fluorescent detection in real-time mode "AmpliSens HCV-Monitor-FL." The use of various consumables for different pathogens makes this method very expensive. Therefore, at the present time, the problem of automatic monitoring of characteristics of drinking water directly within a water steam is particularly acute.

Two resonance control techniques could be particularly instrumental in finding solution of that problem—spectroscopy of Raman scattering and stimulated Brillouin scattering. The utilization of Raman scattering spectroscopy technique requires transferring an enormous amount of energy for extracting an informative signal, which is considerably lower than the noise [3].

Laser-based technology requires no consumables, or reagents are currently being developed [10]. A new method for detection of pathogens in water and water-based solutions is described below. It is based on the diagnostics of nonlinear effects, which comprises two phenomena: an induced luminescence of DNA under the influence of laser radiation and a stimulated Brillouin scattering (SBS) [11]. The following model parameters were selected for the identification of the peak positions of a spectral line corresponding to a pathogen and the difference between two wavelengths corresponding, respectively, to a laser mode maximum and to a peak of a spectral line of a pathogen.

We studied transmission IR spectra of a number of pathogen (salmonella, viruses of herpes genitaler, hepatitis A and C, grippe A and B) solutions and luminescence of nanomarkers. In our experiments, the laser radiation passed through a quartz cell with water solutions of the pathogens, nanosilver, or nanomarkers. We found that exciting radiations with wavelengths 1017 and 810 nm induce the stimulated Brillouin scattering (SBS) in spectra of the water containing DNA. We believe that the power threshold for the onset of this effect is achieved by adding a forced radiation luminescence and laser radiation.

4. Conclusions

The new method, the express analysis of pathogens in water, was developed. It shall be mentioned that the proposed method of express diagnostics allows detection of infectious agents in the water in minutes based on nonlinear effects. This research has, hopefully, laid the foundation for development of a prototype for determination of the content of the genetically modified soy in meat products. The inventive methods can be recommended for DNA diagnostics in medicine ,veterinary sciences and in sanitation . The main advantage of this method is that there is no need for DNA isolation. It is sufficient to create a suspension of the product by centrifugation.

Author details

Tatiana Moguilnaya* and Aleksey Sheryshev

*Address all correspondence to: mogilnay@mail.ru

Moscow Aviation Institute (National Research University), Moscow, Russia

References

[1] Bioluminescence: Wikipedia. February 2017. https://en.wikipedia.org/wiki/Bioluminescence

[2] Starunov VS, Fabelinsky IL. Stimulated Mandelstam-Brillouin scattering and stimulated entropy (temperature) scattering of light. Physics-Uspekhi. 1969;**98**:441-491

[3] Abdelsalam M. Theoretical Studies of Raman Scattering. Stockholm, Sweden: Universitetsservice US-AB; 2011. ISBN 978-91-7415-844-1

[4] Tomilin VI, Mogilnaya Yu T, Kononenko AB. Research of dynamics of signal detection of the laser device at control of pathogenic microorganisms by the SBS-method. Ecological Systems and Devices. 2014;**12**:9-13

[5] Moguilnaya Yu T, Saguitova E, Botikov AG. Instrumentation for non-invasive express-diagnostics bacteriophages and viruses by optical method. Smart Medical and Biomedical Sensor Technology. Providence, Rhode Island, USA: Proceedings of SPIE; 2003;**5621**:18-23

[6] Tomilin VI, Moguilnaya Yu T. Study of stocksic and antistocksic components of laser device's signal for controlling of drinking water parameters. Vestnik of the Bauman Moscow State Technical University. Instrumentation Engineering. 2015;**N2**:83-91

[7] Moguilnay Yu T, Tomilin VA, Bobkov PV. Monitoring of toxicants by SBS in a turbulent flow of water. International Journal Laser Physics. Journal of Physics: Conference Series 414;(2013):012023 DOI: 10.1088/1742-6596/414/1/12023

[8] Mogilnaya T, Bobkov P, Toiling V, Agibalov A. Development of devices for rapid analysis of the presence of toxins in drinking water. Prybory. 2013(1):45-51

[9] http://www.diss.seluk.ru/m-biologiya/30006763-1-moskva-2012-osnovi-polimeraznoy-cepnoy-reakcii-pcr-sostavitelya-cel-posobiya-osnovi-polimeraznoy-cepnoy-reakcii-pcr-pomoch-ov.php

[10] The BioSentry™ Offers State-of-the-Art, Laser-Based Technology to Provide Continuous, Online, Real-time Monitoring for Microorganisms in Water Systems. http://www.inter-line.nl/media/1000116/biosentry_wms_v3.2.pdf [Accessed: January 25, 2017]

[11] Cheglov VA. Can I. Create a Laser on the Genetic Structure? Raman Scattering. // 70 Years of Research. Lebedev Physical Institute. Moscow 2004 year p. 250

Chapter 11

The Aflatoxin Quicktest™—A Practical Tool for Ensuring Safety in Agricultural Produce

Francisco Sánchez-Bayo, Luis de Almeida,
Robert Williams, Graeme Wright,
Ivan R. Kennedy and Angus Crossan

Additional information is available at the end of the chapter

http://dx.doi.org/10.5772/intechopen.71331

Abstract

Contamination of corn, peanuts, milk and dairy products with aflatoxins is a worldwide problem, particularly in subtropical regions where the climatic conditions are ideal for the growth of *Aspergillus flavus*, the fungi that produces these toxins. Developing countries have major difficulties in marketing these products abroad due to the stringent international regulations concerning this carcinogenic toxin. Adding to the problem is the analytical cost involved in monitoring the produce, which require sophisticated instrumentation and qualified personnel, neither of which are available for field testing. The development of a rapid Aflatoxin Quicktest™ provides an effective, reliable and cheaper option for screening levels of aflatoxin above the regulatory thresholds in such produce. The test consists of a lateral flow device (LFD) coated with antibodies specific to aflatoxin B1, although it detects other aflatoxins (i.e. G and M) with high cross-reactivity. Its high sensitivity allows analysis of these toxins in the range 2–40 μg/kg of sample in 15 minutes, plus the time for extraction, which varies among different products. Quantification of the test results is done using a Quick Reader, by comparing the readings of individual tests against a standard curve of the analytes in the same manner as it is done with any other analytical equipment. A validation study was carried out using peanuts from Australia and peanuts and corn from Timor-Leste to assess the performance of the Aflatoxin Quicktest™. Results obtained with the LFD showed a good correlation with the standard analytical measurements by HPLC-fluorescence (r^2 above 0.90 for all cases), indicating the Aflatoxin Quicktest™ is capable of measuring levels of aflatoxins accurately and reliably. Given their ease of use, low cost and fast processing time, the Aflatoxin Quicktest™ can be used for screening agricultural produce in countries that cannot afford the costly alternative of using specialised personnel and equipment.

Keywords: mycotoxins, food, analysis, lateral flow devices, peanuts, maize

1. Introduction

Aflatoxins constitute a major group of mycotoxins produced by certain fungi, mainly *Aspergillus flavus* and *Aspergillus parasiticus*, which grow in soil, decaying vegetation, hay and grains. These fungi can infect various crops — frequently peanuts, maize, other cereals as well as tree nuts — either prior to harvest or under moist conditions in stored agricultural produce, leading to their contamination with aflatoxins [1–3]. Contamination levels can sometimes exceed thousands of parts per billion (ppb, either μg/kg or μg/L) in individual kernels of peanuts or other grains, but given the uneven distribution within a batch of produce an intensive, strategic sampling is required to assess the extent of the contamination [4].

Four main types of aflatoxins are recognised, namely B1, B2, G1 and G2, with aflatoxin B1 and G1 as well as their metabolic product M1 being the most commonly found in agricultural produce (**Figure 1**). In terms of acute toxicity, the oral lethal dose (LD50) of aflatoxin B1 for monkeys is 1.75 mg/kg, and for ducks 1.70–2.45 mg/kg. However, these toxins are also carcinogenic because once ingested they are metabolised by the liver to a reactive epoxide intermediate; as a result, chronic ingestion of small amounts of aflatoxins (i.e. in the ppb range) typically produce liver cancer, so they are classified as strong carcinogens by the International Agency for Research on Cancer (IARC). For example, it has been estimated that 12% of cancer occurrence in Indonesia is in the liver, which is linked to consumption of aflatoxin contaminated food [5]. Livestock animals suffer the same effects, with pigs and chicken being particularly susceptible to these mycotoxins. However, animals can also transform aflatoxins B and G into the M metabolites by hydroxylation in the liver, and these transformation products can appear in eggs as well as in poultry meat [6]. Both aflatoxin M1 and M2 are even more toxic, with LD50 for ducks in the range 0.28–0.32 mg/kg. Ruminant animals fed contaminated fodder are more tolerant, but can also pass M aflatoxins into milk and other dairy products [7–9].

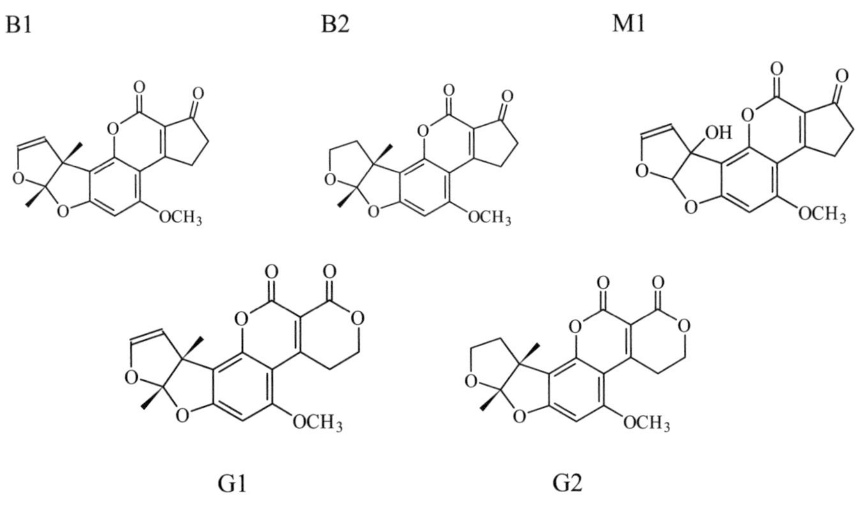

Figure 1. Chemical structures of common aflatoxins found in nuts and grains (B1, B2, G1, G2) or milk (M1) as a by-product.

Contamination of the food supply with aflatoxins poses a serious problem not only for the health effects it causes in people and livestock, but also for trade. Strict regulations have been enacted by the World Health Organisation to prevent trading aflatoxin contaminated produce among countries. The maximum residue limits (MRLs) in grain for human consumption are in the range 2–20 ppb, and for animal feed in the range 20–300 ppb, depending on the country, whereas for milk they can be as low as 0.05 μg/L [10]. In order to meet the international regulations on aflatoxin, countries have to adopt expensive monitoring programs in order to screen their agricultural produce. Screening to detect aflatoxin contamination often relies on fluorescence and has been achieved by reference standards using thin layer chromatography, adsorption on minicolumns [11], high-performance liquid chromatography (HPLC) or liquid chromatography coupled to mass spectrometry (LC-MS) [12, 13]. Unfortunately, many developing countries lack the infrastructure necessary to comply with such regulations even though they often recognise the problem [14]. For example, aflatoxin has been identified as a threat to human health in Timor-Leste [15], and yet some of their agricultural produce could not be marketed in recent years for lack of compliance.

Specific antibodies to aflatoxins have provided an alternative means to conduct ELISA immunoassays [16], which can accurately measure the levels of contamination in grains and nuts. ELISA technologies are more affordable than instrumental analysis such as HPLC-fluorescence or LC-MS, but require a level of analytical skills that may not be found in many developing countries, where the aflatoxin problem is most prevalent [14, 17]. Based on the same immunoassays principles, lateral flow devices (LFD) employing gold nanoparticles have been recently developed [18–20] to be used as rapid methods for screening aflatoxins in food commodities.

One such device [19], the Aflatoxin QuickTest™, provides an effective, reliable and low cost option for screening levels of aflatoxins and meets the regulatory thresholds of agricultural produce. Quantification, as described here, is achieved using a suitable reader and standard curve of the analytes in the same manner as it is done with other analytical equipment. A validation study for quantification using peanuts and maize from Australia and Timor-Leste was carried out in order to assess the performance of the Aflatoxin QuickTest™ and it is presented here for the first time.

This chapter reviews the past research that led to the development of the current Aflatoxin QuickTest™, its use and applications. But before describing how it works, a description of this novel technology is required.

2. Development of antibodies for detection of aflatoxin

2.1. Antibodies for aflatoxin

A polyclonal antibody specific to aflatoxin B1 (AFB1) was developed by Lee et al. [16] using a conjugate of aflatoxin B1-bovine serum albumin (BSA) as antigen. The antibodies were specific to aflatoxin B1, detecting this compound in a mixture of four aflatoxins (B1, B2, G1 and G2), but showed significant cross-reaction with aflatoxin G1 (57–61%) when an individual compound was tested (**Table 1**). This is fortunate, as both aflatoxin B1 and G1 are the two most common aflatoxins found in contaminated produce. Sensitivity of short competitive ELISA assays (15 minutes) showed median inhibition concentration (IC50) values of 21.6 ± 2.7 ppb after a 5-fold dilution of the sample extract – a necessary step to minimise the negative effect of solvent on the antibodies – and a detection range from 4.2 to 99.9 μg/kg sample. This ELISA was able to detect and quantify levels of aflatoxins in peanut, corn, soybean and pistachio samples without significant matrix effects [16].

Furthermore, a validation of the SUNQuik ELISA, which uses the AFB1 antibodies, was carried out using 12 peanut samples that were also analysed by standard HPLC-fluorescence. Levels of total aflatoxins measured by the two analytical methods showed an excellent correlation ($r^2 = 0.938$) over a concentration range 0–1200 μg/kg sample, with no false negatives [21].

2.2. Lateral flow devices for aflatoxins

Whilst the ability of the polyclonal AFB1 antibodies to quantify levels of aflatoxins in grains and nuts was demonstrated, the application of ELISA assays to monitoring surveys requires certain laboratory conditions and appropriate skills by qualified personnel. A simpler method was needed that could be used in field settings by less skilled operators.

In recent years, more convenient procedures based on immunochemistry have been sought for organic contaminants in food and the environment. The lateral flow device (LFD) has been most popular because of its simplicity in design and its automatic function, each LFD unit requiring only a few drops of sample solution for operation. Comprehensive reviews [22–24] have described the lateral flow assay system in depth, covering a broad range of immunoassay procedures and including nucleic acid applications. Many successful ELISAs can be readily converted to LFDs using the same or similar immuno-reagents; important properties established for ELISAs such as the plots of concentration giving 50% inhibition (IC50) perform in a similar manner in LFDs. In essence, a competitive LFD consists of an impervious nitrocellulose strip coated transversal with two lines that contain either a particular target analyte (test line, T) or a general antibody (control line, C). In addition, a sample pad contains colloidal gold

Compound	IC50* (ppb)	%CR
Aflatoxin B1	0.8–6.5	100.0
Aflatoxin G1	1.4–10.8	57.1–60.5
Aflatoxin B2	13.5–55.0	5.9–11.8
Aflatoxin G2	50.1–83.0	1.6–7.8
Aflatoxin P1	>250	<0.3–1.0
Aflatoxin M1	>250	<0.3 to <2.6

*IC50 = median inhibition concentration.

Table 1. Cross reactivity of aflatoxins and metabolites in polyclonal AFB1 assays (after Lee et al. [16]).

nanoparticles conjugated to the specific antibodies of the target analyte (AuNP-IgG); at the other end of the strip there is an absorbent pad (**Figure 2**). The strips are contained within small plastic cassettes that have a well for placing drops of the sample solution and a window to visualise the T and C lines. Conjugates and antibodies on the LFD are usually stable for months when the strips are kept under dry and dark conditions at room temperature, enabling easy transport and storage for use at a later time.

Some authors have successfully described LFDs for aflatoxins that work well with corn [18], grains and feedstuffs [25, 26] and milk [27], but require strip treatment before use. A new LFD for aflatoxins that did not require special pre-treatment was developed by Masinde et al. [19] and has been commercialised as the Aflatoxin Quicktest™ by QuickTest Technologies. The T line in the Aflatoxin Quicktest™ contains aflatoxin-conjugate (AFB1-C) and the C line a non-specific goat anti-rabbit antibody (G-IgG); the sample pad contains gold nanoparticles (~10–15 micron) conjugated to the specific antibodies (AuNP-IgG) developed by Lee et al. for aflatoxin (AFB1).

For running a test, two drops of sample extract are placed over the sample pad, dissolving the AuNP-IgG nanoparticles, which run laterally over the strip towards the absorbent pad. Any aflatoxin present in the sample extract will compete with the AuNP-IgG particles at the T line, where the excess conjugated antigen will bind to them and produce a coloured line. The remaining AuNP-IgG particles will continue moving towards the other end and will bind to the G-IgG at the C line, also producing colour. The time for the competing targets, aflatoxin and AuNP-IgG, to reach an equilibrium is about 15 minutes, although 5 minutes may be sufficient for initial visual detection [19].

The interpretation of the assay is straightforward: an absence of colour at the T line indicates a high concentration of aflatoxins in the sample extract, as it has outcompeted the gold nanoparticles, whereas a full coloured T line indicates the absence of aflatoxins in the sample. A faded line indicates the presence of some aflatoxin in such a way that the less the colour development, the more aflatoxin is present. The coloured C line confirms that the test is valid, that is, when no colour appears at the C line, the test is invalid or the strip is faulty.

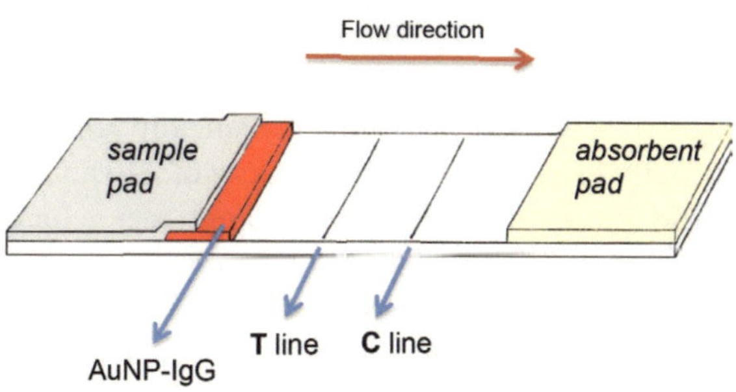

Figure 2. Schematic diagram of a lateral flow device (LFD). A nitrocellulose strip is coated with a solution of a particular target analyte (T line) and a general antibody (C line). The sample pad contains gold nanoparticles conjugated to the specific antibodies of the analyte (AuNP-IgG). The absorbent pad at the other end captures the excess solution flowing across the strip.

The Aflatoxin Quicktest™ can detect aflatoxins at 0.1 μg/L in water or liquid samples that do not require dilution, that is, milk. For solid samples that require extraction (e.g. grain, nuts) with methanol or ethanol, a 10-fold dilution must be applied to avoid serious inactivation of the antibodies; in this case, the limit of detection is at least 1 μg/L or more, depending on the extraction method.

3. Quantification of aflatoxin by the Aflatoxin Quicktest™

The conjugated AuNPs-IgG in the LFD compete with the sample analyte for the same target at the T line in a similar way as in a competitive ELISA assay [21]. Therefore, the amount of immuno-gold attached to the T line is inversely proportional to the level of analyte in the sample and this simple relationship can be used to estimate the analyte concentration when an optical reader that measures reflectance of immuno-gold is available. Reading is typically done for one LFD unit at a time, but instruments with multiple slots for reading test devices are also available, allowing greater sample throughput speed. In practice, readers operate by estimating the ratio of the area under the peaks corresponding to the test and the control line (T/C), because no two strips contain exactly the same amount of gold nanoparticles. A ratio around 1 indicates absence of the analyte, whereas lower values indicate its presence and zero values indicate levels of analyte above the range of detection.

Given the operation of the law of mass action in binding of analytes by specific antibodies, the volume or number of drops added to the sample pad of the LFD is not critical for analysis as the reaction with AuNP-IgG nanoparticles is concentration dependent; the majority of the analyte molecules remain in solution, given the small number of antibody molecules. However, it is preferable to standardise the number of drops to induce reliable lateral flow, with 2 drops being optimal for the Aflatoxin Quicktest™.

As with any other analytical technique, the ratio readings must be compared to a standard curve established beforehand using known concentrations of the target analyte. An example for the Aflatoxin Quicktest™ is presented in **Figure 3**. It should be noted that the shape of the curve is best described by an exponential function, which becomes sigmoidal (with a straight section between two bend ends) when plotted against the logarithm of the aflatoxin concentrations. As in ELISA assays, extreme ratio values either at near zero or at some maximum of the range in LFDs must also be rejected, since accurate estimates can only be made in the straight region of the curve, which is usually found between ratio values of 0.15 and 0.85. Consequently, the working range of Aflatoxin Quicktest™ is in the 0.1–2.0 ppb region for direct sample analysis, but 2.0–40 ppb for solid samples requiring solvent extraction and dilution 10-fold. Repeated measurements of the standard solutions using the Aflatoxin Quicktest™ show good reliability of the assays, with a coefficient of variation of 6.4% within this working range.

Samples that contain aflatoxin levels above the range of detection are diluted and reanalysed. More than one dilution may be needed when the contamination levels are very high. Care is needed to extract only well-mixed grain samples given the extremely uneven distribution of aflatoxin among kernels.

A)

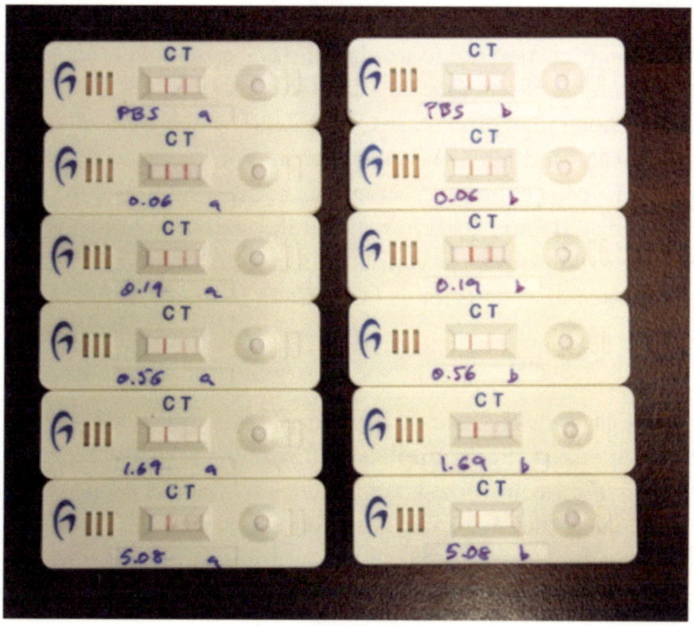

B)

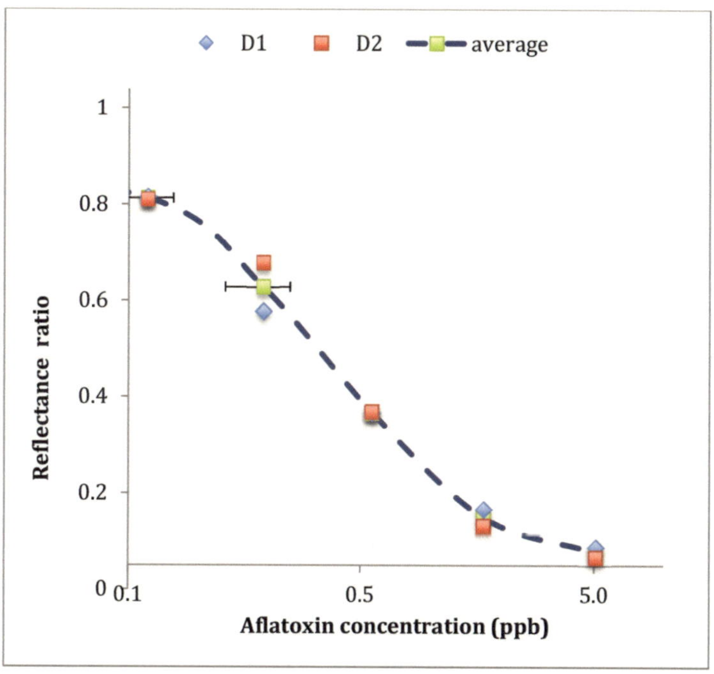

Figure 3. Establishment of standard curves using LFDs. (A) Aflatoxin QuickTest™ cassette strips used at different concentrations of an aflatoxin mixture; (B) standard curve from the reflectance ratio of test- and control-lines. Error bars indicate the 95% confidence intervals of duplicate measurements (D1 and D2) by the optical reader.

4. Validation of the Aflatoxin Quicktest™

Two separate studies were carried out to validate the performance of the Aflatoxin Quicktest™ in analysing peanuts and maize samples for aflatoxin contamination. The first study comprised peanuts samples from Australian growers in Queensland, which were collected during the 2015 and 2016 growing seasons and maize kernels infected with *A. flavus* in a laboratory trial. The second study involved a comprehensive survey of peanuts and maize from markets in Timor-Leste, carried out during 2014 and 2015. In both studies, extracts of the raw samples were analysed using the Aflatoxin Quicktest™ as well as the standard methods of analytical laboratories, that is, HPLC with fluorescence detector or LC-MS/MS, so their results could be compared.

4.1. Australian validation study

From late April 2015, from every load of peanuts delivered into the Kingaroy intake of the Peanut Company of Australia (PCA), duplicate 80% methanol extracts were collected as part of the normal aflatoxin mini-column test conducted at intake. For each load, a separate extraction was performed, such that a duplicate methanol extract was collected for both HPLC (15 ml) and Aflatoxin Quicktest™ (5 ml) aflatoxin analysis. For the 2015 season, about 170 extracts were collected and stored in the fridge (5°C) until the validation study commenced in June of that year.

All 15 ml extracts were analysed by HPLC-fluorescence at the PCA Technical Centre using the company's standard method accredited by National Association of Testing Authorities (NATA, Australia), which included addition of 5% Holaday salt solution to the methanol extract. A selected subset of 13 positive and 12 negative samples randomly chosen was then used in the validation study.

The corresponding subset of 5 ml extracts (n = 25) were analysed in June by the Aflatoxin Quicktest™. For this analysis, 200 μl were taken into an Eppendorf tube and 1.8 ml of phosphate buffer solution (PBS – 50 mM, pH 7.4) added so as to reduce the concentration of methanol to less than 10%. Two drops of the solution were placed on the strip well and left to develop colour for 15 minutes on the laboratory bench, after which time the strips were immediately read using an LFD Quick Reader (Tianjin Jiuding Diagnostics Ltd., China). Samples that produced results above the detection range (2–40 ppb) were diluted further in PBS and reanalysed until their readings fell within this range; all results were calculated taking into account the dilutions factors used for each sample.

Results from the 2015 peanut validation study are shown in **Figure 4A**, where it can be seen the excellent correlation between the HPLC and Aflatoxin Quicktest™ analyses for total aflatoxins ($r^2 = 0.934$ on the logarithmic transformed data).

The same procedure was repeated in 2016, but this time 45 peanut extracts were used in the validation study, which was conducted in October of that year. The results for 2016 (**Figure 4B**) showed also a good correlation between the two analyses ($r^2 = 0.956$), even though a number of samples were well above of the detection range. The results of the second year confirm the validity of the Aflatoxin Quicktest™ as a tool for detecting and measuring total aflatoxin levels in peanuts.

A)

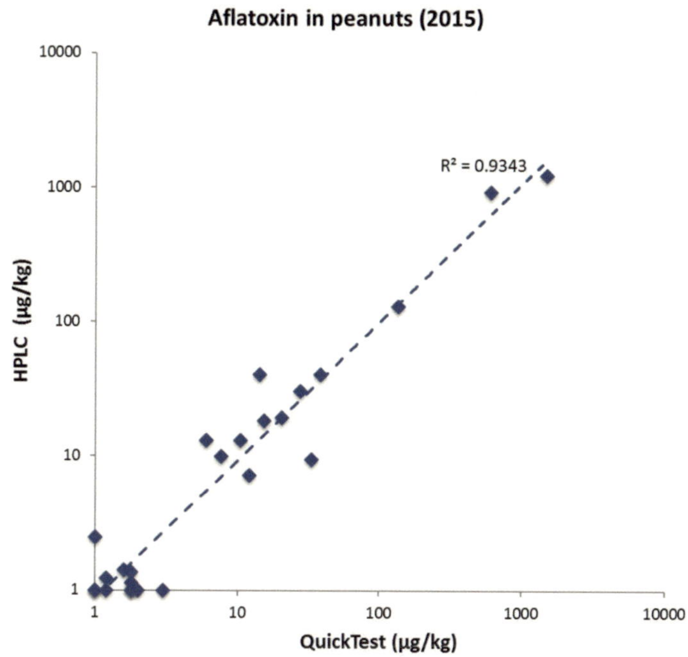

B)

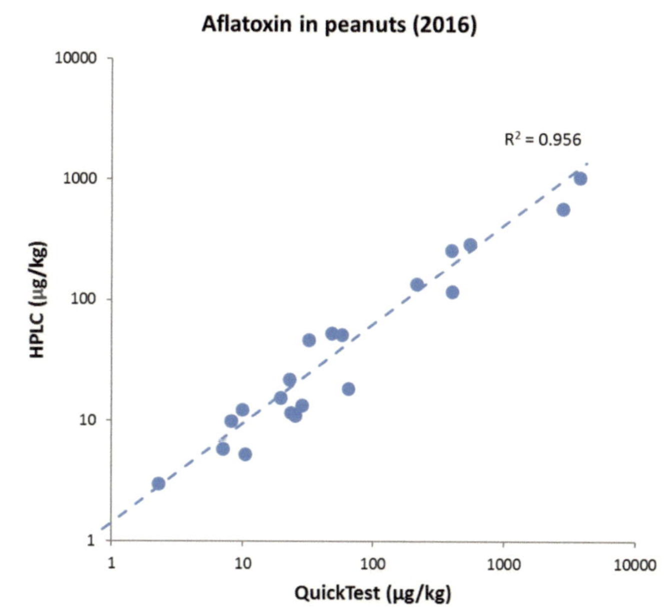

Figure 4. Validation of the Aflatoxin QuickTest™ for peanut samples collected by the Peanut Company of Australia in 2015 (A) and 2016 (B).

In addition to the peanut extracts, 16 samples of maize kernels that had been infected with *A. flavus* in the laboratory were also used for validating the Aflatoxin Quicktest™. The kernels were extracted with a mixture of 80% methanol and 4% Holaday salt solution and analysed first by HPLC-fluorescence at the PCA Technical Centre. The levels of aflatoxins in the kernels were sometimes very high, with the highest reaching 111 mg/kg (ppm). Most of the aflatoxin was found to be G1 (63 ± 27%) and B1 (26 ± 23%), whereas both G2 and B1 were usually below 3%.

Aliquots of the extracts (100 μl) were taken into 900 μl of PBS solution for direct analysis by Aflatoxin Quicktest™, and diluted further in PBS if the readings were above the detection range.

In spite of the high levels of contamination in the maize kernels, which required dilutions of the extracts up to 60,000-fold, a comparison of results by the two analytical methods showed an acceptable correlation for all the aflatoxins in the samples (**Figure 5**, $r^2 = 0.89$). This correlation improved when the results of the Aflatoxin Quicktest™ were compared to the levels of aflatoxin B1 and B2 ($r^2 = 0.97$ and 0.93, respectively) as determined by HPLC, whereas those of aflatoxins G1 and G2 showed lower correlations ($r^2 = 0.86$ and 0.76, respectively). This is in agreement with the differential sensitivity of the antibodies present in the commercial Aflatoxin Quicktest™, which are 100% specific to aflatoxin B1 but less specific to the other forms (see **Table 1**). Aflatoxins B1 and B2 are commonly found in tropical and subtropical regions of the world, whereas aflatoxins G1 and G2 are commonly produced by *A. parasiticus*, a soil species that is rare or absent in South East Asia [28].

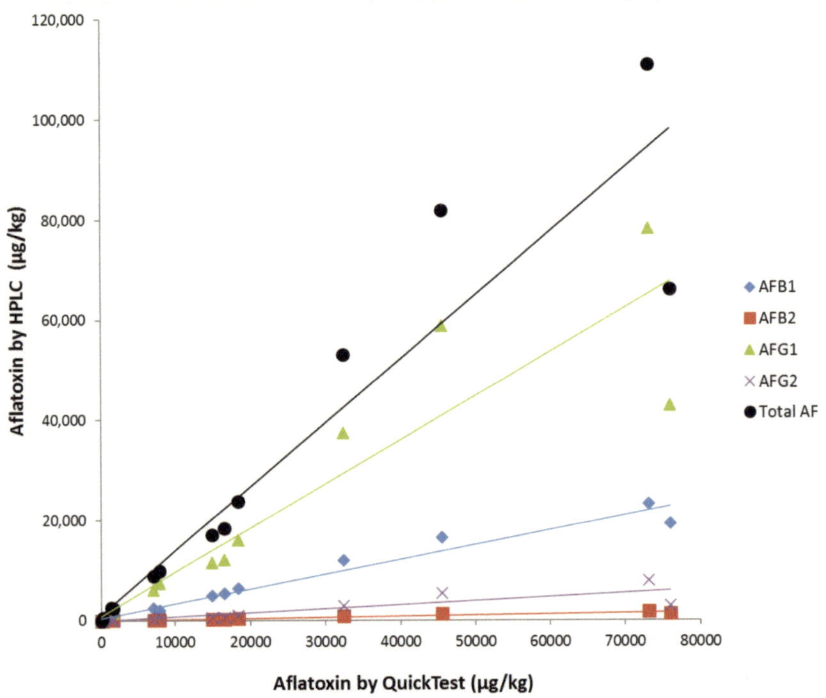

Figure 5. Validation of the Aflatoxin QuickTest™ for maize kernels infected with high levels of aflatoxins: AFB1, AFB2, AFG1, AFG2 and total aflatoxins (AF).

http://dx.doi.org/10.5772/intechopen.71331

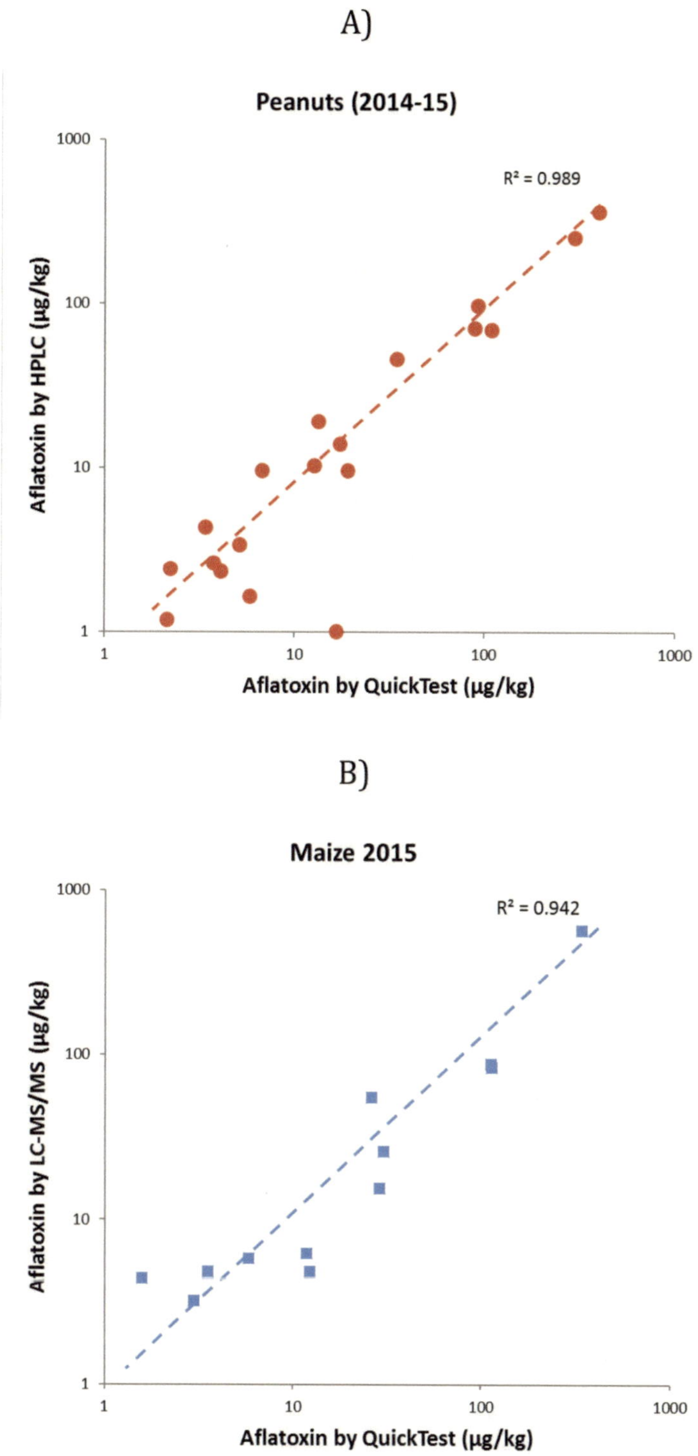

Figure 6. Validation of the Aflatoxin QuickTest™ for peanut (A) and maize (B) samples from Timor-Leste market surveys.

4.2. Timor-Leste validation study

Surveys were conducted in 2013, 2014 and 2015 to collect maize and peanut kernels from markets, seed producers and households in 42 districts of Timor-Leste. A small subset of 33 peanut and 30 maize samples from the two latter years were used for the validation study.

Samples of well-mixed kernels (100 g) were ground using a commercial blender and the meal thus obtained was extracted with 200 ml of 80% methanol containing 4% NaCl in a blender for 3 minutes. The extracts were filtered and 4 ml of supernatant collected for subsequent analysis by both Aflatoxin Quicktest™ and standard analytical methods. All peanut samples were analysed by HPLC-fluorescence at the PCA analytical facilities (Kingaroy, Queensland), whereas only 15 maize samples were analysed by LC-MS/MS at the National Measurement Institute (Sydney, Australia).

Aliquot of the extracts (200 µl) were diluted in phosphate buffer solution (ratio 1:10) to make it ready for Aflatoxin Quicktest™ analysis. Two drops of this solution were added to each strip and allowed to develop colour in 15 minutes. The strips were then read using the Quick Reader, and the results printed and recorded. For readings above 40 ppb, the sample extracts were further diluted and reanalysed again.

The results by both analytical methods were compared in order to validate the Aflatoxin Quicktest™ procedure. The majority of samples showed levels of total aflatoxin below 100 µg/kg. Regression analysis on the sets of peanut (n = 33) and maize samples (n = 15) showed coefficients of determination (r^2) of 0.989 for peanuts (71% aflatoxin B1) and 0.942 for maize (91% aflatoxin B1) (**Figure 6A** and **B**).

In summary, both validation studies were successful, demonstrating the accuracy of the Aflatoxin Quicktest™, which renders results comparable to those obtained by the standard analytical methods in certified laboratories.

5. Advantages of the Aflatoxin QuickTest™

Advantages of the LFD technology are the ease of use, rapid development time, no need for dangerous chemicals, straightforward reading of test results and low cost of the strips. Moreover, very little and inexpensive equipment is required other than a Quick Reader and solvents for the extractions.

This technology is designed to help primary producers screen their produce before selling it in the market. Because the test is very simple and easy to understand, users only require a basic training to become proficient. Thus, local co-operatives, small companies and even farmers can learn it and apply it in their own facilities.

Based on the demonstrated performance of the Aflatoxin QuickTest™ in evaluating aflatoxin contamination in maize and peanuts, the government of Timor-Leste is supporting its use for screening these and other agricultural produce that may be contaminated with this toxin. Local companies may now use this technology to meet international food safety standards for the export market, instead of resorting to the expensive alternative of sending samples to

http://dx.doi.org/10.5772/intechopen.71331

certified laboratories in Indonesia or Australia. Moreover, they can now check the raw produce on site without having to wait weeks until they receive the results from the laboratories. No doubt, this potentially gives them significant competitive advantage in the markets. It is anticipated that application of this technology may allow rapid, accurate and low cost screening of Timorese agricultural produce.

By measuring the levels of aflatoxin in their produce farmers can now manage the problem, whereas lack of awareness of this contamination will only spread the contamination with these toxins among the local population [29], leading to unpleasant health consequences for consumers [5], and probably to a rejection of the products in the market place. Only what can be measured can be managed. In this regard, monitoring of agricultural produce should be followed by practical training sessions where farmers are instructed how to avoid aflatoxin contamination in the first place [1, 30, 31].

So far only grain and nuts have been tested using the Aflatoxin QuickTest™, but it is obvious that other agricultural commodities such as milk and dairy products can also be analysed using this technology. In the case of milk, no extraction may be required, so samples can be used directly for detecting levels of this contaminant in the range 0.1–2.0 μg/L or higher, after diluting by a given factor.

The current Aflatoxin QuickTest™ discussed here uses polyclonal antibodies specific for aflatoxin B1 and G1 (**Table 1**). Different antibodies have also been developed that have variable sensitivities towards other forms of aflatoxin and can be marketed in the near future in accordance with specific market needs.

Author details

Francisco Sánchez-Bayo[1,4]*, Luis de Almeida[2], Robert Williams[2], Graeme Wright[3], Ivan R. Kennedy[4] and Angus Crossan[4]

*Address all correspondence to: francisco.sanchez-bayo@sydney.edu.au

1 School of Life and Environmental Sciences, The University of Sydney, Eveleigh, NSW, Australia

2 Ministry of Agriculture and Fisheries (MAF), Dili, Timor-Leste

3 Peanut Company of Australia (PCA), Kingaroy, QLD, Australia

4 QuickTest Technologies Ltd, Eveleigh, NSW, Australia

References

[1] Rachaputi N, Krosch S, Wright GC. Management practices to minimise pre-harvest aflatoxin contamination in Australian peanuts. Australian Journal of Experimental Agriculture. 2002;**42**(5):595-605

[2] Karaaslan M, Arslanğray Y. Aflatoxins B1, B2, G1, and G2 contamination in ground red peppers commercialized in Sanliurfa, Turkey. Environmental Monitoring and Assessment. 2015;**187**(4):1-9

[3] Kerry R, Ortiz BV, Ingram BR, Scully BT. A Spatio–Temporal investigation of risk factors for aflatoxin contamination of corn in southern Georgia, USA using geostatistical methods. Crop Protection. 2017;**94**:144-158

[4] Whitaker TB, Hagler WM, Giesbrecht F. Performance of sampling plans to determine aflatoxin in farmer stock peanut lots by measuring aflatoxin in high risk grade components. Journal of AOAC International. 1999;**82**:264-270

[5] Tjindarbumi D, Mangunkusumo R. Cancer in Indonesia, present and future. Japanese Journal of Clinical Oncology. 2002;**32**(Suppl_1):S17-S21

[6] Iqbal SZ, Nisar S, Asi MR, Jinap S. Natural incidence of aflatoxins, ochratoxin A and zearalenone in chicken meat and eggs. Food Control. 2014;**43**:98-103

[7] Galvano F, Galofaro V, Galvano G. Occurrence and stability of aflatoxin M1 in milk and milk products: A worldwide review. Journal of Food Protection. 1996;**59**(10):1079-1090

[8] Kamkar A. A study on the occurrence of aflatoxin M1 in Iranian Feta cheese. Food Control. 2006;**17**(10):768-775

[9] Prandini A, Tansini G, Sigolo S, Filippi L, Laporta M, Piva G. On the occurrence of aflatoxin M1 in milk and dairy products. Food and Chemical Toxicology. 2009;**47**(5):984-991

[10] European Commission. Commission decision of 12 Jul 2006 on special conditions governing certain foodstuffs imported from certain third countries due to contamination risks of these products by aflatoxins. Off J Eur Com L. 2006;**49**(L199):21-32

[11] Davidson JI Jr, Dickens JW, Chew V, Sanders TH, Holaday CE, Cole RJ, et al. Performance of the visual, minicolumn and TLC methods in detecting aflatoxin in 20 contaminated lots of farmers stock peanuts. Peanut Science. 1984;**11**:77-83

[12] Whitaker TB, Dorner JW, Giesbrecht FG, Slate AB. Variability among aflatoxin test results on runner peanuts harvested from small field plots. Peanut Science. 2004;**31**:59-63

[13] Blesa J, Soriano JM, Moltó JC, Mañes J. Limited survey for the presence of aflatoxins in foods from local markets and supermarkets in Valencia, Spain. Food Additives and Contaminants. 2004;**21**(2):165-171

[14] Waliyar F, Umeh VC, Traore A, Osiru M, Ntare BR, Diarra B, et al. Prevalence and distribution of aflatoxin contamination in groundnut (*Arachis hypogaea* L.) in Mali, West Africa. Crop Protection. 2015;**70**:1-7

[15] Authors Timor-Leste Food and Nutrition Survey 2013 – Summary of Key Findings and Recommendations. Ministry of Health, Democratic Republic of Timor-Leste; 2015. p. 24

[16] Lee NA, Wang S, Allan RD, Kennedy IR. A rapid aflatoxin B1 ELISA: Development and validation with reduced matrix effects for peanuts, corn, pistachio, and soybeans. Journal of Agricultural and Food Chemistry. 2004;**52**(10):2746-2755

[17] Tran-Dinh N, Kennedy I, Bui T, Carter D. Survey of Vietnamese peanuts, corn and soil for the presence of *Aspergillus flavus* and *Aspergillus parasiticus*. Mycopathologia. 2009;**168**(5):257-268

[18] Anfossi L, D'Arco G, Calderara M, Baggiani C, Giovannoli C, Giraudi G. Development of a quantitative lateral flow immunoassay for the detection of aflatoxins in maize. Food Additives & Contaminants. Part A, Chemistry, Analysis, Control, Exposure & Risk Assessment. 2011;**28**(2):226-234

[19] Masinde L, Sheng W, Xu X, Zhang Y, Yuan M, Kennedy I, et al. Colloidal gold based immunochromatographic strip for the simple and sensitive determination of aflatoxin B1 and B2 in corn and rice. Microchimica Acta. 2013;**180**(9-10):921-928

[20] Luis JM, Kemerait RC Jr. Test strips in the qualitative detection of aflatoxin contamination in peanuts. Peanut Science. 2015;**42**:49-55

[21] Lee NA, Rachaputi NC, Wright GC, Krosch S, Norman K, Anderson J, et al. Validation of analytical parameters of a competitive direct ELISA for aflatoxin B1 in peanuts. Food and Agricultural Immunology. 2005;**16**(2):149-163

[22] Posthuma-Trumpie GA, Korf J, Amerongen A. Lateral flow (immuno)assay: Its strengths, weaknesses, opportunities and threats. A literature survey. Analytical and Bioanalytical Chemistry. 2008;**393**(2):569-582

[23] Xuefei G, Li-Ping X, Shu-Feng Z, Guodong L, Xueji Z. Recent advances in nanoparticles-based lateral flow biosensors. American Journal of Biomedical Sciences. 2014;**6**(1):41-57

[24] Huang X, Aguilar ZP, Xu H, Lai W, Xiong Y. Membrane-based lateral flow immunochromatographic strip with nanoparticles as reporters for detection: A review. Biosensors & Bioelectronics. 2016;**75**:166-180

[25] Zhang D, Li P, Yang Y, Zhang Q, Zhang W, Xiao Z, et al. A high selective immunochromatographic assay for rapid detection of aflatoxin B1. Talanta. 2011;**85**(1):736-742

[26] Shim WB, Yang ZY, Kim JS, Kim JY, Kang SJ, Woo GJ, et al. Development of immunochromatography strip-test using nanocolloidal gold-antibody probe for the rapid detection of aflatoxin B1 in grain and feed samples. Journal of Microbiology and Biotechnology. 2007;**17**(10):1629-1637

[27] Wang J-J, Liu B-H, Hsu Y-T, Yu F-Y. Sensitive competitive direct enzyme-linked immunosorbent assay and gold nanoparticle immunochromatographic strip for detecting aflatoxin M1 in milk. Food Control. 2011;**22**(6):964-969

[28] CAST. Mycotoxins: Risks in Plant, Animal, and Human Systems. Ames, Iowa, USA: Council for Agricultural Science and Technology, Task Force Report 139; 2003, chapter 2.

[29] Cantú-Cornelio F, Aguilar-Toalá JE, de León-Rodríguez CI, Esparza-Romero J, Vallejo-Cordoba B, González-Córdova AF, et al. Occurrence and factors associated with the presence of aflatoxin M1 in breast milk samples of nursing mothers in central Mexico. Food Control. 2016;**62**:16-22

[30] Atanda SA, Aina JA, Agoda SA, Usanga OE, Pessu PO. Mycotoxin management in agriculture: A review. Journal of Animal Science Advances. 2012;**2**(Suppl. 3.1):250-260

[31] Riley RT, Norred WP. Mycotoxin prevention and decontamination - A case study on maize. Food, Nutrition and Agriculture. 1999;**23**:25-32